Clinical Innovation and Technology in Craniomaxillofacial Surgery

Guest Editor

BERNARD J. COSTELLO, DMD, MD, FACS

ORAL AND MAXILLOFACIAL SURGERY CLINICS OF NORTH AMERICA

www.oralmaxsurgery.theclinics.com

Consulting Editor
RICHARD H. HAUG, DDS

February 2010 • Volume 22 • Number 1

SAUNDERS an imprint of ELSEVIER, Inc.

W.B. SAUNDERS COMPANY
A Division of Elsevier Inc.

1600 John F. Kennedy Blvd. ● Suite 1800 ● Philadelphia, PA 19103-2899

www.oralmaxsurgery.theclinics.com

ORAL AND MAXILLOFACIAL SURGERY CLINICS OF NORTH AMERICA Volume 22, Number 1
February 2010 ISSN 1042-3699, ISBN-13: 978-1-4377-1845-4

Editor: John Vassallo; j.vassallo@elsevier.com
Developmental Editor: Theresa Collier

Oral and Maxillofacial Surgery Clinics of North America (ISSN 1042-3699) is published quarterly by Elsevier Inc., 360 Park Avenue South, New York, NY 10010-1710. Months of issue are February, May, August, and November. Business and Editorial Offices: 1600 John F. Kennedy Blvd., Suite 1800, Philadelphia, PA 19103-2899. Periodicals postage paid at New York, NY and additional mailing offices. Subscription prices are $304.00 per year for US individuals, $445.00 per year for US institutions, $140.00 per year for US students and residents, $351.00 per year for Canadian individuals, $530.00 per year for Canadian institutions, $405.00 per year for international individuals, $530.00 per year for international institutions and $190.00 per year for Canadian and foreign students/residents. To receive student/resident rate, orders must be accompanied by name or affiliated institution, date of term, and the *signature* of program/residency coordinator on institution letterhead. Orders will be billed at individual rate until proof of status is received. Foreign air speed delivery is included in all *Clinics* subscription prices. All prices are subject to change without notice. **POSTMASTER:** Send address changes to *Oral and Maxillofacial Surgery Clinics of North America,* Elsevier Periodicals Customer Service, 11830 Westline Industrial Drive, St. Louis, MO 63146. Tel: 1-800-654-2452 (U.S. and Canada); 314-447-8871 (outside U.S. and Canada). Fax: 314-447-8029. E-mail: journalscustomerservice-usa@elsevier.com (for print support); journalsonlinesupport-usa@elsevier.com (for online support).

Reprints. For copies of 100 or more, of articles in this publication, please contact the Commercial Reprints Department, Elsevier Inc., 360 Park Avenue South, New York, NY 10010-1710. Tel.: 212-633-3812; Fax: 212-462-1935; Email: reprints@elsevier.com.

Oral and Maxillofacial Surgery Clinics of North America is covered in MEDLINE/PubMed (*Index Medicus*).

Printed and bound in the United Kingdom
Transferred to Digital Print 2011

Contributors

CONSULTING EDITOR

RICHARD H. HAUG, DDS
Carolinas Center for Oral Health
Charlotte, North Carolina

GUEST EDITOR

BERNARD J. COSTELLO, DMD, MD, FACS
Associate Professor and Program Director,
Chief, Division of Craniofacial and Cleft
Surgery, Department of Oral and Maxillofacial
Surgery, University of Pittsburgh School of
Dental Medicine; Adjunct Faculty, McGowan
Institute for Regenerative Medicine, University
of Pittsburgh Medical Center, Pittsburgh,
Pennsylvania

AUTHORS

FAIZAN ALAWI, DDS
Assistant Professor, Department of Pathology,
University of Pennsylvania School of Dental
Medicine, Philadelphia, Pennsylvania

ERIC J. BECKMAN, PhD
Cohera Medical Inc; Professor, University of
Pittsburgh School of Engineering, Pittsburgh,
Pennsylvania

R. BRYAN BELL, DDS, MD, FACS
Attending Head and Neck Surgeon and
Director of Resident Education, Oral and
Maxillofacial Surgery Service, Legacy Emanuel
Hospital and Health Center; Head and Neck
Surgical Associates; Clinical Associate
Professor, Oregon Health & Science University,
Portland, Oregon

AMOL M. BHATKI, MD
Clinical Instructor, Department of
Otolaryngology Head and Neck Surgery,
University of Pittsburgh School of Medicine,
Pittsburgh, Pennsylvania

ELIZABETH BILODEAU, DMD, MD
Resident, Department of Oral and
Maxillofacial Surgery, University of Pittsburgh
School of Dental Medicine, Pittsburgh,
Pennsylvania

BARTON F. BRANSTETTER IV, MD
Associate Professor of Radiology and
Otolaryngology, University of Pittsburgh
Medical Center, Pittsburgh, Pennsylvania

MICHAEL J. BUCKLEY, DMD, MBA, MS
Private Practice, Greensburg; Adjunct
Associate Professor, University of Pittsburgh
School of Dental Medicine, Pittsburgh,
Pennsylvania

ANDREW CAMPBELL, DDS, FRCD(C)
Former Fellow, Division of Craniofacial and
Cleft Surgery, Department of Oral
and Maxillofacial Surgery, University
of Pittsburgh School of Dental Medicine,
Pittsburgh, Pennsylvania; Private Practice,
Austin, Texas

RICARDO L. CARRAU, MD
Professor, Department of Otolaryngology –
Head and Neck Surgery, Eye and Ear Institute;
Department of Neurological Surgery, University
of Pittsburgh School of Medicine, Pittsburgh,
Pennsylvania

WILLIAM L. CHUNG, DDS, MD
Assistant Professor, Department of Oral and
Maxillofacial Surgery, University of Pittsburgh
Medical Center, Pittsburgh, Pennsylvania

BERNARD J. COSTELLO, DMD, MD, FACS
Associate Professor and Program Director,
Chief, Division of Craniofacial and Cleft
Surgery, Department of Oral and Maxillofacial
Surgery, University of Pittsburgh School of
Dental Medicine; Adjunct Faculty, McGowan
Institute for Regenerative Medicine, University
of Pittsburgh Medical Center, Pittsburgh,
Pennsylvania

ALESSANDRO CUSANO, DDS, MD
Previous Fellow in Microvascular
Reconstructive Surgery, Section of Head Neck
Surgery, Division of Oral and Maxillofacial
Surgery, Department of Surgery, University of
Florida, College of Medicine, Jacksonville,
Florida

SARAH D. DAVIES, DDS, MD
Assistant Professor, Department of Oral and
Maxillofacial Surgery, University of Pittsburgh
School of Dental Medicine, Pittsburgh,
Pennsylvania

THOMAS B. DODSON, DMD, MPH
Visiting Oral and Maxillofacial Surgeon,
Director, Center for Applied Clinical
Investigation, Department of Oral and
Maxillofacial Surgery, Massachusetts General
Hospital; Associate Professor, Department of
Oral and Maxillofacial Surgery, Harvard School
of Dental Medicine, Boston, Massachusetts

SEAN P. EDWARDS, DDS, MD, FRCD(C)
Assistant Professor and Residency Program
Director, Chief, Department of Pediatric
Maxillofacial Surgery, C.S. Mott Children's
Hospital, University of Michigan Health
System, Ann Arbor, Michigan

RUI FERNANDES, DMD, MD, FACS
Assistant Professor, Chief, Section of Head
and Neck Surgery, Director of Microvascular
Reconstructive Fellowship, Division of Oral
and Maxillofacial Surgery, Divison of Surgical
Oncology, Department of Surgery,
University of Florida, College of Medicine,
Jacksonville, Florida

PAUL A. GARDNER, MD
Assistant Professor, Department of
Neurological Surgery, University of Pittsburgh
School of Medicine, Pittsburgh, Pennsylvania

BRAD S. JOHNSON, DMD
Former Chief Resident, Oral and Maxillofacial
Surgery, Broward General Medical Center/
Nova Southeastern University, Fort
Lauderdale, Florida; Private Practice,
Marysville, Tennessee

AMIN B. KASSAM, MD
Professor, Department of Otolaryngology –
Head and Neck Surgery; Department of
Neurological Surgery, University of Pittsburgh
School of Medicine, Pittsburgh, Pennsylvania

PRASHANT KUMTA, PhD
Edward R. Wiedlein Chair, Professor,
Department of BioEngineering; Department
of Chemical and Petroleum Engineering;
Department of Mechanical Engineering and
Materials Science, Swanson School of
Engineering; Department of Oral Biology,
University of Pittsburgh School of Engineering;
Faculty, McGowan Institute for Regenerative
Medicine, Pittsburgh, Pennsylvania

JASON LISS, MD
Fellow, Oculoplastic Surgery, University of
Pittsburgh Medical Center; UPMC Eye Center,
Pittsburgh, Pennsylvania

JOSEPH P. McCAIN, DMD
Professor, Oral and Maxillofacial Surgery,
Broward General Medical Center/Nova
Southeastern University, Fort Lauderdale;
Miami, Florida

MARK W. OCHS, DMD, MD
Professor and Chair, Department of Oral and
Maxillofacial Surgery, University of Pittsburgh
School of Dental Medicine, Pittsburgh,
Pennsylvania

TAO OUYANG, MD
Assistant Professor of Radiology, Penn State
Hershey Medical Center, Hershey,
Pennsylvania

FRED PEDROLETTI, DMD
Chief Resident, Oral and Maxillofacial Surgery,
Broward General Medical Center/Nova
Southeastern University, Fort Lauderdale,
Florida

JOSEPH PETRONE, DMD, MDS, MPH
Chair and Program Director, Department
of Orthodontics, University of Pittsburgh
School of Dental Medicine, Pittsburgh,
Pennsylvania

JOANNE L. PRASAD, DDS
Clinical Assistant Professor, Department of
Diagnostic Sciences, University of Pittsburgh
School of Dental Medicine, Pittsburgh,
Pennsylvania

DANIEL M. PREVEDELLO, MD
Assistant Professor, Department of
Neurological Surgery, University of
Pittsburgh School of Medicine, Pittsburgh,
Pennsylvania

RAMON L. RUIZ, DMD, MD
Medical Director, Department of Pediatric
Craniomaxillofacial Surgery, Arnold Palmer
Hospital for Children; Associate Professor
of Surgery, Department of Surgery, University
of Central Florida College of Medicine,
Orlando, Florida

CHARLES S. SFEIR, DMD, PhD
Director, Center for Craniofacial Regeneration;
Department of Oral Biology, University of
Pittsburgh School of Dental Medicine; Faculty,
McGowan Institute for Regenerative Medicine,
Pittsburgh, Pennsylvania

GAURAV SHAH, BS
Research Associate, Department of Oral and
Maxillofacial Surgery, University of Pittsburgh
School of Dental Medicine, Pittsburgh,
Pennsylvania

CARL H. SNYDERMAN, MD
Professor, Department of Otolaryngology –
Head and Neck Surgery; Department of
Neurological Surgery, University of
Pittsburgh School of Medicine, Pittsburgh,
Pennsylvania

JACQUELINE SOHN, DMD, MDS
Private Practice, Pittsburgh, Pennsylvania

S. TONYA STEFKO, MD, FACS
Assistant Professor, Department of
Ophthalmology, University of Pittsburgh
Medical Center; Director of Oculoplastic,
Esthetic, and Reconstructive Surgery; UPMC
Eye Center, Pittsburgh, Pennsylvania

Contents

Preface   xiii

Bernard J. Costello

Outcomes Research and the Challenge of Evidence-Based Surgery   1

Thomas B. Dodson

> Outcomes research is focused on measuring the results or end products of health
> care interventions, processes, and practices. Data derived from outcomes research
> informs clinical practice, quality assurance, and patient safety activities, and can be
> the nidus for hypothesis-driven, patient-oriented research. This article introduces
> a definition of outcomes research, reviews how outcomes research may guide evi-
> dence-based surgical practice and health care processes, and reviews a model for
> outcomes research.

Prenatal Diagnosis and Treatment of Craniomaxillofacial Anomalies   5

Bernard J. Costello and Sean P. Edwards

> Many advances in health care are built on the evolution of technology. An entirely
> new patient has emerged in fetal medicine, with these advances in prenatal imaging
> allowing one to see and diagnose disease not previously appreciated. Clinicians can
> better plan for the delivery of the neonate, with identified anomalies being optimally
> managed and the impact on the neonate's health minimized. The oral and maxillo-
> facial surgeon offers expertise in the management of craniomaxillofacial anomalies,
> including congenital tumors, facial clefts, craniosynostosis, micrognathia, and other
> congenital abnormalities. The techniques for perinatal care of the patient with cra-
> niofacial abnormalities continue to evolve as the technology improves. The authors
> describe their experience and some of the more common abnormalities with their
> management considerations that may be encountered by the oral and maxillofacial
> surgeon on the fetal diagnosis and treatment team.

Bone Morphogenetic Proteins in Craniomaxillofacial Surgery   17

Sarah D. Davies and Mark W. Ochs

> Craniomaxillofacial surgery has many indications for bone regeneration and aug-
> mentation, ranging from socket preservation to reconstruction of large skeletal de-
> fects. The discovery of bone morphogenetic proteins (BMPs) as osteoinductive
> agents and the subsequent development of commercially available recombinant
> forms of BMPs have offered the potential to replace traditional grafting techniques
> with de novo bone formation. Extensive preclinical and clinical research has focused
> on establishing the safety and efficacy of using recombinant BMPs to regenerate
> bone in the facial skeleton. This article reviews the development and current scien-
> tific basis behind the use of these new biologics.

Regenerative Medicine for Craniomaxillofacial Surgery   33

Bernard J. Costello, Gaurav Shah, Prashant Kumta, and Charles S. Sfeir

> Regenerative medicine has recently seen much activity in basic and translational re-
> search. These advances are now making their way into surgical practice. A conver-
> gence of technologies has afforded opportunities previously not available with
> conventional surgical reconstructive techniques. Patients requiring complex

reconstructive surgery in the craniomaxillofacial region typically benefit from local or regional flaps, nonvascularized grafts, microvascular tissue transfer, or substitute alloplastic materials to restore function and form. In these clinical situations, grafting procedures or alloplastic substitute materials provide best-case replacements for resected, injured, or congenitally missing tissues. However, ideal reconstructive goals, such as a complete return to original form and function, are frequently not completely achieved. Regenerative techniques now in clinical use and at the translational research stage hold promise for custom-tailored constructs with the potential to regenerate tissue in the host without significant donor site morbidity. These techniques may provide better structure, aesthetics, and function than the best currently available options. This article presents the latest concepts in craniomaxillofacial regenerative medicine and reviews the multipronged approach to restoring architecture using novel "smart" multifunctional scaffolds, cellular technologies, growth factors, and other novel regenerative medical strategies.

Cleft Lip and Palate Surgery: An Update of Clinical Outcomes for Primary Repair   43

Andrew Campbell, Bernard J. Costello, and Ramon L. Ruiz

The comprehensive management of cleft lip and palate has received significant attention in the surgical literature over the last half century. It is the most common congenital facial malformation and has a significant developmental, physical, and psychological impact on those with the deformity and their families. In the United States, current estimates place the prevalence of cleft lip and palate or isolated cleft lip at approximately 1 in 600. There is significant phenotypic variation in the specific presentation of facial clefts. Understanding outcome data is important when making clinical decisions for patients with clefts. This article provides an update on current primary cleft lip and palate outcome data.

Orbital Surgery: State of the Art   59

Jason Liss, S. Tonya Stefko, and William L. Chung

Much has been written about the repair of orbital fractures, yet some debate still exists among surgeons with regard to indications for and timing of fracture repair and various surgical techniques. Controversies regarding the surgical maneuvers include the incision, surgical approach, and methods of wound closure. More detailed imaging modalities have allowed clinicians to understand the injuries more completely and plan for and execute more ideal reconstructions. Recent advances in orbital implant materials and the role of endoscopy in orbital fracture repair add to this debate about which techniques would be best for particular injuries. This article discusses these issues and provides the most current literature review regarding the management of various orbital fractures.

Technology in Microvascular Surgery   73

Alessandro Cusano and Rui Fernandes

With the refinement of microvascular technique, free-tissue transfer has emerged as the standard of care in head and neck reconstruction. Success rates and reductions in operative time have reduced "flap take" from being the marker of reconstructive success to being an expectation. Interest has now shifted to improvement of technique, with surgeons placing increasing importance on donor site morbidity, quality of tissue harvested, and esthetic and functional outcomes. Much of the recent success can be attributed to technological advance through improvement in instrumentation and technique and enhancement of the understanding of flap physiology and anatomy. This article reviews some of the recent advances and how they have affected microvascular surgery from preoperative, operative, and postoperative standpoints.

Temporary Skeletal Anchorage Devices for Orthodontics   91

Bernard J. Costello, Ramon L. Ruiz, Joseph Petrone, and Jacqueline Sohn

This article discusses the recent advances and basic concepts of skeletal anchorage devices of various types and reviews the current literature on their use. Temporary skeletal anchorage devices allow orthodontic movements that were previously thought to be difficult if not impossible. Much like the concepts introduced during the beginnings of orthognathic dentofacial teams, treatment that uses skeletal anchorage requires interdisciplinary collaboration and planning with regular interaction, continuing education, and a regular review of the latest relevant literature.

Advances in Head and Neck Imaging   107

Tao Ouyang and Barton F. Branstetter

Imaging plays a key role in dental implantation, management of maxillofacial trauma, facial reconstruction, temporomandibular joint pathology, and evaluation and treatment of neoplasms and infections. In addition to traditional conventional radiography, recent advances in computer tomography, magnetic resonance imaging, and positron emission tomography–computed tomography fusion technology have made radiology an even more vital component of patient care in dental and craniomaxillofacial practice.

Computer-Assisted Craniomaxillofacial Surgery   117

Sean P. Edwards

Computer-assisted surgery (CAS) describes all forms of surgery planning or execution that incorporate various forms of advanced imaging, software, analysis, and planning and, in some cases, rapid prototyping technology, robotics, and image-guidance systems. Innovation is progressing rapidly, and new forms of technology continue to be incorporated and evaluated for their value in improving daily operations. This article reviews imaging, enhanced three-dimensional diagnostics, tactile models, CAS concepts, reconstructive surgery, bone flap shaping, distraction osteogenesis, and orthognathic surgery in relation to craniomaxillofacial surgery.

Computer Planning and Intraoperative Navigation in Cranio-Maxillofacial Surgery   135

R. Bryan Bell

Preoperative computer design and stereolithographic modeling combined with intraoperative navigation provide a useful guide for and possibly more accurate reconstruction of a variety of complex cranio-maxillofacial deformities. Although probably not necessary for routine use, the author's early experience confirms that of other surgeons with more than a decade of experience: computer-assisted surgery is indicated for complex posttraumatic or postablative reconstruction of the orbits, cranium, maxilla, and mandible; total temporomandibular joint replacement; orthognathic surgery; and complex dental/craniofacial implantology. Further study is needed to provide outcomes data and cost-benefit analyses for each of these indications.

Endonasal Surgery of the Ventral Skull Base–Endoscopic Transcranial Surgery   157

Amol M. Bhatki, Ricardo L. Carrau, Carl H. Snyderman, Daniel M. Prevedello,
Paul A. Gardner, and Amin B. Kassam

Skull base surgery is evolving from traditional transfacial and transcranial approaches to the endoscopic endonasal approach, a less intrusive corridor for accessing the ventral skull base. This technique eliminates facial scars, expedites recovery, and obviates brain retraction. The goals of surgical excision, whether palliative or curative, are identical: an approach that is less disruptive to normal tissues. By exploiting the sinonasal corridor, the entire ventral skull base may be accessed to successfully treat benign and malignant lesions. The expanding limits of endoscopic skull base surgery have been accompanied by commensurate innovations in reconstructive techniques that are reliable and have been shown to limit postoperative complications. This article describes the basis for this approach and provides the latest outcome data supporting the current state of the art for endoscopic skull base surgery.

Endoscopic Techniques in Oral and Maxillofacial Surgery   169

Fred Pedroletti, Brad S. Johnson, and Joseph P. McCain

Oral and maxillofacial surgery is entering a new era. Surgeons can use the latest technological advances in equipment in an attempt to improve patient outcomes. Minimally invasive surgery with the use of the endoscope has improved in recent years because of technological advancements in optics and associated instrumentation. Trauma, orthognathic, sialoendoscopy, and temporomandibular joint surgery are commonly performed with the assistance of the endoscope. From an educational standpoint, surgical anatomy and various other principles can easily be taught to trainees with the assistance of the endoscope. The operating surgeon can visualize an area via the endoscope, and instruct regarding the surgical maneuvers on the monitor, without obstructions to view. This technique also allows others in and out of the room to view the image. Endoscopically assisted surgery is gaining popularity and is becoming a tool frequently used by surgeons to assist in and simplify some of the more difficult techniques that often require more extensive surgical exposure for visualization.

Molecular Diagnostics for Head and Neck Pathology   183

Elizabeth Bilodeau, Faizan Alawi, Bernard J. Costello, and Joanne L. Prasad

Molecular diagnostic techniques are quickly finding a role in the detection and diagnosis of tumors, and in predicting their behavior. They may also prove useful in developing new therapeutic approaches to head and neck cancer. The surgeon working in the craniomaxillofacial region should have an understanding of these technologies, their availability in various settings, and how they affect various aspects of treatment, particularly in the detection and treatment of malignancies. This article offers an overview of recent advances in molecular diagnostic techniques, with their implications for diagnosis and management of head and neck tumors.

Adhesive Use in Oral and Maxillofacial Surgery   195

Michael J. Buckley and Eric J. Beckman

Presently, tissue adhesives and sealants have limited use in oral and maxillofacial surgical procedures. Skin closure occurs regularly with cyanoacrylate adhesives. Sealing of dural tears in conjunction with dural closure has been shown to be very successful. With the development of more head and neck reconstructive procedures and cosmetic procedures, demand will increase for better surgical adhesives. Clinical trials are beginning for newly developed adhesives with the chemical characterizations, the safe reabsorptive profile, and the adhesive strength necessary to benefit oral and maxillofacial surgery patients in the near future. Adhesives for bone fixation, while in early development, also show a promising chemical profile and will be of significant benefit to oral and maxillofacial surgical patients.

Index   201

Oral and Maxillofacial Surgery Clinics of North America

FORTHCOMING ISSUES

May 2010

Collaborative Care of the Facial Injury Patient
Vivek Shetty, DDS, Dr Med, Dent and
Grant Marshall, PhD, *Guest Editors*

August 2010

**Alveolar Bone Grafting Techniques in Dental
Implant Preparation**
Peter D. Waite, MPH, DDS, MD, *Guest Editor*

November 2010

**Psychological Issues for the Oral and
Maxillofacial Surgeon**
Hillel Ephros, DMD, MD, *Guest Editor*

RECENT ISSUES

November 2009

**Evaluation and Management of Obstructive
Sleep Apnea**
Scott B. Boyd, DDS, PhD, *Guest Editor*

August 2009

Salivary Gland Infections
Michael D. Turner, DDS, MD, FACS
and Robert Glickman, DMD, *Guest Editors*

May 2009

Current Controversies in Maxillofacial Trauma
Daniel M. Laskin, DDS, MS and
Robert Glickman, DMD, *Guest Editors*

RELATED INTEREST

Dental Clinics of North America, October 2008 (Vol. 52, No. 4)
Contemporary Dental and Maxillofacial Imaging
Steven L. Thomas, DDS, MS and Christos Angelopoulos, DDS, MS, *Guest Editors*

THE CLINICS ARE NOW AVAILABLE ONLINE!

Access your subscription at:
www.theclinics.com

Preface

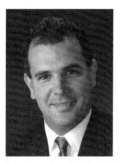

Bernard J. Costello, DMD, MD, FACS
Guest Editor

When one thinks about advances in science or medicine, it is important to put them in perspective within a historical and philosophic context. Ultimately, advances, or even revolutions, are a cumulative enterprise, hopefully with the credit falling to those who laid the groundwork before the sentinel event that defines a particular discovery. It is a process by which invention and discovery often grow out of unsuspected or newly observed phenomena. This process was described by Kuhn as one in which observation occurs, conceptualization happens, assimilation to theory transforms, and discovery arises.[1] This process must take some amount of time. The cumulative occurrences then lead to a change in paradigm that happens as a result of deliberate, but not necessarily long, conceptual assimilation. Often, acceptance of the advancement occurs by violating deeply entrenched expectations (eg, the world is flat). As a result, considerable debate typically surrounds transformative advances.

Understanding how to interpret new surgical techniques and technologies is fundamental to the progression of our specialty. This issue presents some of the most exciting developments in craniomaxillofacial surgery. The genesis of this issue came out of my discussions with colleagues and trainees regarding the changing face of craniomaxillofacial surgery. The changes currently transforming our specialty include technological advancements, shifts in philosophic thought, and renewed efforts at cross-training and collaboration. The topics within this issue are just some of the many advances that we are experiencing within our anatomically defined specialty. At first glance, these topics seem somewhat unrelated,

but they have been chosen to be representative of two main areas of surgical advancement: (1) innovation in technique and or thought (eg, conceptualizing and executing cleft or craniofacial surgical procedures based on outcome data); (2) technological advances that are catapulting our field forward into new territory (eg, development of the endoscope, navigation, or fetal imaging). The very nature of advancements dictates that by the time this issue is published, certain aspects of what is reported will have changed.

The issue starts with Dr Tom Dodson's discussion regarding the importance of evidence-based care and what rigorous analysis means for our specialty. These key concepts override all that we do that is new. Understanding concepts of outcome-based research allow the informed clinician to make the best choices for his/her patients based on solid evidence, and not solely on the opinion of experts. Throughout these articles, this common thread is presented and reminders of the levels of evidence are indicated to clarify the strength of data behind new concepts. Although several classification systems exist for defining what levels of evidence are meaningful, we have chosen a widely used and simple classification system that outlines important concepts of clinical research and reports.

- Level I evidence: prospective, randomized, clinical trials with sufficient power to make clear and strong conclusions
- Level II evidence: lesser quality prospective comparative studies and well-controlled case cohort studies with strong data and excellent study design

Oral Maxillofacial Surg Clin N Am 22 (2010) xiii–xiv
doi:10.1016/j.coms.2009.11.004

- Level III evidence: retrospective comparative studies, case-control observational studies, systematic reviews that include any studies other than Level I or II papers, case series/reports, and expert opinion.

Regrettably, most surgical care has been dictated by Level III evidence. However, as Dr Dodson points out, evidence is mounting. This includes evidence-based outcome data in the areas of dentoalveolar surgery, anesthesia, cleft care, and others. As with all evidence-based decision making, the surgeon must not blindly follow only prospective evidence, but integrate the best available knowledge with individual experience and patient factors to make the best choices possible.

Important then is the conceptual linking of the need for high level evidence with the introduction of new technologies such as image guidance, biologics, or minimally invasive surgery. Does the new innovative thought process or procedure improve the outcome for the patient? How do we assess this question clearly and completely with data? Does the new technology offer a better recovery or improved long-term measurable results? These are questions that can only be completely and definitively answered by Level I evidence. Some of the new technologies and innovations discussed in this issue have considerable evidence, and others are still developing. Either way, rigorous academic analysis and debate is necessary when we consider the usefulness of these new opportunities for our patients.

Surgery has been slowly changing over the past few decades; it is becoming clearer what evidence should guide us in our decision making.[2–4] Gone are the days when surgical giants merely suggested a treatment philosophy or procedure with its almost immediate acceptance. Surgeons, patients, and even payers in today's health care environment are demanding high levels of evidence to justify clinical choices and validate those concepts we have held dear for decades. Standards are pushed higher and patient care is improved.

The work presented here represents a process of assimilation of thought in various exciting new areas, not just one individual or group's eureka moment. The contributors to this issue have unique skills that not only include surgical excellence but also represent exceptional surgical thinking with an ability to transform ideas into new surgical principles. These new ideas are presented to you for further debate and perhaps for assimilation into mainstream practice.

Bernard J. Costello, DMD, MD, FACS
Department of Oral and Maxillofacial Surgery
University of Pittsburgh School of Dental Medicine
Salk Hall, 3501 Terrace Street
Pittsburgh, PA 15261, USA

Pediatric Oral and Maxillofacial Surgery
Children's Hospital of Pittsburgh
Pittsburgh, PA, USA

E-mail address:
bjc1@pitt.edu

REFERENCES

1. Kuhn TS. The structure of scientific revolutions. 2nd edition. London: University of Chicago Press; 1970.
2. Cochrane AL. Effectiveness and efficiency: random reflections on health services. London: Nuffield Provincial Hospitals Trust; 1972. Reprinted in 1989 in association with the BMJ. Reprinted in 1999 for Nuffield Trust by the Royal Society of Medicine Press, London, UK.
3. Gray JAM. Evidence-based healthcare: how to make health policy and management decisions. London: Churchill Livingstone; 1997.
4. Sackett DL, Rosenberg WM, Gray JA, et al. Evidence based medicine: what it is and what it isn't. Br Med J 1996;312(7023):71–2.

Outcomes Research and the Challenge of Evidence-Based Surgery

Thomas B. Dodson, DMD, MPH[a,b,*]

KEYWORDS

- Outcomes research • Quality assurance
- Evidence-based surgical practice
- Patient-oriented research

The purposes of this article are to introduce a definition of outcomes research, to review how outcomes research may guide evidence-based surgical practice and health care processes, and to review a model for outcomes research.

WHAT IS OUTCOMES RESEARCH?

Almost invariably, when the author mentions outcomes research, audiences or readers raise their collective eyebrows quizzically as if to ask, "What does that mean?" It is an excellent question. In general, outcomes research focuses on the end products or results of health care practices, interventions, and processes.

As practiced, however, outcomes research means different things to different people. To some, outcomes research means developing clinical benchmarks or practice guidelines. To others, outcomes research is used for quality assurance and patient safety activities. To others still, outcomes research tries to explain variability in clinical practice or linking types of care to outcomes. Regardless of an individual's definition of outcomes research, outcomes research has similar goals (eg, improve the patient care or the health care process) and uses similar clinical epidemiologic investigative tools.

At the Center for Applied Clinical Investigation (CACI) based in the Department of Oral and Maxillofacial Surgery at Massachusetts General Hospital, outcomes research is one area of focus. Outcomes researchers at CACI measure what happened and why it happened.

CACI's outcomes research activities are grouped into two areas. First, researchers want to estimate how often events of interest occur, that is, what happened. Frequency, incidence, or survival estimates of outcomes are measured for patient care activities (eg, nerve repair, complications after third molar surgery, or implant survival).[1–5] This information is used to inform clinical care and practice.

Equally important is estimating the results of health care processes or practices (eg, satisfaction with telephone follow-up after dentoalveolar procedures or following nerve repair, frequency of completed consent forms, or length of hospitalization after orthognathic surgery).[6–8] This information can be used for benchmarking, patient education, or improving quality or safety processes.

Article preparation was supported by the Massachusetts General Hospital Department of Oral and Maxillofacial Surgery's Center for Applied Clinical Investigation and Education and Research Fund and Massachusetts General Physician Organization.

[a] Center for Applied Clinical Investigation, Department of Oral and Maxillofacial Surgery, Massachusetts General Hospital, 55 Fruit Street, Warren Building Suite 1201, Boston, MA 02114, USA
[b] Department of Oral and Maxillofacial Surgery, Harvard School of Dental Medicine, 188 Longwood Avenue, Boston, MA 02115, USA
* Center for Applied Clinical Investigation, Department of Oral and Maxillofacial Surgery, Massachusetts General Hospital, 55 Fruit Street, Warren Building Suite 1201, Boston, MA 02114.
E-mail address: tbdodson@partners.org

Oral Maxillofacial Surg Clin N Am 22 (2010) 1–4
doi:10.1016/j.coms.2009.10.004
1042-3699/10/$ – see front matter © 2010 Elsevier Inc. All rights reserved.

oralmaxsurgery.theclinics.com

The Center's second outcomes research activity focuses on identifying factors or variables associated with the outcome (ie, why did the event of interest happen?). These factors can be classified as prognostic (ie, associated with a favorable outcome or result) or risk (ie, associated with an unfavorable outcome or result). For example, one could look at factors associated with implant survival (prognostic) or implant failure (risk).[9] The factors associated with an outcome of interest are then categorized as immutable (eg, age or sex) or potentially modifiable (eg, perioperative antibiotic use). Immutable factors may be used to predict prognosis or risk for outcomes of interest. Modifiable factors may be used to improve outcomes.

USING OUTCOMES RESEARCH TO ENHANCE AND GUIDE EVIDENCE-BASED SURGICAL PRACTICE AND HEALTH CARE PROCESSES
Enhancing Evidence-based Surgical Practice

Systematic collection of outcome data can inform clinical practice. Frequency, incidence, or survival data can be used be used to inform patients of the likelihood of a good (or bad) result. For example, these types of data can be used to inform the average patient about the likelihood for postoperative infection or nerve injury after third molar surgery or the chance that an implant will survive.

As noted above, factors associated with outcomes are identified and grouped into two categories: immutable (eg, age and sex) or modifiable (eg, tobacco use, implant length, timing of implant loading, use of antibiotics). Since immutable variables cannot be changed, data regarding these variables can be used to inform the patient of prognosis or risk. For example, an older patient may have an increased risk for intra- or postoperative complications associated with third molar surgery. One cannot change the patient's age, but can use that information to help set treatment or prognosis expectations.

In contrast, modifiable variables may be used to enhance prognosis or decrease the risk for an adverse outcome. Modifying tobacco use may affect the risk of postoperative complications. As such, the clinician may suggest that a patient stop smoking before implant insertion to improve the likelihood of implant survival or decrease the risk for a postoperative inflammatory complication.

Modifiable variables can be used to generate additional studies to test a hypothesis that changes in the modifiable variable results in changes the outcome. Absent additional data, one should be quite cautious in translating the findings from an outcomes study directly to patient care. In most cases, outcomes studies are not designed to identify variables associated with the outcome of interest. These findings are valuable "side-effects" of the study. As such, biases in study sample selection, incomplete data collection, subject follow-up, or variable definitions could produce spurious associations. Instead, new, controlled trials should be implemented, guided by hypotheses arising from the outcomes research, to confirm or refute the observed relationship between the factor and outcome of interest.

Enhancing Evidence-based Healthcare Processes

Outcomes research can improve or inform health care processes. Outcomes research may be used to establish benchmarks and used as a quality assurance or safety activity. For example, national statistics suggest that the frequency of patients who are extremely or moderately satisfied with their deep sedation, general anesthesia experience is 94.9%.[10] Individual clinicians or practices may survey their patients' satisfaction with deep sedation, general anesthesia and compare the results to a prespecified target or nationally established benchmark. Adverse deviations from the target or benchmark may prompt a review of clinical protocols, and suggest changes, implementation of a new clinical protocol, and iterative measures of the outcome to see if the changes result in achieving or exceeding the benchmark.

Absent a prespecified national benchmark, the practice may survey its patients to establish its own baseline frequency of some outcome of interest (eg, use of two identifiers for patient identification). Once the baseline is established, the practice may repeat the survey on a regular basis to confirm that the baseline target is being achieved. If the target is consistently achieved, a new target may be specified or a different outcome evaluated.

Outcomes research can be used for patient education. Estimates of a practice's or specialties' frequency of inferior alveolar nerve injury or surgical site infection after third molar removal may be valuable information because, when conveyed to patients, it may to help them determine the best management choice for third molars.

A MODEL FOR OUTCOMES RESEARCH

Fig. 1 summarizes CACI's outcomes research cycle. The first step is to generate a research question. There are two excellent sources to generate research questions. The first is the

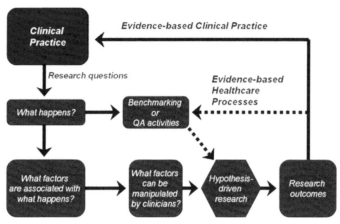

Fig. 1. Models for outcomes research.

investigator's clinical practice. A practical alternative source is a regulatory or licensing body.

Generically, the research question takes the following form, "Among patients with (some clinical problem of interest), what is the frequency of (an outcome of interest) and what factors or variables are associated with (the outcome of interest)?" A specific question could be, "Among patients receiving dental implants in my practice, what is the one-year survival rate and what prognostic factors are associated with survival?"

To answer the question, the investigator will need to determine a study design and choose a clinically relevant sample. For many outcomes research purposes, retrospective or cross-sectional study designs work are excellent for generating preliminary data or benchmarks. Use of retrospective or cross-sectional data allows the investigator to generate quickly a study sample and a database. However, as noted previously, because of well-known biases associated with retrospective or cross-sectional studies, one should exercise caution in translating these findings to patient care.

To maximize data collection efforts, the study should be designed to address the two primary goals of outcomes research, estimating the frequency of outcome of interest and identifying factors associated with the outcome. For purposes of benchmarking activities, one may only be interested in the frequency estimates and use these estimate to establish targets or benchmarks as part of quality assurance exercises. For clinical practice, the investigator will try to identify modifiable variables associated with the outcome. In the latter circumstance, these factors can be converted into new clinical questions and generate new hypothesis-driven research usually in the form of a prospective, controlled clinical trial. The

results from well-designed, controlled clinical trials may then feed back to improve clinical practice. A side effect of outcomes research may be observations that generate biologic questions answered in basic research laboratories.

Quality assurance or patient safety studies used to generate targets or benchmarks need not be limited to generating descriptive statistics alone. These types of projects can be readily adapted to become hypothesis-driven outcomes research. One can just as easily identify factors associated with achieving targets and then manipulate them to enhance the likelihood of reaching future targets.

SUMMARY

Outcomes research is a special case of patient-oriented research activities. Its focus is measuring the frequency of outcomes and identifying factors associated with outcomes. The goals of outcomes research are to improve clinical care and health care processes and practices.

REFERENCES

1. Chuang SK, Perrott DH, Susarla SM, et al. Risk factors for inflammatory complications following third molar surgery. J Oral Maxillofac Surg 2008;66: 2213–8.
2. Susarla S, Kaban LB, Donoff RB, et al. Does early repair of lingual nerve injuries improve functional sensory recovery? J Oral Maxillofac Surg 2007;65: 1070–6.
3. Bui CH, Seldin EB, Dodson TB. Types, frequencies, and risk factors for complications following third molar extraction. J Oral Maxillofac Surg 2003;61: 1379–89.

4. Chuang SK, Tian L, Wei L-J, et al. Kaplan-Meier analysis of dental implant survival: a strategy for estimating survival with clustered observations. J Dent Res 2001;80:2016–20.

5. Susarla SM, Dodson TB. How well do clinicians estimate third molar extraction difficulty? J Oral Maxillofac Surg 2005;63:191–9.

6. Human ET, Juvet LM, Nastri A, et al. Changing patterns of hospital length of stay following orthognathic surgery. J Oral Maxillofac Surg 2008;66:492–7.

7. Susarla S, Kaban LB, Donoff RB, et al. A comparison of patient satisfaction and objective assessment of neurosensory function after trigeminal nerve repair. J Oral Maxillofac Surg 2005;63:1138.

8. Lam NP, Kaban LB, Donoff RB, et al. Patient satisfaction after trigeminal nerve repair. Oral Surg Oral Med Oral Pathol 2003;95:538–43.

9. Chuang SK, Wei L-J, Douglass CW, et al. Risk factors for dental implant failure: a strategy for the analysis of clustered failure time observations. J Dent Res 2002;81:572–7.

10. Perrott DH, Yuen J, Andresen R, et al. Office-based ambulatory anesthesia: an overview of the clinical practice of oral and maxillofacial surgeons in the United States. J Oral Maxillofac Surg 2003;61:983–95.

Prenatal Diagnosis and Treatment of Craniomaxillofacial Anomalies

Bernard J. Costello, DMD, MD, FACS[a,b,]*,
Sean P. Edwards, DDS, MD, FRCD(C)[c]

KEYWORDS

- Cleft • Micrognathia • Prenatal diagnosis
- Fetal facial anomalies

Encountering the fetus as a patient has become a reality. Advances in prenatal imaging allows one to see and diagnose malformations and disease not previously appreciated. With this information, clinicians can better plan for the delivery of the neonate such that any identified anomalies are optimally managed and the impact on the neonate's health minimized. The oral and maxillofacial surgeon can play a key role by offering expertise in the immediate and staged management of craniomaxillofacial anomalies, including congenital tumors, facial clefts, craniosynostosis, micrognathia, and other developmental abnormalities. Understanding the natural course of these congenital abnormalities allows the experienced oral and maxillofacial surgeon to work in an interdisciplinary fashion to provide care to this new population of patients.

FETAL DIAGNOSIS AND TREATMENT: INTERDISCIPLINARY TEAM CARE

Much like the dynamics in a well-balanced and effective cleft/craniofacial team, the fetal diagnosis and treatment team can offer a unique opportunity for a very high level of care that thrives on interdisciplinary collaboration. This is particularly important in planning for and delivering a child with an anomaly that may have an impact on the child's health or survival. Fetal diagnosis and treatment teams may be comprised of specialists from a wide variety of disciplines. These teams usually include practitioners from genetics, neonatology, maternal-fetal medicine/obstetrics, radiology, medical ethics, and social work, and other pediatric specialists with expertise in each of the body systems.

The oral and maxillofacial surgeon has an integral role on such teams and may be of assistance in developing a differential diagnosis of a lesion or syndrome, which may affect the management of the fetus at birth. Abnormalities of the craniomaxillofacial structures can have an immediate effect on the viability of a neonate because of their impact on the airway or on swallowing. Some anomalies require an early management protocol during the first days of life. Others require a staged reconstruction, and careful planning with the family is essential for the best outcome. The careful treatment of these anomalies requires training and experience. As with many clinical issues that traverse the scope of various specialties, the decision-making regarding treatment is best accomplished in an interdisciplinary format.

[a] Craniofacial and Cleft Surgery, Department of Oral and Maxillofacial Surgery, University of Pittsburgh School of Dental Medicine, 3471 Fifth Avenue, Suite 1112, Pittsburgh, PA 15213, USA
[b] Pediatric Oral and Maxillofacial Surgery, Children's Hospital of Pittsburgh, Pittsburgh, PA, USA
[c] Pediatric Oral and Maxillofacial Surgery, Division of Oral and Maxillofacial Surgery, Department of Surgery, University of Michigan Medical Center, MI, USA
* Corresponding author. Craniofacial and Cleft Surgery, Department of Oral and Maxillofacial Surgery, University of Pittsburgh School of Dental Medicine, 3471 Fifth Avenue, Suite 1112, Pittsburgh, PA 15213.
E-mail address: Bjc1@pitt.edu

Oral Maxillofacial Surg Clin N Am 22 (2010) 5–15
doi:10.1016/j.coms.2009.10.003

The authors have encountered several abnormalities that benefit from the involvement of a specialist trained in craniomaxillofacial deformity.[1] Because this is a relatively new field, the total number of referrals to the center increased dramatically over a 6-year period as the community became more aware of the resources of the team (**Fig. 1**).

The total number of patients with prenatal diagnoses determined by the University of Pittsburgh Fetal Diagnosis Treatment Team was 1782 for a 6-year period. Of these anomalies, 304 were anomalies that had craniomaxillofacial implications. Clefts were 4% of the total anomalies seen over the 6-year period. Masses accounted for 3%, and other craniofacial anomalies accounted for 11%. Some of the other craniofacial anomalies included micrognathia, midfacial hypoplasia, nasal abnormalities, and facial asymmetry. The most common craniomaxillofacial abnormalities were cleft lip and palate, cervical or oral masses, micrognathia, and various craniofacial anomalies with facial dysmorphology, typically seen on ultrasonography.[2] The number of patients with particular diagnoses increased in certain categories (**Fig. 2**). This was probably based on the increased experience of ultrasonographers and the team. Increasing referrals over 6 years probably had an effect on the types of anomalies sent to the team for evaluation.

The importance of interdisciplinary care cannot be overemphasized. The antenatal diagnosis of a malformation, lesion, or syndrome carries with it a great deal of social, ethical, and medical management issues, none of which are easily separated from the other. In the end, several patients are being treated. Although the health of the developing fetus is of considerable concern, the health of the mother cannot be separated from it. A diagnosis of a prenatal abnormality will bring stress and anxiety and tax the coping skills of any family. Interdisciplinary teams must function as a resource to help them throughout the process on every level.

The fetal diagnosis team can offer several levels of care, depending on the severity of the disorder identified. Some anomalies, such as a cleft lip, will often require no special antenatal intervention although additional testing may be warranted. However, antenatal diagnosis does offer the opportunity to relay important information about care of children with cleft deformities when the family is not overwhelmed by having a new baby at home. The fetal diagnosis and treatment team may elect to refer the parents, prenatally, to a cleft and craniofacial surgeon and team so that parents may take advantage of the resources the team can offer.

When a fetus presents with multiple or complex anomalies, delivery of the child with coordinated management of all involved specialties is facilitated. Certain anomalies will present an immediate threat to the viability of the fetus in utero or at the time of delivery. These may be managed with fetal procedures or via a myriad of postnatal procedures such as the EXIT (ex utero intrapartum therapy) and possibly ECMO (extracorporeal membrane oxygenation). These techniques have been developed over recent years and continue to be refined.[1–7]

The implementation of these procedures becomes part of a delivery plan formulated by the team. This plan deals with family logistics of getting the mother and baby where they need to be and arranging that needed specialists and resources are immediately available for the delivery. Other issues to be resolved include team members that would need to be present at the delivery, equipment that will be necessary, and determination of the optimal anesthetic plan. Plans should also be made for appropriate neonatal care and for critical care for the mother if necessary. These deliveries can be very complex and time spent working out details and different scenarios that may arise can be invaluable in achieving a successful outcome. Such teams are the ideal format for continual data gathering, outcomes assessment, system development, and amelioration. This process starts with detailed prenatal care.

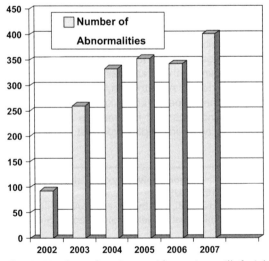

Fig. 1. Number of patients with craniomaxillofacial deformities referred to the University of Pittsburgh fetal diagnosis treatment team from 2002 to 2007.

Prenatal Care

Prenatal care is a complex process of screening, diagnostic tests, physical examinations, and

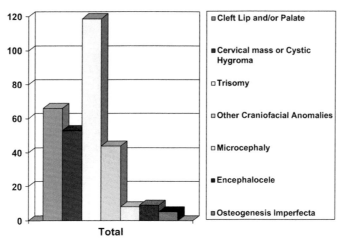

Fig. 2. Type of craniomaxillofacial deformities that patients who were treated at the University of Pittsburgh fetal diagnosis treatment team from 2002 to 2007.

counseling that functions as a form of preventative medicine designed to ensure the health of the fetus and mother alike. The complexity of this process depends on the identification of maternal factors that increase the risk for developing an anomaly, such as advanced age, family history, and maternal exposures. Typically, this care involves, at a minimum, an ultrasonography of the fetus to look for more common anomalies. If a significant family history or other important information exists, then additional visits for ultrasonographic imaging may be indicated. Additional testing (eg, chorionic villus sampling (CVS) or amniocentesis for karyotyping, fluorescent in situ hybridization analysis, or DNA analysis) may be offered.

Integral to this scheme and essential to the prenatal diagnosis of a fetal anomaly is imaging. In general, prenatal imaging serves several generally agreed on functions:

1. Confirming the presence of an intrauterine pregnancy
2. Estimating gestational age via a series of fetal measurements
3. Confirming suspected multiple gestations
4. Evaluating growth of the fetus and detect aberrancies therein
5. Evaluating the cause of vaginal bleeding
6. As a procedural aid for CVS, amniocentesis, or percutaneous umbilical blood sampling
7. Evaluating uterine anomalies and pelvic masses.

Detailed ultrasonography in the second trimester has become a routine part of pregnancy. This ultrasonography should occur when the fetus is large enough to detect anomalies

with a fair sensitivity and early enough to permit further investigations without excessive risk to the fetus when an anomaly is discovered. This age range is generally accepted to be 18 to 20 weeks. There is some controversy as to the necessity of routine prenatal ultrasonography but it seems that at least 70% of pregnant women undergo the procedure.[6–8] Ultrasonography is not merely aimed at the detection of fetal anomalies; it also plays an important role in this complex process of prenatal care. Computed tomography is not a recommended choice for imaging because of the possible effects of radiation on the fetus during early development. Magnetic resonance imaging (MRI) may be considered for special imaging needs described later in the article.[9,10]

Ultrasonography

Ultrasonography is a noninvasive, negligible-risk intervention that has become a standard component of prenatal care in much of the developed world.(**Figs. 3** and **4**) First introduced to obstetric care in the 1950s, the technology has gone through several advances that have allowed it to assume the prominent role it plays today. Gray-scale imaging and real-time sonography became available in the 1970s permitting differentiation of tissue planes and useful image capture of the constantly moving fetus (**Fig. 5**). Color and Doppler examinations were added in the 1980s and most recently, ultrahigh resolution with 3-dimensional (3D) real-time rendering has emerged.[11–15]

Three-dimensional imaging is essentially the 2-dimensional images acquired as a sweep or volume (see **Fig. 5**B). The acquired data can then

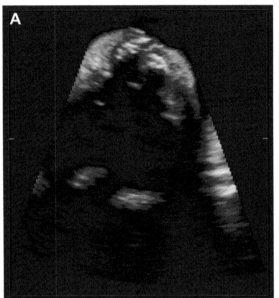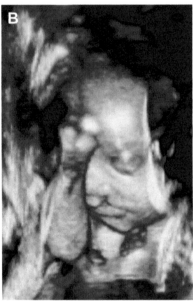

Fig. 3. (*A*) Two-dimensional ultrasonography in axial view of the maxilla showing the greater and lesser segments of a unilateral cleft lip and palate. Usually only the anterior palate is able to be visualized using this technique. (*B*) Three-dimensional ultrasonography of a child with a left-sided unilateral cleft lip and palate.

be displayed in any arbitrary plane or as a surface-rendered image.[11,13–18] This necessary range of freedom exists because it would be impossible with current technology to manually scan a fetus in the typical X, Y, and Z axes given the constraints imposed by fetal position and movement. The advantage of being able to manipulate this data becomes apparent when one considers that profile views of the face were obtained previously by simple probe positioning and effort of the ultrasonographer and could easily be subverted by fetal arm position. Computerized manipulation of this data can then be used to provide surface-rendered images. When these images are displayed in cinematic sequence, the technology has been referred to as "four-dimensional" ultrasonography.[9,14]

From a practical standpoint, most ultrasonographic examinations are real-time, 2-dimensional (2D) images that may be acquired in transabdominal, transvaginal, or transperineal fashion. As expected, it is neither possible nor practical to search every fetus for every anomaly possible. Instead, most examinations are general fetal surveys to confirm and document the fetal number, measure and confirm gestational age, document fetal well-being, and detect any obvious anomalies. That said, if an anomaly is detected or if a fetus is thought to be at an elevated risk of developing of certain anomalies, then a high-level examination can be performed.

Fetal MRI

Fetal MRI is becoming an increasingly popular modality for the more complete evaluation of fetal anomalies already noted on ultrasonography (see **Fig. 5**C). This popularity has arisen because of its safety and improvements in MRI technology. First applied to examine the developing fetus in 1983, the technique was slow and required sedation to slow the movement of the fetus to diminish the resultant artifact.[9] Currently, single-shot fast spin-echo T2-weighted images are the workhorse of fetal MRI. This technique allows acquisition of single slices in less than one second, minimizing the effect of fetal motion. Contrast is avoided because gadolinium, categorized as a pregnancy class C drug, is known to cross the placenta and may be absorbed by the fetus.

Fast fetal MRI does not supplant ultrasonography as a screening tool, and in fact, an ultrasonography is necessary. The objectives of fetal MRI, outlined by Sandrasegaran and colleagues[10] include

1. Confirming equivocal ultrasonography findings so that a confident decision for pregnancy management may be considered
2. Detecting other anomalies that may change fetal prognosis or maternal management
3. Helping in planning fetal surgery when necessary
4. Helping to plan the delivery, including the site of delivery, that is, tertiary versus community hospital, mode of delivery, level of neonatal

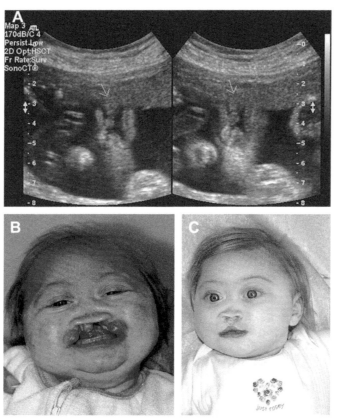

Fig. 4. (A) Two-dimensional ultrasonography of a bilateral cleft lip and palate (B) The child from Fig. 4A who also has semi-lobar holoprosencephaly (C) Postoperative result of the child from Fig. 4B.

care required, and individuals who need to be present at the delivery.

The study is usually performed with the mother supine, although in later stages of pregnancy, she would be placed in left decubitus to minimize caval compression. Sedation is avoided. A typical study can take 20 minutes to complete, depending on the image sequences required for the given lesion; however, the time is decreasing with better technology.[10]

The technique is useful for evaluation of central nervous system structural anomalies. It also has an important role in differentiating cystic lesions from solid masses and therefore, an important role in the evaluation and treatment planning of various craniofacial, cervical, thoracic, and abdominal lesions.

FETAL INTERVENTIONS AND PERINATAL THERAPIES
Parental Support and Counseling

One of the most satisfying interactions that a specialist on the fetal diagnosis treatment team

can provide is the early support for parents of a fetus with a congenital anomaly. The opportunity to discuss the details and expectations inform and empower the family during this difficult time. Misconceptions can be dispelled and important information for pregnancy management and delivery is considered. Important issues, such as the location of delivery and availability of various practitioners for coordinated care, are discussed up front. An essential aspect of this process is genetic counseling. The information gathered can be used to inform the parents about possible associated genetic disorders and the likelihood of having more children with similar anomalies. Confirmatory prenatal testing through CVS or amniocentesis can be considered. Testing is available for various entities, and the list is quickly expanding. Genes have been identified for many of the craniofacial dysostosis syndrome variants (eg, Apert, Crouzon, and Pfeiffer syndromes), Treacher Collins, velocardiofacial, and Sticker syndromes, and many others. The utility of testing is best determined in conjunction with an experienced geneticist as these tests are expensive. In many cases, pedigree analysis and a morphologic analysis of

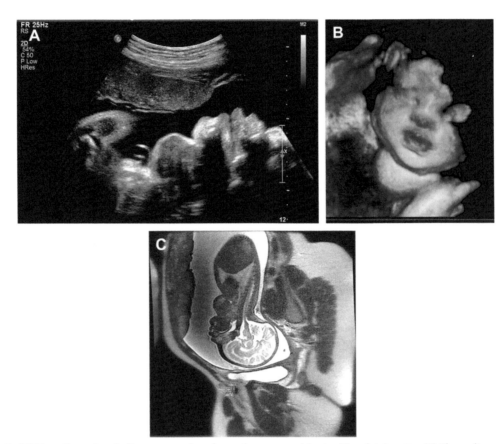

Fig. 5. (*A*) Two-dimensional ultrasonography of a neck mass consistent with a fetal goiter (*B*) Three-dimensional ultrasonography of a neck mass (fetal goiter from Fig. 5A) (*C*) Fetal MRI study of the fetus from Fig. 5A, B with a fetal goiter.

probands in the family results in a clear phenotypic diagnosis without the risk or expense of testing.

Fetal Interventional Procedures and Surgery

The current technology and neonatal support techniques do not allow for safe fetal repair and reconstruction of most anomalies in the craniomaxillofacial region. Thus, fetal surgery and other interventional procedures are generally reserved for life-threatening abnormalities that can be addressed in the later part of fetal development. As described later, abnormalities that involve the airway may require intervention to support the child during the early moments of birth. With rare exceptions, most fetal craniomaxillofacial abnormalities may be addressed at some point after birth (**Fig. 6**). In these cases, the risk is generally too great to warrant fetal intervention, although this may change as perinatal technology and technique improves. Unfortunately, technologic advances can be associated with morbidity, and this can be the case with fetal intervention procedures, such as

selective reduction of nonviable multiples. This is precisely why an experienced team of individuals is required to make careful decisions regarding the utility of various approaches as this area expands.

EXIT

The primary purpose of the EXIT procedure is to maintain uteroplacental blood flow to the newly born child when it would otherwise be compromised by structural or neoplastic lesions of the face, neck, and thorax.[3–5] Maintenance of this supply of oxygenated blood permits an airway to be secured in a safe orderly fashion, avoiding emergency intubations or more serious outcome. When successfully applied, normal blood gases can be maintained for close to one hour with the technique. There are several keys to the successful application of the technique, beginning with the recognition of a threatening lesion. Equally important is the assembly of the EXIT team and rehearsal of the process. Also important from a physiologic perspective,

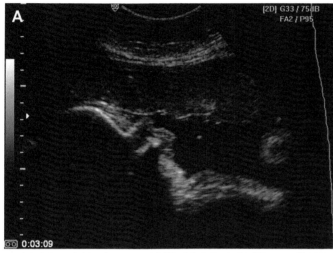

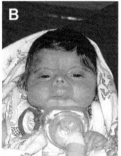
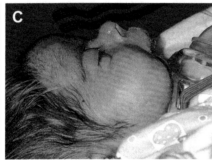

Fig. 6. (A) Two-dimensional ultrasonography of a child with micrognathia (B) Frontal view of a patient who was diagnosed with severe micrognathia in the prenatal period. An EXIT procedure was performed and the tracheostomy was performed in conjunction with pediatric surgery and otolaryngology when initial attempts at intubation failed. The process was carefully orchestrated at each step by the fetal diagnosis team before the birth, allowing for a seamless delivery of care. (C) Lateral view.

is deep, normotensive general anesthesia preventing intrauterine contraction, cessation of placental blood flow, and uteroplacental separation. With the neonate delivered via cesarean section, an airway can be established via conventional laryngoscopy, rigid endoscopy, fiberoptic intubation, or tracheostomy. When an airway cannot be obtained, ECMO can be considered in the so-called EXIT-to-ECMO scenario. This technique allows oxygenated blood to be circulated within the newborn using an external circuit when the lungs cannot be ventilated and oxygenated. A highly orchestrated and coordinated team with experience is required to successfully cannulate the fetal circulation, care for the mother, and seamlessly provide timely intervention throughout this process. The fetus with anticipated airway obstruction from micrognathia, oral/pharyngeal and cervical tumors, or other airway obstructions is a candidate for this procedure. Definitive treatment of the obstruction is not necessary in most cases and can be delayed to allow for a more coordinated treatment approach after a detailed assessment (**Fig. 7**).

CRANIOMAXILLOFACIAL ANOMALIES
Cleft Lip and Palate

Cleft lip and palate is the most common, major craniofacial anomaly in the United States. It should come as no surprise that it is the most commonly diagnosed fetal craniofacial abnormality, usually diagnosed quite easily after 16 weeks on routine screening ultrasonography. Additional imaging later in the pregnancy may be indicated to reassess fetal growth and check for other anomalies. Despite improvements in imaging technology, false-positive results for clefting have been reported using ultrasonography when the umbilical cord is overlying the lip of the fetus.[19,20]

The antenatal diagnosis of a cleft lip gives parents the chance to gather information regarding the condition (see **Figs. 3** and **4**). Parents have the opportunity to meet with a cleft team that could help them prepare for the birth of their child and any treatment they may need. Doing so in the prenatal period affords the surgeon a more receptive audience, as opposed to the new, overwhelmed parents faced with an unanticipated cleft deformity. Such advance opportunities permit the clinicians to dispel any misconceptions

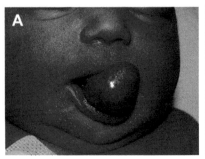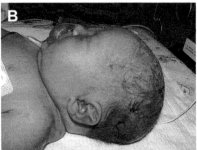

Fig. 7. (*A*) A granular cell tumor seen on ultrasonography in the prenatal period. The mass does not obstruct or compromise the airway in any way. (*B*) Lateral view.

regarding cleft deformities and their treatment and assess the resources and coping skills of the parents and their families. Instruction in specific feeding techniques and other important information can prepare the parents for the early care after birth. The authors routinely have a discussion with the parents on complete and comprehensive interdisciplinary care of children with clefts during this consultation.

Genetic counseling is helpful in dispelling unwarranted concerns regarding the genetic basis of most facial clefting and affords an opportunity to provide accurate information regarding these issues. Additional anomalies may prompt a more detailed fetal cardiac ultrasonography or other evaluations. In certain instances additional testing may be warranted in children with a suspected syndromic diagnosis. Screening for disorders, such as Down, Stickler, and velocardiofacial syndrome, is considered with prenatal DNA analysis. As additional gene loci information and DNA analysis becomes available for different disorders, this practice will increase in frequency. Postnatal repair at approximately 3 months is the standard of care for most centers. Prenatal attempts at repair are too dangerous with the current technologies and techniques of maternal and fetal medicine. Theoretically, there is no advantage to the prenatal repair of cleft lip or palate.

MICROGNATHIA

Micrognathia, whether as an isolated condition or as part of a defined syndrome, can present with significant airway and feeding difficulties, and this warrants special discussion. It is becoming much more common for ultrasonographers to diagnose a significantly hypoplastic mandible during routine screening examinations, and measurements of mandibular length can be compared with standards and norms for gestational age (see **Fig. 6**). Visualizing the mandible is somewhat technique-sensitive and requires

a skilled ultrasonographer with adequate experience to visualize the mandible in the true sagittal plane.[14] Incomplete and parasagittal views may result in a false-positive result for hypoplasia of the mandible even when using 3D sweeping techniques. The diagnosis of a hypoplastic mandible should alert clinicians to consider other anomalies that may be associated with a syndromic diagnosis (eg, Nager, Cornelia de Lange, or Sticker syndromes).[17] MRI adds little to the diagnostic capabilities of ultrasonography for this anomaly.

The small mandible can cause retroplacement of the tongue and floor of the mouth resulting in airway obstruction that may require immediate intervention. Management of airway obstruction associated with micrognathia is generally tiered based on severity. After birth, mild cases may be managed with positional therapy and prone feedings. More severe cases may benefit from temporary nasal stenting, tongue-lip adhesion, distraction osteogenesis, or tracheostomy.

If a severely hypoplastic mandible is noted prenatally, then consideration should be given to an EXIT procedure. If the airway is obstructed after birth, then airway support techniques need to be considered. Maternal circulation can be sustained in the early moments after birth to assess whether intubation is possible or if tracheostomy is required. The more long-term airway management can then be considered. Mild cases may be managed with positional therapy, temporary nasal airway placement, or prone feeding as needed. Other long-term management techniques for more complicated airway obstruction may include long-term tracheostomy, early distraction osteogenesis, or other techniques, after a thorough evaluation has been performed. Early experience at the authors' institution has shown that distraction osteogenesis in the truly syndromic population is not as successful when compared with the nonsyndromic population and that many patients have multilevel airway compromise (ie, tracheomalacia, subglottic stenosis, epiglottic collapse, or other anomalies). For many of these patients, a gastric tube may be necessary to allow for appropriate nutrition because swallowing is usually adversely affected.

CERVICAL MASSES AND ORAL/PHARYNGEAL MASSES

Various congenital lesions may present in the oral cavity. These may include vascular lesions, neoplasms, hamartomas, dental anomalies, or salivary gland lesions.[21,22] Most lesions are best dealt with at some point after birth if they require intervention. Rarely do they require intervention at birth because of airway obstruction, but this is precisely where perinatal intervention may be most helpful. Screening ultrasonography examinations with supplemental MRI scans are the norm for these types of anomalies.

Congenital lesions of the vascular system including arteries, veins, and lymphatics, are fairly common. Although the nomenclature of these lesions is controversial, their management challenges are universally accepted. Most are lymphatic-based lesions with some being mixed in nature. Rarely, arteriovenous malformations are encountered and may present unique challenges because of their potential for exsanguinating episodes. All of these lesions can be considerably deforming and may also impact the airway of the newborn. In many instances the airway is patent and not affected, but preparations should be made to ensure appropriate and timely intervention when necessary.

Other lesions may present in the oral cavity at birth. The granular cell tumor is fairly common. These lesions can resemble teratomas, congenital rhabdomyomas, or other lesions causing concern on initial ultrasonography (see **Fig. 7**). Prenatal or postnatal imaging differentiates between most of these lesions, and their management usually includes excision. Congenital ranulas present in the oral cavity and are fluid-filled. Usually, the echogenicity and signal characteristics of these lesions are quite different when imaged with ultrasonography or MRI. Doppler ultrasonography can also aid in this differentiation because some lesions do not have a significant blood supply.

Teratomas require additional attention due to their sometimes impressive presentation. Overall, teratomas are relatively common, with a prevalence of approximately 1 in 4000 births.[22,23] However, they usually occur in the sacral and coccygeal regions. Lesions occurring in the head and neck represent only 2% of these, and generally, they are cervical or nasopharyngeal in origin. Teratomas, by definition, are tumors containing all three germ layers; they may contain hair and teeth and are variably surfaced by a somewhat normal-appearing skin. They are sometimes confused with a failed or severely malformed twin fetus.

The epignathic tumor is a teratoma protruding from the oral cavity and is a potential cause of postnatal airway obstruction and feeding difficulties. Most of these lesions do not present an immediate airway concern, but a significant percentage do present with clinically important airway obstruction. After a complete ultrasonographic evaluation, a fetal MRI is helpful in evaluating the density of the lesion and its anatomic boundaries. Doppler ultrasonography may be helpful in appreciating the relative vascularity of the lesion. Many of these lesions are pedunculated and easily removed. Even the more posterior oral-pharyngeal teratomas can be easily managed with skilled endoscopic technique and image guidance when pedunculated.

As with other large lesions in the oral/pharyngeal region, an EXIT procedure may be necessary to ensure adequate ventilation and oxygenation. ECMO is rarely necessary, except in rare instances of lower cervical lesions that physically obstruct access to the trachea, precluding tracheotomy.

Teratomas or epignathic tumors may or may not obstruct the airway, but usually they are easily removed with a fairly simple surgical procedure because they are often pedunculated. Many of the intraoral posterior lesions arise from the cranial base and physically obstruct the palatal shelves; this creates a wide cleft palate. Molding devices can be used to reshape the maxilla or mandible if significant deformity exists. Individualized planning is necessary to watch the growth and development of the maxillofacial structures and then act in the early stages of life when functional problems arise, such as speech or feeding issues.

Other Craniofacial Anomalies

Craniosynostosis is the premature fusion (usually prenatal) of the natural-forming growth sutures of the skull, causing the potential for a reduced cranial vault size and an abnormal shape.[20,24] The particular shape abnormality and degree of possible increase in intracranial pressure is dependent on the type and location of suture fusion. These anomalies can be isolated or syndromic. Nonsyndromic, single-suture craniosynostosis is difficult to diagnose with ultrasonographic images unless the dysmorphology is particularly severe.[18,25] Occasionally, if a fontanel region is involved, as with sagittal craniosynostosis, the suture and missing fontanel may be visualized with 3D ultrasonographic images. Head-shape abnormalities can be due to molding and related to intrauterine positioning or oligohydramnios. In these instances, because the resultant head shape is deformational in etiology rather than sutural, it can be addressed after birth with a molding helmet or band instead of surgery.

The craniofacial dysostosis syndromes are more commonly appreciated with ultrasonographic evaluation because of the more severe dysmorphology. Cranial vault abnormalities, such as turricephaly (tower skull), clover-leaf anomaly, and severe orbital-midfacial hypoplasia seen in children with syndromic craniosynostosis, are more apparent on ultrasonographic images. The most common forms of syndromic craniosynostosis include Crouzon, Apert, Saethre-Chotzen, and Pfeiffer syndromes that usually exhibit bicoronal craniosynostosis or other multiple suture fusions. Occasionally, fetuses can present with total midfacial hypoplasia, but without craniosynostosis, which can occur with several of the craniofacial dysostosis syndromes or with other anomalies, such as Down syndrome. Similar issues may present with fetuses diagnosed with Down syndrome, achondroplasia, or other developmental size discrepancies of the maxillofacial structures. DNA analysis may be helpful in determining the exact diagnosis before birth if it is not evident based on family history or parent testing.

Other craniofacial abnormalities, such as encephaloceles, central dermoids, congenital gliomas, or other lesions preventing craniofacial fusion, may be diagnosed in the prenatal period.[26] Detailed evaluation with high quality 2D and 3D ultrasonographic images provides the most important information for clinical decision-making. MRI is usually not necessary for most lesions in this category. Once the child is born and stabilized, interdisciplinary care involves reconstruction of the dysmorphology once some growth has been achieved.

SUMMARY

The oral and maxillofacial surgeon is an important part of a comprehensive interdisciplinary fetal diagnosis and treatment team, providing expertise for patients with various craniomaxillofacial anomalies. A detailed diagnosis using appropriate imaging and directed studies is helpful in planning the delivery and care of the child. Several other diagnoses are possible with prenatal imaging, and other diagnostic tools may be used beyond what is discussed in this article. The capabilities are expanding quickly as is the technology used for diagnosis. The new window into the state of the fetus as a patient offers unique opportunities

for care. Prenatal care also involves the education of the family regarding specific issues that are likely to be important after birth, including the staged reconstructive needs of the child over the long term.

REFERENCES

1. Costello BJ, Edwards SP. Fetal diagnosis and treatment for craniofacial anomalies. J Oral Maxillofac Surg 2008;66(10):1985–95.
2. Wagner W, Harrison MR. Fetal operations in the head and neck area: current state. Head Neck 2002;24:482–90.
3. Hirose S, Farmer DL, Lee H, et al. The ex utero intrapartum treatment procedure: looking back at EXIT. J Pediatr Surg 2004;39:375 [discussion].
4. Hirose S, Harrison MR. The extra utero intrapartum treatment (EXIT) procedure. Semin Neonatol 2003; 8:207–14.
5. Bouchard S, Johnson MP, Flake AW, et al. The EXIT procedure; experience and outcome in 31 cases. J Pediatr Surg 2002;37:418–26.
6. Gonclaves LF, Romero R. A critical appraisal of the RADIUS study. Fetus 1993;3:7–18.
7. Hartnick CJ, Barth WH, Cote CJ, et al. A pregnant woman with a large mass in the fetal oral cavity. N Engl J Med 2009;360(9):913–21.
8. Crane JP, LeFevre ML, Winborn RC, et al. A randomized trial of prenatal ultrasonographic screening: impact on the detection, management, and outcome of anomalous fetuses. Am J Obstet Gynecol 1994; 171(2):392–9.
9. Prayer D, Brugger PC, Prayer L. Fetal MRI: techniques and protocols. Pediatr Radiol 2004;34(9): 685–93.
10. Sandrasegaran K, Lall C, Aisen AA, et al. Fast fetal magnetic resonance imaging. J Comput Assist Tomogr 2005;29(4):487–98.
11. Johnson DD, Pretorius DH, Budorick NE, et al. Three-dimensional ultrasound of the fetal lip and primary palate: three-dimensional versus two-dimensional ultrasound. Radiology 2000;217:236–9.
12. Baba K, Satoh K, Sakamoto S, et al. Development of an ultrasonic system for three-dimensional reconstruction of the fetus. J Perinat Med 1989;17:19–24.
13. Hamper UM, Trapanatto V, Sheth S, et al. Three-dimensional ultrasound: preliminary clinical experience. Radiology 1994;191:397–401.
14. Pretorius DH, Nelson TR. Fetal face visualization using three-dimensional ultrasound. J Ultrasound Med 1995;14(5):349–56.
15. Mertz E, Weber G, Bhlmann F, et al. Application of transvaginal and abdominal three-dimensional ultrasound for detection or exclusion of malformations of the fetal face. Ultrasound Obstet Gynecol 1997;14: 237–43.

16. Lee W, McNie B, Chaiworapongsa T, et al. Three-dimensional ultrasonographic presentation of micrognathia. J Ultrasound Med 2002;21:775–81.

17. Ansart-Franquet H, Houfflin-Debarge V, Ghoumid J, et al. Prenatal diagnosis of Nager syndrome in a monochorionic-diamniotic twin pregnancy. Prenat Diagn 2009;29(2):187–9.

18. Pretorius DH, Nelson TR. Prenatal visualization of cranial sutures and fontanelles with three-dimensional ultrasonography. J Ultrasound Med 1994; 13(11):871–6.

19. Grandjean H, Larroque D, Levi S, the Eurofetus Study Group. The performance of routine ultrasonographic screening of pregnancies in the Eurofetus Study. Am J Obstet Gynecol 1999;181:446–54.

20. da Silva Dalben G. Termination of pregnancy after prenatal diagnosis of cleft lip and palate-possible influence on reports of prevalence. Oral Surg Oral Med Oral Pathol Oral Radiol Endod 2009;107(6):759–62.

21. Chervenak FA, Isaacson G, Blakemore KJ, et al. Fetal cystic hygroma: course and natural history. N Engl J Med 1984;309:822.

22. Chervenak FA, Isaacson G, Touloukian R, et al. The diagnosis and management of fetal teratomas. Obstet Gynecol 1984;94:94.

23. Holt JE, Weaver RG. Dermoids and teratomas of the head and neck. Ear Nose Throat J 1979;58:520–31.

24. Ruiz RL, Ritter AM, Turvey TA, et al. Nonsyndromic craniosynostosis: diagnosis and contemporary surgical management. Oral Maxillofac Surg Clin N Am 2004;16:447–63.

25. Itoh S, Nojima M, Yoshida K. Usefulness of magnetic resonance imaging for accurate diagnosis of Pfeiffer syndrome type II in utero. Fetal Diagn Ther 2006;21: 168–71.

26. Posnick JC, Costello BJ. Dermoid cysts, gliomas, and encephaloceles: evaluation and treatment. Atlas Orl Maxillofac Surg Clin of NA 2002;10:85–99.

Bone Morphogenetic Proteins in Craniomaxillofacial Surgery

Sarah D. Davies, DDS, MD*, Mark W. Ochs, DMD, MD

KEYWORDS

- Craniomaxillofacial surgery • Bone morphogenetic proteins
- Grafting • Facial skeleton

The field of craniomaxillofacial surgery has many indications for bone regeneration and augmentation. Specific applications include extraction socket preservation, alveolar cleft grafting, and reconstruction of defects of the maxilla, mandible, and cranium. Traditionally, craniofacial surgeons relied on alloplasts, xenografts, allografts, or autogenous bone to accomplish these goals. In addition, clinicians have sought to use guided bone regeneration and distraction osteogenesis to create bone in the craniofacial skeleton. Success of grafting materials varies according to the physiologic properties of osteoconduction, osteogenesis, and osteoinduction and the placement technique, surgical application, and physical characteristics of the graft.[1] Small defects with adequate amounts of native bone at the margins may be satisfactorily reconstructed with an osteoconductive material.[1] Osteoconductive agents support bone growth by providing a scaffold for bone apposition. Osteoinduction describes a biologic response where chemical mediators induce recipient stem cells to differentiate into mature bone forming cells, whereas osteogenesis describes the ability of the graft to produce new bone from live bone cells within the graft itself.[2] Alloplasts serve as biologically inert space maintainers, which provide osteoconduction. Their utility is limited, however, due to inability to grow, lack of resorption, and potential for infection or extrusion.[3] Mineralized or demineralized allografts supply an osteoconductive milieu and provide a varying but often limited amount of osteoinductive potential.[1] Additional disadvantages of allografts include immunologic reactions, fear of disease transmission, and slow incorporation by creeping substitution.[2,4] Autogenous grafts have long been considered the gold standard for many craniofacial bone augmentation and replacement applications. Autogenous bone provides osteogenic activity, an osteoconductive environment, and the presence of some level of cells and growth and differentiation factors resulting in osteoinduction. Autogenous grafting has shortcomings, however, such as donor site morbidity, increased operative time, insufficient quantities of available bone, and variable success rates of incorporation.[1,3] The need to develop alternatives to traditional bone grafting led researchers to investigate use of osteoinductive agents in bone for de novo bone regeneration.

HISTORY

In 1965 Marshall Urist implanted bovine dimineralized bone matrix (DBM) intramuscularly in rats and rabbits and noted ectopic bone production at the implant sites.[5,6] He attributed the process to presence of a bone matrix protein, which chemotactically attracted pluripotent mesenchymal cells

Department of Oral and Maxillofacial Surgery, University of Pittsburgh School of Dental Medicine, 3471 Fifth Avenue, Suite 1112, UPMC Kaufman Building, Pittsburgh, PA 15213, USA
* Corresponding author.
E-mail address: Sdemarco7@aol.com

Oral Maxillofacial Surg Clin N Am 22 (2010) 17–31
doi:10.1016/j.coms.2009.10.007

and induced bone formation locally.[5,7] Urist named the responsible substance, bone morphogenetic protein (BMP). Subsequent isolation and cloning of additional related proteins allowed clear demonstration that BMPs are independently osteoconductive.[7] BMPs are members of the transforming growth factor-beta superfamily and elicit cellular effects through induction of heteromeric complexes of type I and type II serine/threonine receptors.[8] In addition to bone formation, BMPs play a role in development of virtually all organs and tissues, including the nervous system, somites, lungs, kidneys, skin, and gonads and in establishing the embryonic body plan.[8] Currently, approximately 20 different members of the BMP supergroup have been identified; however, only a subset are able to singly promote osteoinduction.[9] These include BMP-2 through -7 and BMP-9.[10] Naturally occurring BMP, collected through purification of DBM, is available in minute quantities.[11] Using molecular biology techniques, human homologs of bovine BMP coding sequences were acquired and mammalian cells were engineered to express each protein in a purified form.[1] Therefore, using recombinant gene technology, a large, uniform supply of a specific BMPs can be generated.[11] Currently, recombinant human BMPs (rhBMP)-2 and rhBMP-7 are the most extensively studied and are commercially available for specific indications.

BIOLOGIC ACTIVITY

Kang and colleagues[12] demonstrated possible increased osteogenic potential of BMP-6 and BMP-9 in an orthotopic ossification model in mice; however, these factors have not been investigated significantly in preclinical or clinical trials. After ectopic implantation, rhBMPs stimulate a sequence of events typical of endochondral bone formation: recruitment of mesenchymal cells, differentiation to chondrocytes, chondrocyte hypertrophy, calcification of cartilage matrix, osteoblast differentiation and bone formation, and eventual remodeling of newly formed bone and marrow creation (**Fig. 1**).[10] Osteoinductivity of individual rhBMPs has a steep dose-response curve, with low doses resulting in little cartilage and bone formation and increasing concentrations eventually resulting in direct (intramembranous) ossification.[1,10] The concentration of the BMP at the site of implantation is more crucial than the total dose of BMP administered.[10] In addition, preclinical studies have demonstrated that the therapeutic dose of BMP multiplies with advancement from rodents to higher-level mammals and

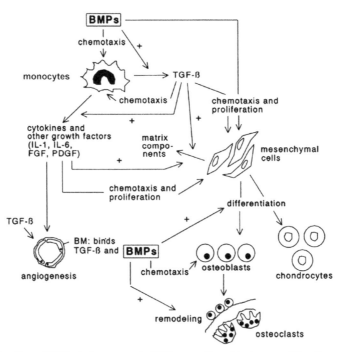

Fig. 1. Mechanism of action of BMPs in bone repair. BMPs recruit and induce proliferation of mesenchymal cells, which differentiate into chondrocytes and osteoblasts. +, stimulating effect. (*Reprinted from* Termaat MF, Den Boer FC, Bakker FC, et al. Bone morphogenetic proteins. Development and clinical efficacy in the treatment of fractures and bone defects. J Bone Joint Surg Am 2005;87(6):1367–78; with permission.)

nonhuman primates.[10] The suggested human therapeutic doses (0.88 mg/mL of sterile water for rhBMP-7 and 1.50 mg/mL of sterile water for rhBMP-2) were derived from nonhuman primate studies and verified in clinical orthopedic studies.[8,10] The doses of rhBMP required to induce bone formation in humans is orders of magnitude higher than endogenous concentrations of BMPs.[7,10] Requirements for supraphysiologic doses may be secondary to the tightly regulated signaling pathways and brisk local and systemic clearance of BMP in higher species.[10] In addition, the potency of the resident BMP assortment may be superior to singly applied rhBMP.[7]

CARRIER MATERIALS

Because BMP acts locally, the protein must be transferred to the implantation site via a carrier matrix, which prevents prompt rhBMP clearance. Hollinger and colleagues[13] reported that less than 5% of rhBMP remains at the implantation site when using solely a buffering delivery system but combining rhBMP with gelatin foam, collagen, or calcium phosphate pastes increases the retention by 5% to 15%. Ideally a matrix allows a predictable rate of release of the factor and continues to emit protein for an adequate duration.[7] A burst release of rhBMP to first recruit mesenchymal cells to the site of implantation followed by sustained release to differentiate the osteoprogenitor cells toward osteoblast phenotype seems to be the preferred kinetics.[7] Furthermore, the delivery system must serve as a scaffold with pores large enough ($>100 \mu m$) to allow cellular infiltration and vascular in growth. The scaffold also provides a template onto which initial bone deposition can occur.[6,8] An ideal delivery system is biocompatible, biodegradable in a predictable manner, stable with sterilization, and malleable and provides sufficient compressive and tensile strength.[6,8] The optimal matrix design depends ultimately on the type and amount of tissue being regenerated and the weight-bearing requisites of the application.[1,8] Carrier materials can be classified into four major subgroups: natural polymers, inorganic materials, synthetic polymers, and composites.[1,8] Although BMP has been combined with matrices from all of these categories in various preclinical and clinical studies, currently only three carriers are approved for clinical use.[8] The approved carriers include type 1 absorbable collagen sponge (ACS), particulate bone-derived type 1 collagen matrix, and a combination of rhBMP-7 delivered in the particulate collagen matrix combined with carboxymethyl cellulose.[8]

Collagen-based carriers have received the most attention because of the historical safety profile, excellent biocompatibility, degradation into physiologic products, intermediate rhBMP release rate kinetics, and positive effects on wound healing.[6] One commercially available product consists of freeze-dried rhBMP-2 reconstituted with sterile water at the time of surgery and applied evenly to a type 1 ACS. The high porosity of ACS allows it to assume the same volume as the rhBMP-2 solution applied to it; therefore, the volume of rhBMP-2 solution used equates to the volume of defect it is able to fill.[9] The ACS degrades over 2 to 4 weeks in vivo and the half-life of rhBMP-2 is 2.5 days with detectable levels at the surgical site for 3 weeks.[9] Even if rhBMP is applied in an osteoconductive matrix with appropriate scaffold properties, a devascularized surgical locale lacking responsive osteoprogenitor cells may cause bone formation to fail.[11]

CLINICAL STUDY AND SAFETY

In preclinical and clinical research, rhBMP has shown a positive safety profile. With the use of supraphysiologic doses of rhBMP required to promote bone formation in studies, no harmful systemic or direct toxic effects attributable to BMP have been reported in the literature.[9] A preclinical study examining direct intravascular injection (5.3 mg/kg) and orthotopic implantation (1.6 mg/kg) of rhBMP at levels 1000 times those used clinically saw no adverse effects.[14] In addition, human studies using rhBMP-2 for alveolar ridge augmentation, maxillary sinus augmentation, and spinal fusion have exposed no harmful consequences.[14] After intravenous administration in the nonhuman primate, the half-life of rhBMP-2 is 6.7 minutes. When rhBMP-2 is implanted with ACS, the slow release results in minimal levels rhBMP-2 detectable in the systemic circulation, and what enters the circulation is rapidly cleared. Similarly, clinical investigations of rhBMP-7 in long bone defects, spine fusion, and thoracolumbar fusions have revealed no adverse systemic events.[14] Human studies have also failed to identify any major local toxicity of rhBMP-2 or rhBMP-7. In animal studies, rhBMP-2 caused fibrous, cartilaginous, and bony tissue growth at sites of intravenous administration; however, this was attributed to extravascular escape near venous injection sites.[14] Several clinical studies and case reports have described a greater amount of local edema at rhBMP implant sites versus controls in the postoperative period.[15] The increased edema is thought to be secondary to recruitment and influx of mesenchymal cells by the rhBMP grafts.

Although BMP and BMP receptors have been observed in tumors, there are no data to indicate they are carcinogenic.[8,14] Manufacturer preclinical safety studies of rhBMP-2 showed inhibitory effects on human osteosarcoma, prostate, lung, and tongue carcinoma cell lines.[8] rhBMP-7 has no mutogenic or cytotoxic effects on bacterial or mammalian cells in published genotoxicity studies.[16]

Immunogenicity of rhBMP-2 is reportedly low but may be higher in ACS carriers. Clinical spinal fusion trials found antibodies to rhBMP-2 developed in only 0.7% of 137 patients, similar to the occurrence in controls (0.8%). Higher incidences of antibody formation to type 1 bovine collagen have been described, yet titers have been low, and there have been no adverse effects systemically or on local healing. Friedlaender and colleagues[17] found 10% of patients treated with rhBMP-7 for tibial nonunion developed antibodies to the protein, and additional studies reported an incidence of antibody formation up to 38%. Titers again were low and transient, and no harmful outcomes were reported.

The risk of bony overgrowth caused by rhBMP has been a concern when used in spinal fusion due to the proximity to neural elements and risk of inadvertently fusing adjacent levels. Data presented in animal and human studies reveal that restenosis can take place if rhBMP contacts raw bone surfaces, such as laminectomy sites or decompressed nerve foramina. Therefore, leakage of rhBMP beyond the direct application site may lead to fusion of adjacent levels. Recommendations for use in spinal applications include avoidance of placement on raw bone edges and use of appropriate carriers to retain rhBMP to the specified fusion area. In a study by Paramore and colleagues, rhBMP-7 was intentionally implanted into the subarachnoid space of dogs and the dura closed over the defect. All animals treated with rhBMP-7 showed bone growth in the subdural space, whereas none of the control animals formed bone in this area. The investigators reported no clinical or histopathologic characteristics of neurotoxicity in either group.[18] Similar studies for rhBMP-2 have not been reported. The implications of possible rhBMP-induced bony overgrowth in craniofacial applications are less clear than in spinal fusions. When rhBMP is used for cranial reconstruction, however, the possibility of subdural bone formation in the setting of dural tears must be considered and care taken to avoid this complication.

Currently, two rhBMPs with coupled delivery systems have been granted Food and Drug Administration (FDA) approval. OP-1 (Stryker Biotech, Hopkinton, Massachusetts) contains rhBMP-7 plus bovine collagen and is reconstituted with saline to create a paste. Carboxymethylcellulose may be added to form putty. The INFUSE (Medtronic Sofamor Danek USA, Memphis, Tennessee) graft includes freeze-dried rhBMP-2 that is reconstituted with saline and then injected onto an ACS.[9] The FDA-approved applications for the rhBMPs are as follows. OP-1 may be used as an alternative to autogenous grafts in recalcitrant long bone nonunions when using autograft is not feasible and alternatives have failed. It may also be used as an alternative to autograft in medically compromised patients who require revision posterolateral lumbar spinal fusion and autogenous bone or when marrow harvest is unachievable or is not expected to promote fusion. INFUSE bone graft has FDA approval for spinal fusion in skeletally mature patients with degenerative disc disease at one level from L2 to S1. The INFUSE must be used in conjunction with the LT-CAGE Lumbar Tapered Fusion Device or the INTER FIX RP Threaded Fusion Device. INFUSE also has premarket approval for use in the treatment of acute, open tibial shaft fractures. OP-1 and INFUSE are contraindicated for use in patients who are pregnant, have allergies to any materials contained in the graft, have infection present in proximity to the surgical incision, have had a tumor removal in the area of implantation, or who are skeletally immature.

The FDA-approved INFUSE for use in sinus augmentation and alveolar ridge augmentation associated with extraction sockets in March 2007. The approval for maxillofacial applications was based on five clinical studies, which included 312 patients. Alveolar ridge defects result from periodontal disease, trauma, tooth loss, and endodontic failures. When the alveolar bone lacks appropriate height and width, restoration with conventional prosthodontics or implants in an esthetic and functional manner becomes more challenging. Preservation of the alveolar ridge after tooth extraction offers a means to avoid future ridge augmentation procedures and ensure adequate quality and quantity of bone exists for dental restoration.[19] Cochran and colleagues reported on 12 patients who received rhBMP-2/ACS at 0.43 mg/mL in extraction sockets or alveolar ridge augmentation. They were treated with endosseous implants in the augmented areas and bone core samples of the grafted region were obtained for histologic analysis. Three-year follow-up results found that all implants placed were stable and without clinical or radiographic complications, and bone biopsies showed normal bone formation. The investigators concluded that rhBMP-2/ACS could be safely used in extraction sites and for localized alveolar ridge augmentation and that dental implants placed in the grafted regions are stable and functional.[20] The pivotal study supporting use of rhBMP-2/ACS for ridge preservation was a randomized, masked, placebo-controlled, multicenter clinical study reported by Fiorellini and colleagues[21] in 2005, which looked at two sequential cohorts of 40 patients (with a total of 95 defects). The patients required localized ridge augmentation/preservation of maxillary teeth (premolar and anterior) with greater than or equal to 50% buccal bone loss of the extraction socket. Each patient was randomized to receive 0.75 mg/mL or 1.50 mg/mL rhBMP-2/ACS, placebo (ACS alone), or no treatment in a 2:1:1 ratio. Surgical procedure included the following steps: full-thickness periosteal flaps, extraction of teeth, perforation of socket walls with round bur, placement of placebo or rhBMP-2 as strips into the socket and a larger piece placed over the entire site, and a tension-free flap closure. Efficacy parameters included CT-based measurement of alveolar bone height and width of various levels of the extraction socket at baseline and 4 months after treatment and, secondarily, whether or not adequate bone volume was attained to place dental implants. In addition, bone densities of native bone and treatment areas were calculated with reference to a standard density block. Results indicated that sockets treated with 1.5-mg/mL rhBMP-2/ACS achieved significantly greater bone augmentation versus controls. Sufficiency of bone for dental implant placement was almost twice as high in the rhBMP-2 groups compared with placebo and no treatment sites (**Figs. 2 and 3**).[21]

CLINICAL APPLICATIONS

Patients with edentulous posterior maxillas often have atrophied alveolar ridges and pneumatization of the maxillary sinuses, which compromise the amount of bone available for dental implant placement. Performing sinus floor augmentation with several graft materials has proved successful in resolving this problem over the past several decades. Autogenous bone, allogeneic bone, xenografts, and a combination of materials have been used in maxillary sinus floor augmentation with varying degrees of success. There are shortcomings to each of these methods; however, the availability of rhBMP-2 grafts offers a new method to induce de novo bone formation in the maxillary sinus floor. Initially, rhBMP-2 was investigated as an alternative to traditional maxillary sinus augmentation materials in animal models.

Kirker-Head and colleagues described using an rhBMP-2/ACS sinus implant in a goat model with a buffer/ACS implant serving as a contralateral control. CT was used to monitor bone formation over a 12-week period and histologic evaluation of bone was performed. The rhBMP-2 implants retained a comparatively stable volume after surgery and demonstrated a time-dependent increase in mineralization. The control implants did not mineralize and completely resorbed after 4 weeks.[22] Additionally, Hanisch and colleagues[23] demonstrated significantly greater vertical bone gain in nonhuman primate maxillary sinuses associated with rhBMP-2/ACS implants compared with ACS alone. In comparing rhBMP-2/ACS to autogenous particulate bone and marrow graft as maxillary sinus augmentation materials in a rabbit model, Wada and colleagues[24] found no statistical difference between the histometric volume or histologic character of the bone formed in the grafted areas.

Feasibility studies evaluating the use of rhBMP-2/ACS for human maxillary sinus augmentation began with Boyne's study published in 1997.[25] RhBMP-2/ACS was implanted into the sinuses of 12 patients with inadequate bone height in the posterior maxilla (**Figs. 4 and 5**). In 11 patients available for follow-up evaluation, mean bone height achieved after grafting was 8.51 mm, and there were no serious immunologic or adverse events associated with the procedure.[25] In a follow-up phase II study, Boyne and colleagues[15] assessed the safety and efficacy of two concentrations (0.75 mg/mL and 1.50 mg/mL) of rhBMP-2 used in human maxillary sinus augmentation to induce sufficient bone for implant placement. They also looked at the success rate of implants placed in the induced bone after 36 months of function. These results were compared with maxillary sinuses augmented with bone graft and subsequent implants placed in these sites. The mean increase in alveolar ridge height at 4 months post surgery was comparable between the groups (ranging 9.5 mm to 11.3 mm). Bone density was significantly greater after the first 4 months in the bone graft cohort and greater in the 1.50-mg/mL group than the 0.75-mg/mL patients, but bone density equalized in the treatment groups after 6 months of implant functional loading. Overall, implant survival rates after 36 months of functional loading were 81%, 88%, and 79% for the bone graft, 0.75-mg/mL, and 1.50-mg/mL treatment groups, respectively. The investigators concluded that both concentrations of rhBMP-2 are safe for maxillary augmentation procedures and induce a similar amount of bone formation as bone graft, but the higher concentration of rhBMP-2 induces bone formation at a faster rate than the lower

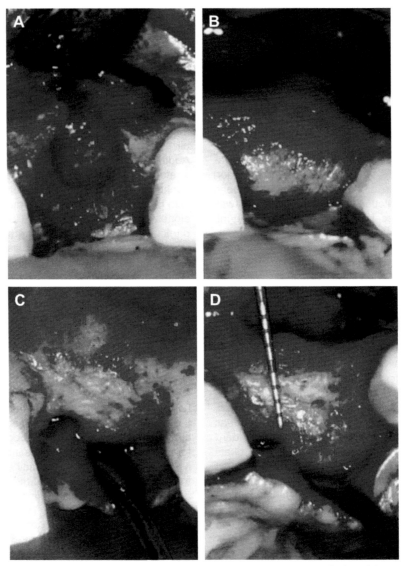

Fig. 2. (*A*) Extraction site (tooth #9) exhibiting greater than 50% buccal bone height loss. (*B*) Treatment site with 1.5-mg/mL rhBMP-2/ACS contour to reconstruct alveolar ridge. (*C, D*) Extraction site after 4 months of healing. (*Reprinted from* Fiorellini JP, Howell TH, Cochran D, et al. Randomized study evaluating recombinant human bone morphogenetic protein-2 for extraction socket augmentation. J Periodontol 2005;76(4):605–13; with permission from the American Academy of Periodontology.)

concentration. The rhBMP-2 was successful in inducing bone in the maxillary sinus that could support placement and long-term functional loading of dental implants.[15]

Using the 1.5-mg/mL rhBMP-2 dose suggested by the previous study, Li and colleagues evaluated the osteogenic pathways of rhBMP-2 and autogenous bone graft in 190 maxillary sinus augmentation surgeries. Dental implants were placed into the grafted areas 6 to 15 months after augmentation and bone core biopsies were harvested at that time. Trabecular bone volume was similar between the BMP and bone graft sites; however,

the BMP-treated areas had statistically greater amount of lamellar bone and trabecular number than the bone grafted group. In addition, nonviable bone granules were detected in 16% of the bone graft patients. The study provided conclusive evidence that BMP-2–induced bone formation is an osteoinductive process and bone graft–induced osteogenesis is an osteoconductive development.[26] Additional reports by Spagnoli, Chandler, and Li's group have promoted the importance of providing the research defined concentration of 1.5 mg/mL rhBMP-2 at the interface of the defect being treated and the surrounding tissues where

No Treatment　　　　　**ACS Alone**　　　　　**1.5mg/ml rhBMP-2/ACS**

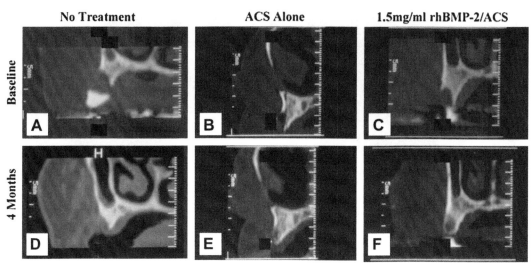

Fig. 3. Baseline (*A–C*) and 4 months post treatment (*D–F*). CT scans for no treatment (tooth #5) (*A, D*), ACS alone (tooth #10) (*B, E*), and 1.5 mg/mL rhBMP-2/ACS (tooth #4) (*C, F*). (*Reprinted from* Fiorellini JP, Howell TH, Cochran D, et al. Randomized study evaluating recombinant human bone morphogenetic protein-2 for extraction socket augmentation. J Periodontol 2005;76(4):605–13; with permission from the American Academy of Periodontology.)

the BMP can have the most chemotactic and vascular field effect. The lower concentration of 0.75 mg/mL may then be used at the core of the defect.[27] These investigators have also suggested that using rhBMP-2 in combination with allogeneic or autogenous grafts in maxillary sinus augmentation will maintain the efficacy of the BMP-induced bone formation while allowing the total dose of BMP required to be reduced. This may be a more cost-effective alternative.

Although currently, rhBMP-2 has FDA approval for the craniofacial region for sinus augmentation and extraction socket grafting, many studies and case reports have investigated the protein's utility for bone induction in other craniofacial applications. In the dentoalveolar region, rhBMP-2 has been considered in grafting periodontal defects, peri-implant defects, supra-alveolar ridge defects, and peri-implantitis–induced bone loss (**Fig. 6**). Sigurdsson and colleagues[28] looked at the potential bone formation elicited by rhBMP-2 with various carriers applied to a supra-alveolar periodontal defect model in dogs. Defects in contralateral jaw quadrants in six dogs were assigned to receive

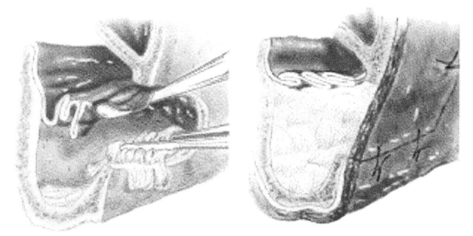

Fig. 4. Medical illustrations of surgical procedure implanting rhBMP-2/ACS. (*Reprinted from* Boyne PJ, Lilly LC, Marx RE, et al. De novo bone induction by recombinant human bone morphogenetic protein-2 (rhBMP-2) in maxillary sinus floor augmentation. J Oral Maxillofac Surg 2005;63(12):1693–707; with permission.)

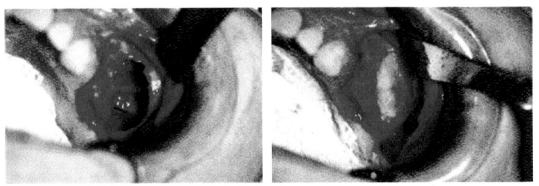

Fig. 5. Clinical photographs of surgical procedure implanting rhBMP-2/ACS. (*Reprinted from* Boyne PJ, Lilly LC, Marx RE, et al. De novo bone induction by recombinant human bone morphogenetic protein-2 (rhBMP-2) in maxillary sinus floor augmentation. J Oral Maxillofac Surg 2005;63(12):1693–707; with permission.)

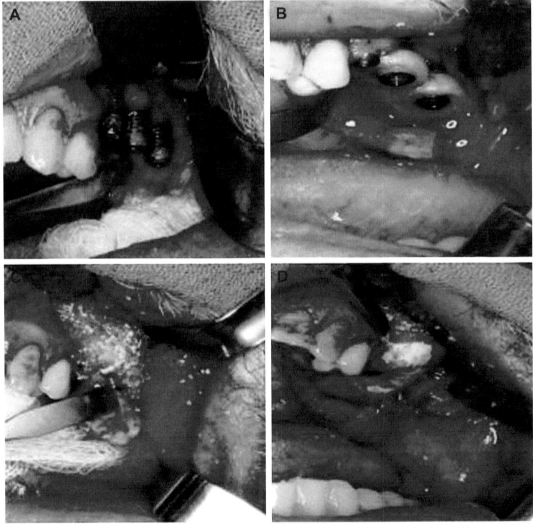

Fig. 6. (*A*) Maxillary left implants with peri-implantitis–induced bone loss. Shown after débridement and cleansing with etchant. (*B*) INFUSE strips placed circumferentially around implants. (*C*) Bovine-derived hydroxyapatite, DBM, and infuse strips packed into bony def. (*D*) Large INFUSE strip placed over composite graft.

rhBMP-2 combined with DBM, ACS, Bio-Oss (Geistlich Pharma AG, Wolhusen, Switzerland), DL-polylactic acid granules (PLA), 50:50 polylactic acid–polyglycolic acid copolymer (BEP), or a DBM control. Histologic evaluation of the implanted site was undertaken after 8 weeks of healing. Outcomes depended on the carrier: Bio-Oss failed to resorb and obstructed bone formation; PLA showed poor bone quantity and quality with many macrophages at the site; BEP supported good bone quality but variable bone quantity; the DBM implant exhibited wide bone formation with quality comparable to the surrounding resident bone; and the ACS handled well but lacked ability to maintain space and allowed limited bone formation when used as an onlay graft. The investigators concluded that carrier system requirements differ depending on the graft indication and graft site. Sites requiring space definition and maintenance may necessitate rhBMP-2 to be coupled with a carrier that resists compression from surrounding tissues to demarcate the shape of the rhBMP-2–induced bone.[29]

In another dog model of supra-alveolar peri-implant defects, Sigurdsson and colleagues[30] revealed that rhBMP-2/ACS could induce significant alveolar bone production when used as an onlay supported by the dental implants. RhBMP-2/ACS at 0.43 mg/mL or buffer/ACS was implanted into 5-mm, supra-alveolar, peri-implant defects in contralateral quadrants in five dogs. At 16 weeks, the defects treated with rhBMP-2 showed statistically greater bone formation along the exposed implant surface than controls; however, the bone layer formed was thin. Thus, the carrier system was thought ineffective in preserving space for sufficient bone volume to form.[30] Sigurdsson and colleagues later demonstrated that rhBMP-2 in a freeze-dried DBM/autologous blood carrier may provide clinical utility to graft alveolar ridge defects where dental implants are subsequently to be placed. Bilateral 5- to 6-mm supra-alveolar ridge defects in five dogs were treated with an unsupported onlay graft of 0.2-mg/mL rhBMP-2/DBM/blood. Nonsubmerged 10-mm dental implants were placed into the induced bone at 8 and 16 weeks. Histometric analysis at 24 weeks found that rhBMP-2–induced bone covered 90% of the bone-anchoring surface of the implants, and similar amounts of bone-implant contact were seen in the induced versus native bone (approximately 55%).[31] Hanisch and colleagues showed that rhBMP-2/ACS yielded bone fill and dental implant re-osseointegration in an induced peri-implantitis model in Rhesus monkeys. Ligature-induced peri-implantitis was created around hydroxyapatite coated titanium implants in the posterior mandible and maxilla of four adult monkeys over an 11-month period. The defects were débrided surgically and the implant surfaces disinfected before placing rhBMP-2/ACS at 0.4 mg/mL as a graft or buffer/ACS as a control in the contralateral jaw. After 16 weeks of healing, the rhBMP-2/ACS grafted sites showed three times more vertical bone gain than controls and qualitatively appeared to be reosseointegrated.[32] When rhBMP-2/ACS is used as an inlay to treat space-preserving alveolar ridge defects, it has been shown to be successful in augmenting bone with and without guided bone regeneration membranes in animal models.[4] Therefore, intrabony and saddle-type defects may be more amenable to treatment with the rhBMP-2/ACS construct than larger critical size supra-alveolar defects that require compression resistance.

Reconstruction and osseous regeneration of large traumatic, congenital, and pathologic critical-size defects of the facial skeleton continue to challenge craniomaxillofacial surgeons. A critical-size defect refers to a bony defect that does not spontaneously heal and form osseous union without adjunctive methods.[33] Several types of autogenous grafts including vascularized flaps and free bone grafts have been used in large craniofacial reconstructions over the past several decades, yet an ideal bone grafting procedure remains to be discovered.[4,34] Development of the commercially available recombinant BMPs gave hope that bone inductors could successfully regenerate large continuity defects in the facial bones without the need for bone grafting.[35] Toriumi and colleagues reconstructed 3-cm, full-thickness, canine mandibular defects stabilized with stainless steel plates using rhBMP-2 with bone matrix carrier, carrier without rhBMP, or no implant. Due to the presence of stiff, mineralized bone across the defects, reconstruction plates were removed after 10 weeks in the rhBMP grafted dogs, and the animals were allowed to chew a solid diet. The mandibular defects in the control groups displayed nominal bone regeneration and remained grossly mobile. At 6 months, the rhBMP implants were 68% replaced with mineralized bone; however, fewer than 4% of the control sites were mineralized, according to histomorphometric analysis.[36]

Boyne and colleagues conducted several studies using a nonhuman primate model of hemimandibulectomy defects to evaluate the potential of rhBMP-2 to regenerate bone in these areas. In the first arm of the study, 2.2-cm resections of the mandibular body were performed bilaterally in seven animals, and then rhBMP-2 in a collagen carrier was placed into the defects supported by titanium mesh. Doses of rhBMP ranged from 0.2 mg to 0.8 mg per site and four sites were grafted with cortico-cancellous bone as a control. The alveolar ridge completely regenerated in all animals within 5 to 6 months.[37] In a second group of four adult monkeys, partial mandibulectomies were performed from symphysis to third molar region and the defect was stabilized with titanium mesh before placing the rhBMP-2 graft. Two dental implants were placed into the regenerated alveolar ridges after a 5-month healing period. After an additional 4 months, the implants were functionally loaded and the animals placed on a soft diet. After 6 months of function, histomorphometric analysis and photomicrographs of the specimens revealed increased density in the bone surrounding the titanium implants versus the density seen in the rhBMP-induced bone in the previous study where no implants were placed. The investigators concluded that the improvement and preservation of bone density after implant placement signified the long-term stability of rhBMP-2 regenerated critical-sized mandibular defects.[35,38]

To better document the ability of rhBMP-2 to induce intramembranous bone formation in a critical-sized facial bone defect, Carstens and colleagues[34] looked at regeneration of a 10-cm mandibular defect in a porcine model. A subperiosteal trapezoidal defect was created in the mandibular body and stabilized with a titanium reconstruction plate. RhBMP-2/ACS was inserted in the periosteal chamber using two sponges (4 cm × 3 cm) containing an rhBMP-2 concentration of 1.5 mg/mL. Radiographs were taken monthly, and after 3 months the regenerated bone was analyzed histologically. Grossly, the defect had completely consolidated and bone was seen between the lateral edge of the plate and the periosteum. Radiographically, the bone showed progressive ossification over the 3-month period, with complete ossification at 90 days. Histologically, woven bone was present throughout the defect but with increasing levels of replacement by lamellar bone occurring at the periphery. The typical process of membranous ossification was observed in the rhBMP-induced bone.[34]

In addition to regeneration of large mandibular defects with directly applied rhBMP, prefabrication of bone grafts using rhBMP-7 had been investigated. Terheyden and colleagues implanted rhBMP-7 with a xenogenic bone block carrier into the latissimus dorsi muscle of miniature pigs to create a preformed vascularized bone graft. Using microsurgical anastomosis and fixation with miniplates, the grafts were used to reconstruct mandibular defects. Contralateral defects were reconstructed with direct implantation of rhBMP-7 on xenogenic bone mineral carrier. The preformed bone grafts maintained viability, and the investigators described a superior reconstructive outcome for the prefabricated sites based on histologic CT assessment.[39,40]

Alveolar clefts are a further example of craniomaxillofacial critical-size defects for which rhBMP may be useful. The standard treatment usually involves autogenous grafting, although several other methods, including human banked bone, bovine bone mineral, and alloplasts, are occasionally used.[41] Use of autogenous particulate marrow cancellous bone from the iliac crest remains a successful technique for regenerating bone in the osseous cleft defect. Effective reconstruction using rhBMP would avoid a second operative site and potentially decrease rehabilitation costs.[42] Boyne and colleagues created a simulated bilateral cleft model in six young nonhuman primates to assess the ability of rhBMP-2 to induce bony regeneration in the cleft site. Maxillary surgical defects were produced via ostectomy and oral antral fistulas were fashioned by inverting the oral mucosal flap to the nasal mucosa. Three months after fabricating the clefts, the sites were reopened. One side was grafted with 0.43-mg/mL rhBMP-2/ACS and the opposite side was treated with ACS alone or particulate marrow bone to serve as a control. At the end of 3 months, the thickness of the cortical bone in the regenerated areas was similar between the rhBMP and particulate marrow sites, and histomorphometric analysis found no statistical difference in the amount of new bone formed on each side.[35,42] Chin and colleagues presented a series of 43 human patients undergoing repair of 50 cleft sites using rhBMP-2. Of these children, 37 presented with 44 typical unilateral or bilateral clefts. The alveolar cleft repairs followed standard surgical closure of oronasal fistulas followed by creation of chambers to contain the grafts by advancing mucosal flaps. The rhBMP-2 was reconstituted to a concentration of 1.5 mg/mL and applied to an ACS before being packed into the cleft sites. Postoperative radiographs depicted consolidated bone in the former alveolar clefts and eruption of teeth into the constructed bone (**Figs. 7** and **8**). Teeth were observed to respond normally to orthodontic forces.[41]

A similar technique was employed by Dickinson and colleagues[43] in their comparison of rhBMP-2/ACS versus iliac cancellous bone grafting of alveolar clefts in skeletally mature adult patients, who predictably have inferior outcomes relating to alveolar bone grafting than younger cleft patients. Twenty-one adult unilateral cleft lip and palate patients were randomized to have alveolar cleft reconstruction with rhBMP-2/ACS or iliac crest

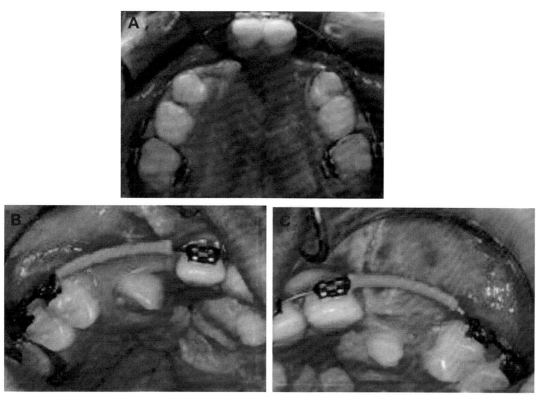

Fig. 7. (A) Bilateral alveolar clefts and oronasal fistula preoperative (B) Reconstructed right alveolus, 15 months postoperative (C) Reconstructed left alveolus, 15 months postoperative. (Reprinted from Chin M, Ng T, Tom WK, et al. Repair of alveolar clefts with recombinant human bone morphogenetic protein (rhBMP-2) in patients with clefts. J Craniofac Surg 2005;16(5):778–89; with permission.)

cancellous graft. In the experimental group, the rhBMP-2 sponge was divided into two portions, with the larger portion placed into the cleft defect and the smaller portion positioned as support under the alar base. In addition, a gelfoam block was used with the collagen sponge to maintain space, if necessary. Bone healing was evaluated clinically and with panoramic 3-D reconstruction and periapical views. The rhBMP-2 group had 95% of the alveolar defect filled with new bone compared with 63% in the iliac crest group based on volumetric analysis. Although the bone

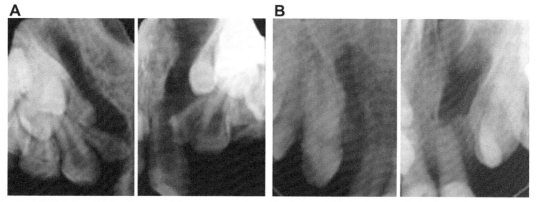

Fig. 8. (A) Right and left alveolar clefts, preoperative. (B) Right and left alveolar clefts, bone formation at 15 months postoperative. (Reprinted from Chin M, Ng T, Tom WK, et al. Repair of alveolar clefts with recombinant human bone morphogenetic protein (rhBMP-2) in patients with clefts. J Craniofac Surg 2005;16(5):778–89; with permission.)

formation in the iliac crest group is considerably lower in this study than in historical reports of standard autogenous alveolar cleft grafting, the bone fill in the rhBMP-2 group seems dramatic. Radiographic mineralization was also superior in the experimental sites. Iliac crest grafted patients had 50% complication rate versus 11% in the rhBMP-2 group. The complication rate in the iliac crest group is considerably higher than in previous reports and the 11% rate is similar or slightly increased when compared with traditional autogenous iliac crest bone grafting for alveolar cleft reconstruction. The mean total cost of the bone graft procedure was $21,800 as opposed to $11,100 for the rhBMP-2 implant in this adult cohort.[43] Although the previous study suggests that rhBMP may have superior results to autogenous grafting in adult alveolar clefts, FDA approval has not been granted for the use of BMPs in the pediatric population. rhBMP effects on growth of the skeleton, development and eruption of teeth, and effects on recurrence or malignant transformation of pathologic lesions have not been thoroughly evaluated.

RhBMP has been particularly interesting to pediatric craniomaxillofacial surgeons as a potential solution to the reconstructive difficulties faced with the developing facial skeleton. There is generally a limited supply of bone for autogenous grafts, which are currently the gold standard for reconstruction of congenital defects and traumatic losses.[3] By age 2 years, the dura loses potential to spontaneously regenerate large calvarial defects, and the diploic space is not sufficiently developed to allow split-thickness grafting until approximately age 10.[3] In addition, bone substitutes have been evaluated in multiple studies, but bone regeneration is less consistent than with autografts and some materials lack compatibility with the growing craniofacial skeleton.[3] Although rhBMPs seem to be a promising option for use in pediatric craniomaxillofacial reconstruction, questions remain with regard to their short- and long-term effects on the growing bones and neural development.[3] Limited preclinical studies looking at neurotoxicity of rhBMP-2/ACS used in cranial defects and spinal laminectomy procedures with dural puncture found no adverse effects on neural tissues.[3,44]

Springer and colleagues[45] conducted a study of autogenous bone and rhBMP-7 in critical-size cranial defects in infant minipigs and evaluated the volume and shape of regenerated bone and any disturbance on cranial development. After 4 months of healing, animals treated with particulate iliac bone retained minor bony gaps and had significantly less bone volume on the experimental

side versus native bone. The group implanted with rhBMP-7–composite collagen plus carboxymethylcellulose showed complete continuity and no substantial difference in bone volume in treated versus unoperated areas. The diameters of the skulls increased by 16.4%; however, no interference with centrifugal expansion was observed.[45] Although performed in mature versus growing animals, Sheehan and colleagues studied rhBMP-2/ACS–induced healing of critical-size cranial defects in the nonhuman primate. The rhBMP-2 grafted defects achieved 71% ($\pm$12%) closure after 6 months whereas the untreated defects obtained 28% ($\pm$11%) closure.[44] Smith and colleagues[46] have recently published their results of using rhBMP-2/ACS for the restoration of large calvarial defects in a rabbit model. The investigators created 15 × 15 mm critical-size defects in the rabbit skull maintaining an intact dura. The defects were treated with no repair, ACS alone, or rhBMP-2/ACS at 0.43 mg/mL. The edges of the ACS were in direct contact to bone edges laterally and the dura inferiorly. After 6 weeks, CT data demonstrated 32.8% ossification in untreated sites, 34.4% with ACS, and 96.9% ossification in the rhBMP-2–implanted defects. Healing seemed to occur in a concentric fashion in the rhBMP-2–treated defects and, according to cross-sectional CT and histologic data, had architecture similar to native bone.[44] Variability in the percentages of ossification and healing rates of the rhBMP-2–treated cranial defects between the Sheehan and Smith studies may be related to the dose of rhBMP-2 used or the decreased responsiveness of higher-order animals to given concentrations of rhBMP.[46] Additional studies in large animal models and nonhuman primates would be beneficial in determining the efficacy of rhBMP-2 for human cranial reconstruction. Carstens and colleagues[34] have presented data recently with their use of BMP-2 to successfully graft 22 human calvarial defects and results were hopeful.

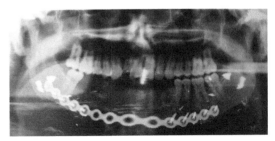

Fig. 9. Panoramic image showing large continuity defect of mandible after gunshot wound, débridement, stabilization with reconstruction plate, and failed initial graft.

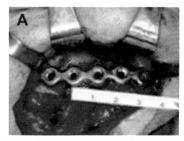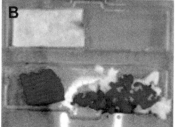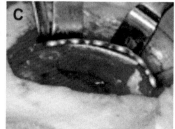

Fig. 10. (A) Defect exposed from extraoral approach. (B) INFUSE, corticocancellous iliac crest block graft, and INFUSE mixed with cancellous marrow bone from iliac crest. (C) Placement of INFUSE and cancellous bone into "chamber" created by autogenous block graft, titanium reconstruction plate, and titanium mesh.

The abundance of preclinical and clinical research involving rhBMP-2 has proved that it can be used to safely induce production of vascularized, viable trabecular bone in the craniomaxillofacial skeleton, and the bone favorably responds to functional loads.[27] The ACS carrier's capacity to concentrate the rhBMP at the graft site for a sufficient amount of time, benign tissue response, and complete resorption are key components. Furthermore, the environment must provide adequate supply of mesenchymal stem cells from periosteum, muscle, or bone marrow to be recruited by the rhBMP-2 graft.[34] In more challenging locations with less protection from tissue compression or a paucity of donor stem cells, other mechanisms to support the defect "chamber" and provide mesenchymal cells to the area must be provided. In some cases, titanium plates or mesh may be used to support the local soft tissues whereas the rhBMP regenerated bone forms and matures. Alternatively, use of compression resistant carriers for the rhBMP-2 may be used. Several nonhuman primate studies and prospective randomized clinical trials in the spinal literature have demonstrated efficacy of RhBMP-2 coupled with a type 1 bovine collagen sponge impregnated with biphasic calcium phosphate ceramic granules (15% hydroxyapatite and 85% β-tricalcium phosphate), which acts as a longer-lasting scaffold than ACS alone.[9,27] In addition, a combination of rhBMP-2 with autograft or allogenic grafts may provide enough bulk to prevent compression by local soft tissues, and autogenous bone can provide a source of mesenchymal stem cells to the area.

In a recent clinical case from the authors' institution, INFUSE was mixed with autogenous cancellous marrow and placed in conjunction with a corticocancellous iliac crest block graft and titanium mesh chamber to reconstruct a large posttraumatic mandibular continuity defect. The patient had sustained a gunshot wound and subsequently underwent débridement, radial forearm flap for intraoral soft tissue coverage, and a failed attempt at reconstruction by another service with INFUSE bulked with MASTERGRAFT (Medtronic, Sofamor Danek USA, Memphis, Tennessee) encased between rib grafts (**Figs. 9** and **10**). In some instances where extensive loss of periosteum and muscle occur, such as gunshot wounds and cancer resections, a stem cell source must be procured from a distant area.[34] Carstens and colleagues[34] suggest harvesting a vascularized galeal-subgaleal fascia flap based on the superficial temporal artery, which can be tunneled beneath the zygomatic arch, as a source for oral cavity reconstruction in such cases. When lack of soft tissue envelope exists, Carstens has described using distraction osteogenesis to expand the periosteal chamber; rhBMP-2/ACS can then be placed into the expanded pocket to generate bone of the desired size and shape.[47] A multitude of potential uses of rhBMP to facilitate reconstruction of the craniomaxillofacial skeleton continues to be developed. Future research looking at improved carriers, optimal concentration and dosing at different sites, and combination grafts will better define the current FDA-approved uses. The potential availability of additional recombinant BMPs with ability to induce more robust and mature ossification may further enhance current clinical applications.

REFERENCES

1. Wozney JM. Overview of bone morphogenetic proteins. Spine 2002;27(16 Suppl 1):S2–8.
2. Kalfas IH. Principles of bone healing. Neurosurg Focus 2001;10(4):E1.
3. Smith DM, Cooper M, Mooney MP, et al. Bone morphogenetic protein 2 therapy for craniofacial surgery. J Craniofac Surg 2008;19(5):1244–59.
4. Wikesjo UM, Sorensen RG, Wozney JM. Augmentation of alveolar bone and dental implant osseointegration: clinical implications of studies with rhBMP-2. J Bone Joint Surg Am 2001; 83(Suppl 1(Pt 2)):S136–45.

5. Urist MR. Bone: formation by autoinduction. Science 1965;150(698):893–9.
6. Geiger M, Li RH, Friess W. Collagen sponges for bone regeneration with rhBMP-2. Adv Drug Deliv Rev 2003;55(12):1613–29.
7. Li RH, Wozney JM. Delivering on the promise of bone morphogenetic proteins. Trends Biotechnol 2001;19(7):255–65.
8. Vaibhav B, Nilesh P, Vikram S, et al. Bone morphogenic protein and its application in trauma cases: a current concept update. Injury 2007;38(11):1227–35.
9. Vukicevic S, Sampath KT. Bone morphogenetic proteins: regeneration of bone and beyond. Boston. Basel: Birkhauser Verlag; 2004. p. xi, 310.
10. Termaat MF, Den Boer FC, Bakker FC, et al. Bone morphogenetic proteins. Development and clinical efficacy in the treatment of fractures and bone defects. J Bone Joint Surg Am 2005;87(6):1367–78.
11. Lane JM. Bone morphogenic protein science and studies. J Orthop Trauma 2005;19(Suppl 10):S17–22.
12. Kang Q, Sun MH, Cheng H, et al. Characterization of the distinct orthotopic bone-forming activity of 14 BMPs using recombinant adenovirus-mediated gene delivery. Gene Ther 2004;11(17):1312–20.
13. Hollinger JO, Uludag H, Winn SR. Sustained release emphasizing recombinant human bone morphogenetic protein-2. Adv Drug Deliv Rev 1998;31(3):303–18.
14. Poynton AR, Lane JM. Safety profile for the clinical use of bone morphogenetic proteins in the spine. Spine 2002;27(16 Suppl 1):S40–8.
15. Boyne PJ, Lilly LC, Marx RE, et al. De novo bone induction by recombinant human bone morphogenetic protein-2 (rhBMP-2) in maxillary sinus floor augmentation. J Oral Maxillofac Surg 2005;63(12):1693–707.
16. Orui H, Imaizumi S, Ogino T, et al. Effects of bone morphogenetic protein-2 on human tumor cell growth and differentiation: a preliminary report. J Orthop Sci 2000;5(6):600–4.
17. Friedlaender GE, Perry CR, Cole JD, et al. Osteogenic protein-1 (bone morphogenetic protein-7) in the treatment of tibial nonunions. J Bone Joint Surg Am 2001;83-A(Suppl 1(Pt 2)):S151–8.
18. Paramore CG, Lauryssen C, Rauzzino MJ, et al. The safety of OP-1 for lumbar fusion with decompression—a canine study. Neurosurgery 1999;44(5):1151–5 [discussion: 1155–6].
19. Howell TH, Fiorellini J, Jones A, et al. A feasibility study evaluating rhBMP-2/absorbable collagen sponge device for local alveolar ridge preservation or augmentation. Int J Periodontics Restorative Dent 1997;17(2):124–39.
20. Cochran DL, Jones AA, Lilly LC, et al. Evaluation of recombinant human bone morphogenetic protein-2 in oral applications including the use of endosseous implants: 3-year results of a pilot study in humans. J Periodontol 2000;71(8):1241–57.
21. Fiorellini JP, Howell TH, Cochran D, et al. Randomized study evaluating recombinant human bone morphogenetic protein-2 for extraction socket augmentation. J Periodontol 2005;76(4):605–13.
22. Kirker-Head CA, Nevins M, Palmer R, et al. A new animal model for maxillary sinus floor augmentation: evaluation parameters. Int J Oral Maxillofac Implants 1997;12(3):403–11.
23. Hanisch O, Tatakis DN, Rohrer MD, et al. Bone formation and osseointegration stimulated by rhBMP-2 following subantral augmentation procedures in nonhuman primates. Int J Oral Maxillofac Implants 1997;12(6):785–92.
24. Wada K, Nimi A, Watanabe K, et al. Maxillary sinus floor augmentation in rabbits: a comparative histologic-histomorphometric study between rhBMP-2 and autogenous bone. Int J Periodontics Restorative Dent 2001;21(3):252–63.
25. Boyne PJ, Marx RE, Nevins M, et al. A feasibility study evaluating rhBMP-2/absorbable collagen sponge for maxillary sinus floor augmentation. Int J Periodontics Restorative Dent 1997;17(1):11–25.
26. Li JZ, Li H, Hankins GR, et al. Different osteogenic potentials of recombinant human BMP-6 adeno-associated virus and adenovirus in two rat strains. Tissue Eng 2006;12(2):209–19.
27. Vukicevic S, Sampath KT. Bone morphogenetic proteins: from local to systemic therapeutics. Boston. Basel: Birkhäuser; 2008. p. xi, 343.
28. Sigurdsson TJ, Nygaard L, Tatakis DN, et al. Periodontal repair in dogs: evaluation of rhBMP-2 carriers. Int J Periodontics Restorative Dent 1996;16(6):524–7.
29. Nevins M, Kirker-Head MA, Nevins M, et al. Bone formation in the goat maxillary sinus induced by absorbable collagen sponge implants impregnated with recombinant human bone morphogenetic protein-2. Int J Periodontics Restorative Dent 1996;16(1):8–19.
30. Sigurdsson TJ, Fu E, Tatakis DN, et al. Bone morphogenetic protein-2 for peri-implant bone regeneration and osseointegration. Clin Oral Implants Res 1997;8(5):367–74.
31. Sigurdsson TJ, Nguyen S, Wikesjo UM. Alveolar ridge augmentation with rhBMP-2 and bone-to-implant contact in induced bone. Int J Periodontics Restorative Dent 2001;21(5):461–73.
32. Hanisch O, Tatakis DN, Boskovic MM, et al. Bone formation and reosseointegration in peri-implantitis defects following surgical implantation of rhBMP-2. Int J Oral Maxillofac Implants 1997;12(5):604–10.
33. Wikesjo UM, Kean CJ, Zimmerman GJ. Periodontal repair in dogs: supraalveolar defect models for evaluation of safety and efficacy of periodontal reconstructive therapy. J Periodontol 1994;65(12):1151–7.

34. Carstens MH, Chin M, Li XJ. In situ osteogenesis: regeneration of 10-cm mandibular defect in porcine model using recombinant human bone morphogenetic protein-2 (rhBMP-2) and Helistat absorbable collagen sponge. J Craniofac Surg 2005;16(6):1033–42.

35. Boyne PJ. Application of bone morphogenetic proteins in the treatment of clinical oral and maxillofacial osseous defects. J Bone Joint Surg Am 2001; 83(Suppl 1(Pt 2)):S146–50.

36. Toriumi DM, Kotler HS, Luxenberg DP, et al. Mandibular reconstruction with a recombinant bone-inducing factor. Functional, histologic, and biomechanical evaluation. Arch Otolaryngol Head Neck Surg 1991;117(10):1101–12.

37. Boyne PJ. Animal studies of application of rhBMP-2 in maxillofacial reconstruction. Bone 1996;19(Suppl 1):83S–92S.

38. Boyne PJ, Nakamura A, Shabahang S. Evaluation of the long-term effect of function on rhBMP-2 regenerated hemimandibulectomy defects. Br J Oral Maxillofac Surg 1999;37(5):344–52.

39. Terheyden H, Knak C, Jepsen S, et al. Mandibular reconstruction with a prefabricated vascularized bone graft using recombinant human osteogenic protein-1: an experimental study in miniature pigs. Part I: prefabrication. Int J Oral Maxillofac Surg 2001;30(5):373–9.

40. Terheyden H, Jepsen S, Rueger DR. Mandibular reconstruction in miniature pigs with prefabricated vascularized bone grafts using recombinant human osteogenic protein-1: a preliminary study. Int J Oral Maxillofac Surg 1999;28(6):461–3.

41. Chin M, Ng T, Tom WK, et al. Repair of alveolar clefts with recombinant human bone morphogenetic protein (rhBMP-2) in patients with clefts. J Craniofac Surg 2005;16(5):778–89.

42. Boyne PJ, Nath R, Nakamura A. Human recombinant BMP-2 in osseous reconstruction of simulated cleft palate defects. Br J Oral Maxillofac Surg 1998;36(2):84–90.

43. Dickinson BP, Ashley RK, Wasson KL, et al. Reduced morbidity and improved healing with bone morphogenic protein-2 in older patients with alveolar cleft defects. Plast Reconstr Surg 2008; 121(1):209–17.

44. Sheehan JP, Sheehan JM, Seeherman H, et al. The safety and utility of recombinant human bone morphogenetic protein-2 for cranial procedures in a nonhuman primate model. J Neurosurg 2003; 98(1):125–30.

45. Springer IN, Yahya A, Solveig K, et al. Bone graft versus BMP-7 in a critical size defect–cranioplasty in a growing infant model. Bone 2005;37(4): 563–9.

46. Smith DM, Afifi AM, Cooper GM, et al. BMP-2-based repair of large-scale calvarial defects in an experimental model: regenerative surgery in cranioplasty. J Craniofac Surg 2008;19(5):1315–22.

47. Carstens MH, Chin M, Ng T, et al. Reconstruction of #7 facial cleft with distraction-assisted in situ osteogenesis (DISO): role of recombinant human bone morphogenetic protein-2 with Helistat-activated collagen implant. J Craniofac Surg 2005;16(6): 1023–32.

Regenerative Medicine for Craniomaxillofacial Surgery

Bernard J. Costello, DMD, MD, FACS[a,b,]*, Gaurav Shah, BS[c],
Prashant Kumta, PhD[b,d,e,f,g], Charles S. Sfeir, DMD, PhD[b,g,h]

KEYWORDS

- Regenerative medicine • Scaffolds
- Tissue engineering • Stem cells

There is a need for surgeons to use predictable reconstructive techniques in patients with complex injury, congenital malformation, or defects from ablative surgery. To date, reconstructive goals have note been met by even the best of reconstructive surgeons using the latest techniques.[1] Typically, traditional techniques focus on providing tissue from the local anatomic region to compensate for the lost tissue or from another region of the body to retrofit this anatomy to the desired form. The craniofacial region has various specific functional demands, such as protection of the brain and optic tracts, breathing, mastication, speech, and hearing. The craniofacial region is also important for social acceptance and self-esteem.[2] To achieve success, a surgeon must be mindful of the functional and aesthetic requirements in planning for reconstructions.

Regenerative medicine and tissue engineering aim to provide custom constructs that become integrated fully into the local anatomy and have ideal form and function once they are in the host. Regenerative medicine can be used to recruit local tissues to produce the desired tissue, ideally in aesthetically and functionally useful structure and form. The use of commercially available recombinant bone morphogenic protein (BMP) products is an example of this concept.[3] Today, proteins can be delivered to "grow" bone at a given site and regenerate lost bony tissue.[4] However, these concepts are being taken several steps further. Examples of current strategies include a biodegradable scaffold embedded with stems cells to produce bone regeneration after mandibular resection, or advanced calcium phosphate-based cements that are biomimetic and tailored with

[a] Division of Craniofacial and Cleft Surgery, Department of Oral and Maxillofacial Surgery, University of Pittsburgh School of Dental Medicine, 3471 Fifth Avenue, Suite 1112, Pittsburgh, PA 15213, USA
[b] McGowan Institute for Regenerative Medicine, Pittsburgh, PA, USA
[c] Department of Oral and Maxillofacial Surgery, University of Pittsburgh School of Dental Medicine, 3471 Fifth Avenue, Suite 1112, Pittsburgh, PA 15213, USA
[d] Department of Bioengineering, Swanson School of Engineering, University of Pittsburgh School of Engineering, Pittsburgh, PA, USA
[e] Department of Chemical and Petroleum Engineering, Swanson School of Engineering, University of Pittsburgh School of Engineering, Pittsburgh, PA, USA
[f] Department of Mechanical Engineering and Materials Science, Swanson School of Engineering, University of Pittsburgh School of Engineering, Pittsburgh, PA, USA
[g] Department of Oral Biology, University of Pittsburgh School of Engineering, Pittsburgh, PA, USA
[h] Center for Craniofacial Regeneration, University of Pittsburgh School of Dental Medicine, Pittsburgh, PA, USA
* Corresponding author. Division of Craniofacial and Cleft Surgery, Department of Oral and Maxillofacial Surgery, University of Pittsburgh School of Dental Medicine, 3471 Fifth Avenue, Suite 1112, Pittsburgh, PA 15213.
E-mail address: bjc1@pitt.edu

Oral Maxillofacial Surg Clin N Am 22 (2010) 33–42
doi:10.1016/j.coms.2009.10.009

nanofunctional attributes offering the capability to temporally release proteins or genes that drive the regenerative process locally.[5–9]

The exponential growth in technologies related to this field has propelled the possibilities forward, and new reconstructive options are now becoming a reality. The convergence of several different technologies has been instrumental in contributing to the recent developments in this area. This article discusses these advances—the basic concepts of regenerative medicine for the craniomaxillofacial region.

REGENERATIVE MEDICINE: A NEW INTERDISCIPLINARY FIELD

The basic premise of regenerative medicine or tissue engineering is that a practitioner could provide a new construct to replace lost tissue whether that tissue be bone, skin, mucosa, tendon, cartilage, heart muscle, liver, entire solid organs, or composite tissues.[10,11] Various terms have been used to describe activities involved in repairing and regenerating tissues, wholly or partly by using cells, proteins, matrices, signaling molecules or other strategies. Regenerative medicine, reparative medicine, and tissue engineering have been used, somewhat interchangeably, to describe these activities over the past several decades. As with many advances, the process of defining these efforts is more accurately described as an incremental process and systematic discovery, rather than a specific sentinel event or seminal published work. Many discussions, papers, and symposia have contributed to current understanding of the field. However, one can point to several areas of growth to explain the direction today in the area of craniofacial regeneration.[12–14]

Thus far, biomaterials have been used as replacement tissues, and grafting is performed to reconstruct defects in the craniofacial region. Synthetic vascular grafts, resorbable collagen matrix, synthetic bone cements, and allogeneic transplants have been used as replacement tissues for those that were diseased, lost to injury, or lacking in some way due to congenital deformity.[10,12–16] In some cases, autogenous grafts could be used to replace lost tissue. These techniques have worked reasonably well but have considerable disadvantages. When Urist[4] first produced exogenous bone with the help of bone morphogenic protein, it became clear that it is possible to engineer a process within tissues using the local milieu and its complex cellular signaling environment to produce a desired tissue response. Although these attempts have been directed at producing only some bone at a few

select locations, they have been the first successful attempts at tissue engineering in the craniofacial region. Other tissues, including skin and bone, have also been repaired or regenerated using various techniques, such as expanded neonatal cell lines and stem cell transplants (**Figs. 1** and **2**).[17] The recent challenge has been to combine various technologies to control the response in a particular defect. Currently, a collision of bioscience, bioengineering, biomaterials science, and clinical surgery is occurring in an attempt to find workable constructs or bioreactors to produce regenerated tissue.

BASIC PRINCIPLES OF REGENERATIVE MEDICINE

Regenerative medicine or tissue engineering is an interdisciplinary, translational field that applies the principles of bioengineering to the development of biologic substitutes that restore, maintain, or improve tissue function.[10] To regenerate new tissues within a specific environment, 3 basic tools are required: the cells, a scaffold, and the signaling molecules. Some or all of these may be provided by the engineered construct. In some instances, proteins, signaling molecules, and/or matrices may be used to drive the body's response in the desired direction for regeneration. Several concerted efforts in the craniomaxillofacial region are being explored using various techniques, such as bone regeneration with proteins, cellular technologies, synthetic matrices, and vascular biomimetic systems.

Bone Regeneration

The area of regenerative medicine that has received the most attention for the craniomaxillofacial region is bone regeneration with cellular techniques, biomaterial replacement, or signaling molecule use. Autogenous grafting has been considered the standard for bone replacement in the craniomaxillofacial region over the years. Surgical specialists have been looking for bone substitutes to avoid donor site morbidity and provide a more convenient way to regenerate defects, whether they are from congenital deformities, acute trauma, chronic nonunion, or resection of pathology. Allogeneic bone grafts are suitable to some extent for more simple defects, but they still have several drawbacks, such as the cost, the less than ideal mechanical properties, the risk of disease transmission, and the need to procure the material from limited cadaveric specimens. For most craniomaxillofacial defects of significance, allografts and xenografts have little purpose if one compares outcomes with

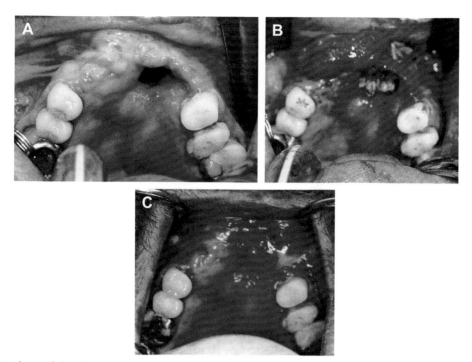

Fig. 1. (*A–B*) An adult with a large, unrepaired unilateral cleft of the maxilla and alveolus. His fistula is symptomatic and closure has previously been attempted by several surgeons. He consented to the use of cultured neonatal cells on a bilaminar collagen membrane in conjunction with a revision palatoplasty. The fistula was closed without evidence of recalcitrant fistula.

autogenous sources. Grafting a maxillary/alveolar cleft site is typically performed with autogenous bone from the iliac crest. Previous attempts to use allogeneic bone grafts or xenografts have not had the success rates seen with autogenous grafting, and as a result, these techniques are not often used. Any option must surpass the success of autogenous grafting while providing a solution that also limits morbidity.[18,19]

To engineer a substitute, it is necessary to regenerate bone in a manner by which the materials can survive through the initial phases of healing and implantation. This generally means that bone must form reasonably quickly and that the typical cellular, biochemical, and biomechanical challenges must be overcome in a given region. For example, the cranial vault is essentially a non–weight-bearing and nonfunctional bone when compared with the mandible. A critical size defect of the cranial vault is likely to sustain less biomechanical force than a critical size defect of the mandible. Although the cranium and mandible have excellent blood supply in the region, bacterial contamination is much more of an issue in the mandible than in most areas of the cranium. Consequently, the 3-dimensional (3D) construct that provides the structural support for the reconstruction must be suited to meet the

biomechanical demands and provide an appropriate environment for regeneration. Autogenous grafting has done this fairly well, but even microvascular tissue transfer often fails to provide the ideal 3D structure that completely restores the defect back to full functionality and meets the aesthetic demands. Procedures that have provided BMP-2 to a defect site in the craniomaxillofacial region often produce bone, but in an unpredictable fashion. These reconstructions frequently lack the desired 3-dimensional structure. New efforts are aimed at designing novel 3D functional scaffolds exhibiting all the desired biofunctional attributes of biocompatibility, bioactivity, safety, and internal and external micro- and macrostructure combined with the desired spatial and temporal pharmacokinetic transport response. Consequently, novel biocompatible scaffolds are available that serve as a home for cells or proteins while also serving as smart delivery systems to address some of these shortcomings (**Fig. 3**).

Scaffolds

Tissue in the craniomaxillofacial region is varied in composition, but in its simplest definition, it consists of a matrix and various cell types.[20] The matrix represents a 3D structure or scaffold for cells, which provides them with a specific

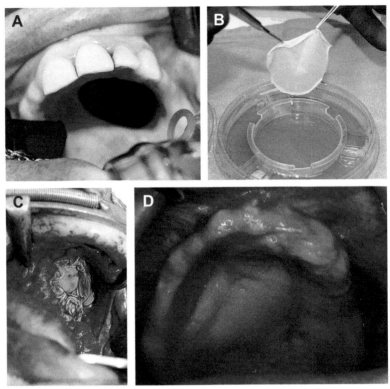

Fig. 2. (*A–D*) A woman with a chronic fistula from cocaine use and presumed granulomatosis disorder who failed multiple attempts by other surgeons for closure of a large oral-nasal-antral fistula and also refused temporalis flap or microvascular tissue transfer techniques. She consented to the use of cultured and expanded neonatal cells on a bilaminar collagen membrane in conjunction with a single-layered closure of mucosa on the oral side. The wound healed completely without any evidence of even a small fistula.

environment and architecture for a given functional purpose.[21] The structure also serves as a reservoir of water, nutrients, cytokines, and growth factors. When one applies these concepts to tissue engineering in the craniofacial skeleton to restore function or regenerate the bone tissue, the scaffold will act as a temporary matrix or template for cell proliferation, extracellular matrix deposition, bone regeneration, and remodeling until the mature bony tissue is regenerated.[10,22,23] During this process, the scaffold acts as a template for the vascularization.[24,25] Recently, various new materials have been used as a matrix for bone regeneration including ceramics, synthetic and natural polymers, and composites.[20] Examples have included demineralized bone, collagen, proteins, fibrin, and various forms of calcium phosphate.[10,20] Nanostructured forms of calcium phosphates can bind and condense plasmid DNA and attach growth factors, including 3D architectures of tailored natural polymer-based gels and cements, exploiting the enhanced bioactivity and resorption potential. These novel cements are also being studied as next-generation systems for tissue engineering.[26–29]

The scaffolds ideally need to accomplish several goals that include biocompatibility, appropriate mechanical strength, and appropriate degradation. If a material lacks biocompatibility, then it elicits host responses that destroy the materials.[30] The surface of the scaffolds must also support appropriate cell interaction. Because proliferation of most mammalian cell types is anchorage-dependent, scaffolds must provide a suitable surface for cell attachment, proliferation, differentiation, and migration.[31] This can be achieved by the use of materials that are derived from or mimic the microphysiologic environment.[20,26–29]

A scaffold must also have adequate tensile and compressive strengths in a given functional environment. These requirements might vary in different areas of the craniomaxillofacial complex. For example, a zygomatic bone or cranial vault reconstruction does not typically require that the construct endure a heavy functional load. However, the mandible routinely requires substantial strength to endure various loads in multiple directions and dimensions. It is essential that the scaffold exhibit acceptable tensile and compressive strengths to be able to execute the biologic

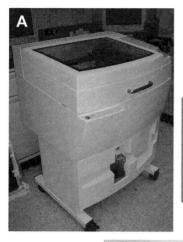

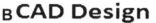

CAD Design

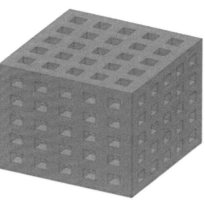

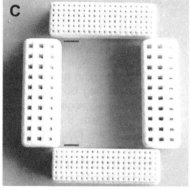

Fig. 3. (*A–C*) A 3D ink-jet printer that can print various materials, including metal structures or calcium phosphate cement material, from standard imaging software. Digital Imaging and Communications in Medicine (DICOM) images can be imported into the software where the scaffolding can be adjusted or redesigned for printing. Custom constructs can be printed for use with proteins, cells, or other materials for regenerating tissues.

cues needed for regeneration. In vitro, the scaffolds should also have sufficient mechanical strength to withstand hydrostatic pressures and maintain the spaces required for cell ingrowth and matrix production.[32] In vivo, the mechanical properties of the implanted construct should ideally match those of living bone, so that an early mobilization of the reconstructed site can occur.[23]

Additionally, the degradation rate should be matched with the regeneration rate of the newly forming tissue in an optimal fashion, such that the time for regeneration of the defect tissue adequately matches the time for complete degradation of the scaffold. The scaffold should also exhibit nontoxic degradation. For example, polylactic acid constructs typically degrade by hydrolysis via the Krebs cycle and release carbon dioxide and water as their by-products.

Porosity and interconnectivity are also important for an efficient and effective diffusion of nutrients and gases. These properties aid in the appropriate removal of metabolic waste resulting from the cells that regenerate into the scaffold. Because of metabolic demands of the bone, high rates of mass transfer are expected to occur with the regenerative process. The scaffold must have

a structure that allows for efficient removal of these waste products.[33] The pore size of scaffold material also plays an important role in cell proliferation and cell distribution throughout tissue regeneration.[34] Some have suggested an optimal pore size between 200 and 400 μm.[35] Others have suggested that pore sizes up to 200 μm in polyester membranes result in the best bone ingrowth.[36] The size of the pore has a significant effect on its mechanical integrity and its ability to perform under functional demands.[21] Pores and voids disrupt the continuity of the solid phase and subsequently lower the solid phase density. This weakening of the solid phase and reduced mass density across the surface and bulk results in defects at the atomic and molecular levels, causing the material to fail more easily under reduced stresses in comparison to the denser (less porous) material. There is considerable work in progress to maximize the strength of the solid phase while maintaining porosity in the range of 70% with biologically acceptable pore sizes. Thus far, this has been a challenge when combining materials science and clinical applicability of bone substitutes, scaffolds, and various materials used in regenerative approaches.

Growth factors

Growth factors are proteins produced by cells that act as signaling molecules on an appropriate cell to carry out a desired function. These proteins activate the cellular communications network and influence functions, such as cell proliferation, matrix deposition, and differentiation of tissues.[37] Growth factors have been shown to play a key role in bone and cartilage formation, fracture healing, and the repair of other musculoskeletal tissues.[38] Abnormalities in the genes that code for these proteins cause various craniofacial skeletal dysostoses (ie, Apert syndrome, Crouzon syndrome, and the achondroplasia syndromes). The binding of a growth factor to its receptor initiates intracellular signaling that will lead to different events, such as the promotion or prevention of cell adhesion, proliferation, migration, and differentiation. This typically occurs by upregulating or downregulating the synthesis of proteins and receptors.[38–40] Hence, these molecules are recognized as fairly important for tissue formation and may play an important role in regenerative medical approaches.

If one looks at bone regeneration strategies, much like other tissues, bone has a wide variety of growth factors that are active in its formation and remodeling processes. BMPs, transforming growth factor beta (TGF-β), fibroblast growth factors, insulin growth factor I and II, and platelet-derived growth factors are the most commonly studied. Several of these have been evaluated for their inductive potential in regenerative medical adjuncts.[3–7,38–42]

In 1965, Urist[4] made the observation that demineralized bone matrix could produce bone formation when placed in subcutaneous tissue. This capability was later attributed to BMP.[4,42] Currently, the BMPs are grouped into the TGF-β superfamily because of their similarities in protein structure and sequence homology. BMPs are closely associated with the bone matrix, and they are expressed during the early phases of fracture healing.[43] Their role is to recruit mesenchymal stem cells to the healing site and then differentiate them into the osteogenic lineage for bone deposition. Although there are many BMPs described, BMP-2, -4, -6 and -7 are the best studied in craniofacial biology and are considered to have the most potential for regeneration.[40,44,45]

CELLULAR APPROACHES

Cells are important during the integration of materials used for reconstruction and for the long-term viability of any implanted material or device. These cells may be provided initially with the "graft" or recruited into the construct during the early regenerative process. Different tissues and sizes of defects will have different demands, and the interaction of the cells, signaling molecules, and scaffold are vastly different for soft tissue, bone, and other complex tissues. As the scaffold changes or is resorbed in the regenerative process, the cellular components are likely to change in various ways. The sequence of these events can be complicated and represent a major challenge when designing regenerative techniques for the craniomaxillofacial region. Various cellular technologies and approaches have been used to achieve regeneration in this region.

One way to provide cells to a defect is simple bone marrow autotransplantation. Free and nonvascularized, bone grafts have been the mainstay of reconstruction for various craniomaxillofacial defects for decades. These techniques were some of the very first to be used in bone tissue engineering. These procedures were tried as an empiric approach and at the time, seemed ideal for regenerating bone, because bone marrow is rich in osteoprogenitor cells and osteogenic precursors, with the ability to secrete BMPs.[22] The procedure involves procuring bone marrow from a donor site (eg, iliac crest, cranium, rib, tibia, or mandible) and transplanting it into the defect site with enough soft tissue coverage to allow the local tissues to eventually provide vascular supply to the graft. Autogenous grafting is fairly simple and inexpensive and has limited morbidity in most cases. However, the limited sources and relative scarcity of osteogenic cells after aging, disease, and irradiation ultimately limits its widespread use for all defects or compromised sites.[46,47] Additionally, these types of grafting procedures rarely heal in a manner that achieves the ideal 3D structure to replace the defect.

Mesenchymal Stem Cell Technology

Mesenchymal stem cells (MSCs) are immature and undifferentiated cells that are obtained from bone marrow and the periosteum. They have the capacity to achieve extensive replication without differentiation and they possess multilineage developmental potential, making them a powerful source of cells.[48,49] MSCs can be subdivided into adult stem cells (ASCs) and embryonic stem cells.(ESCs). ESCs are usually isolated from the inner wall of the preimplantation blastocysts. These embryonic cells in the early developmental stages are more proliferative and are pluripotent because of their indefinite amplification without the risk of dedifferentiation.[50] ASCs reside in the fully differentiated or adult tissues. ASCs have been procured from the bone marrow, periosteum, muscle, fat, brain, dental pulp, and skin.[51–58] Ethical issues, immune rejection uncertainty, and uncontrolled differentiation make embryonic stem cell use challenging.

Besides their differentiation potential, MSCs have other important attributes. It has been suggested that these cells may possess unique immune effects that may render them either immune-privileged or may play immunosuppressive roles, which would make them suitable for allogeneic or xenogeneic transplantation. An important issue clinicians face when using MSCs is how to induce them, while controlling their differentiation, into the desired cell type. Crucial to this process is the clear understanding and reproducibility of methods to isolate desired populations of MSCs. The process by which these cells undergo expansion and differentiation into different cell lineages is quickly being understood, such that cell lineages that produce bone, fat, cartilage, muscle, and tendon can now be produced.

These techniques have been used to regenerate bone in cranial vault defects, cartilage in fetal tracheas, and cardiac muscle after acute myocardial infarction.[59–63] Today, considerable work is focused on these concepts and on using these technologies to provide live cells to a craniomaxillofacial wound defect to regenerate tissues without a significant immune response.

Differentiated Osteoblasts

These cells are committed mesenchymal cells that have been directed down the osteogenic lineage to push the cell type closer to the final type desired. Using this type of approach has the potential advantage of achieving rapid repair of defects, because the cells are already differentiated. The main disadvantage is that they have a limited capacity for proliferation, because they are able to perform only a certain number of replication cycles before the problem of dedifferentiation arises. The presence of these cells may drive the process locally and recruit additional cells from the host to continue the process.

Perivascular cells

Recent research has shown that human perivascular cells possess multilineage progenitor properties. These perivascular cells, pericytes in particular, were purified from skeletal muscle, pancreas, adipose tissue, and other organs and were demonstrated to be myogenic in vivo and ex vivo, regardless of their tissue of origin.[64–66] These human perivascular cells when sorted from diverse human tissues and cultured over the long term have the ability to produce adherent, multilineage progenitor cells that exhibit the features of MSC.

Stem cell biology is changing rapidly, and the understanding of stem cell differentiation or dedifferentiation of somatic cells is expanding greatly. Recent advancement in research has transformed mature skin cells into pluripotent cells by inserting just 4 genes, *Oct3/4*, *Klf4*, *Sox2*, and *c-Myc*, into the cell nucleus. These cells were called induced pluripotent stem cells.[64–66] Although more basic research is required to acquire basic knowledge about these cells, they are considered to be a major therapeutic possibility. Cellular therapy is changing rapidly and future use of these advanced technologies for craniofacial regeneration holds great promise for patients.

VASCULAR REGENERATION

One of the most intriguing aspects of tissue engineering has been the challenge of encouraging neo-vascularization, particularly for large defects. Although it has become straightforward to provide a large mass of cells to a defect in a given scaffold, providing adequate blood supply to sustain those cells throughout the "graft" has proven to be difficult. Providing a conduit for application of growth factors within a wound for temporal release throughout the regenerative process has also been challenging. Various approaches have been considered to address these concerns. Much is understood about the process of normal vascular development, neoangiogenesis in the adult, and also about the genes that are involved in vascular development.[67,68] There is a complex dynamic that occurs during vascular development including extrinsic influences, flow physics, hypoxia, and other factors.[69,70] Many scientists working in this area think that once the issue of vascular regeneration is adequately addressed, it will provide a new opportunity for regenerative medicine.

The process of neovascularization involves the interaction of endothelial cells and their formation of a primitive blood-vessel plexus that becomes a network of arteries, veins, and their associated capillaries. This process is thought to be tightly regulated with various signal pathways and involves the interaction of the local environment and the regulation of genes important in vascular development. The vascular endothelial growth factors (VEGFs) involved in this process are thought to drive this system forward in the proper manner. As such, the simple deposition of one particular type of VEGF at a high concentration within a wound is not likely to reproduce a complex vasculature system. The temporal release of these and other factors in the proper environment makes it challenging to creating a vasculature that could support a regenerative tissue construct. Additionally, there are several pathologic processes that probably involve inappropriate VEGF upregulation, such as arteriovascular malformations, tumor growth, and aneurysm formation. Understanding this complex mechanism is the key to developing a tissue-engineered construct that will have appropriate vascular support.

VEGF seems to have a key role in the tissue development and regenerative processes. It has been well described as a part of the cascade controlling bone development during the promotion of vascular structures, particularly in the process of bone healing by acting on bone-forming cells.[68,71,72] Taking advantage of this growth factor has proven to be more challenging that just delivering it to a site with the expectation that vascular tissues will regenerate. There are dose effect concerns, and the importance given to the temporal release of factors during a healing/regeneration phase is appropriate. Krebsbach and colleagues[73] have reported some interesting work in this area, including the use of a VEGF-based scaffold that showed improved neovascularization and bone regeneration in a critical-size rat calvarial defect exposed to radiation. Continued work in this area is likely to produce factors that optimize vascular proliferation and also give clinicians ways to optimize vasculature within tissue-engineering constructs.

SUMMARY

Regenerative medicine is poised to have a major impact on craniomaxillofacial surgery in the near future. Signaling molecules and proteins are being used to drive local tissues to produce bone. Cellular technologies are providing some options for regeneration of tissues in the craniomaxillofacial skeleton and are poised to have a major impact on the field. Novel materials are being evaluated for improved scaffolds, with better functionality to serve as delivery systems of growth factors, proteins, and genes in a controlled efficient manner, better mechanical properties, and improved biocompatibility. The understanding of neovascularization is helping tailor approaches to designing regenerated tissues in the craniomaxillofacial region. Advances in the understanding of signaling molecules, scaffolds, and cellular technology are already affecting regenerative possibilities, and many of these technologies are being evaluated in large animal models. Surgeons who

work in the craniomaxillofacial region must have a clear understanding of these concepts.

REFERENCES

1. Rodriguez ED, Bluebond-Langner R, Park J, et al. Preservation of contour in periorbital and midfacial craniofacial microsurgery: reconstruction of the soft tissue elements and skeletal buttresses. Plast Reconstr Surg 2008;121(5):1738–47.
2. Adams GR. The effects of physical attractiveness on the socialization process. In: Lucker GW, Ribbens KA, McNamara JA, editors. Psychological aspects of facial form craniofacial growth series monograph no. 11. Ann Arbor (MI): University of Michigan Press; 1981. p. 25–47.
3. Carter TG, Brar PS, Tolas A, et al. Off-label use of recombinant human bone morphogenetic protein-2 (rhBMP-2) for reconstruction of mandibular bone defects in humans. J Oral Maxillofac Surg 2008; 66(7):1417–25.
4. Urist MR. Bone formation by autoinduction. Science 1965;150:893–9.
5. Terheyden H, Knak C, Jepsen S, et al. Mandibular reconstruction with a prefabricated vascularized bone graft using recombinant human osteogenic protein-1: an experimental study in miniature pigs. Part I: prefabrication. Int J Oral Maxillofac Surg 2001;30:373.
6. Terheyden H, Warnke P, Dunsche A, et al. Mandibular reconstruction with a prefabricated vascularized bone graft using recombinant human osteogenic protein-1: an experimental study in miniature pigs. Part II: transplantation. Int J Oral Maxillofac Surg 2001;30:469.
7. Terheyden H, Menzel C, Wang H, et al. Prefabrication of vascularized bone grafts using recombinant human osteogenic protein-1. Part 3: dosage of rhOp-1, the use of external and internal scaffolds. Int J Oral Maxillofac Surg 2004;33:164.
8. Warnke PH, Springer I, Wiltfang J, et al. Growth and transplantation of a custom vascularised bone graft in a man. Lancet 2004;364:766.
9. Warnke PH, Wiltfang J, Springer I, et al. Man as living bioreactor: fate of an exogenously prepared customized tissue-engineered mandible. Biomaterials 2006;27:3163.
10. Langer R, Vacanti JP. Tissue engineering. Science 1993;260:920–6.
11. Evans CH, Palmer GD, Pascher A, et al. Facilitated endogenous repair: making tissue engineering simple, practical, and economical. Tissue Eng 2007;13(8):1987–93.
12. Haseltine WA. The emergence of regenerative medicine: a new field and a new society. J Regen Med 2001;2:17–23.

13. Tissue engineering. Selected papers from the ucla symposium of tissue engineering. Keystone, Colorado, April 6–12, 1990. J Biomech Eng 1991;113(2): 111–207.

14. Bell E. Tissue engineering, an overview. In: Bell E, editor. Tissue engineering: current perspectives. Boston: Birkhäuser; 1993. p. 3–15.

15. Matsuda T, Akutsu T, Kira K, et al. Development of hybrid compliant graft: rapid preparative method for reconstruction of a vascular wall. ASAIO Trans 1989;35(3):553–5.

16. 19th Annual UCLA symposium: tissue engineering. [abstracts]. J Cell Biochem Suppl 1990;14E: 227–56.

17. Eaglstein WH, Falanga V. Tissue engineering and the development of Apligraf a human skin equivalent. Adv Wound Care 1998;11(Suppl 4):1–8.

18. Costello BJ, Kail M. Alveolar/maxillary bone grafting. In: Laskin D, editor. Problem solving in oral and maxillofacial surgery. Hanover Park (IL): W.B. Saunders; 2007. p. 144–5.

19. Ruiz R, Costello BJ. Contemporary management of cleft lip and palate. Fonseca's oral and maxillofacial surgery. Philadelphia (PA): Elsevier; 2009.

20. Salgado AJ, Coutinho OP, Reis RL. Bone tissue engineering: state of the art and future trends. Macromol Biosci 2004;4:743–65.

21. Kneser U, Schaefer DJ, Munder B, et al. Tissue engineering of bone. Minim Invasive Ther Allied Technol 2002;11:107–16.

22. Laurencin CT, Ambrosio AMA, Borden MD, et al. Tissue engineering: orthopaedic applications. Annu Rev Biomed Eng 1999;1:19–46.

23. Hutmacher DW. Scaffolds in tissue engineering bone and cartilage. Biomaterials 2000;21:2529–43.

24. Deporter DA, Komori N, Howley TP, et al. Reconstituted bovine skin collagen enhances healing of bone wounds in the rat calvaria. Calcif Tissue Int 1988;42:321.

25. Murata M, Huang BZ, Shibata T, et al. The design of scaffolds for use in tissue engineering. Part I. Traditional factors. Tissue Eng 2001;7(6):679–89.

26. Olton D, Li J, Wilson ME, et al. Nanostructured calcium phosphates (NanoCaPS) for non-viral gene delivery: influence of the synthesis parameters on transfection efficiency. Biomaterials 2007;28:1267–79.

27. D Olton. Fundamental studies on the synthesis, characterization, stabilization and trafficking mechanisms of nanostructured calcium phosphates (NanoCaPs) for non-viral gene delivery [PhD dissertation]. Pittsburgh (PA): Carnegie Mellon University; August 2008.

28. Hsu-Feng Ko. Design, synthesis and optimization of nanostructured calcium phosphates (NanoCaPS) and Natural polymer based 3-D non-viral gene delivery systems [PhD dissertation]. Pittsburgh (PA): Carnegie Mellon University; October 2008.

29. A Roy, H Wu, FS Picard, et al. Novel synthetic bone for orthopaedic and craniofacial regeneration, Biomedical Engineering Society, Annual Meeting. Pittsburgh (PA), October 7–10, 2009: 86.

30. Yang S, Leong KF, Du C, et al. The design of scaffolds for use in tissue engineering. Part I. Traditional factors. Tissue Eng 2001;7:679.

31. Gomes ME, Salgado AJ, Reis RL, Polymer-based systems on tissue engineering, replacement and regeneration. The Netherlands: Kluwer, Dordrecht 2002. p. 221.

32. Leong KF, Cheah CM, Chua CK. Solid freeform fabrication of three dimensional scaffolds for engineering replacement. Tissues and organs. Biomaterials 2003;24:3262.

33. Freed LE, Vunjak-Novakovic G. Culture of organized cell communities. Adv Drug Deliv Rev 1998;33:15.

34. Di-Silvio L, Gurav N, Tsiridis E. Tissue engineering, bone. In: Koller MR, Palsson BO, editors. Encyclopedia of biomaterials and biomedical engineering. New York: Marcel Dekker Pubs; 2004. p. 1500–7.

35. Burg KJ, Porter S, Kellam JF. Biomaterial developments for bone tissue engineering. Biomaterials 2000;21(23):2347–59.

36. Pineda LM, Busing M, Meinig RP, et al. Bone regeneration with resorbable polymeric membranes. III. Effect of poly(L-lactide) membrane pore size on the bone healing process in large defects. J Biomed Mater Res 1996;31(3):385–94.

37. Gerstenfeld LC, Cullinane DM, Barnes GL, et al. Fracture healing as a post-natal developmental process: molecular, spatial, and temporal aspects of its regulation. J Cell Biochem 2003; 88:873–84.

38. Giannoudis PV, Pountos I. Tissue regeneration. The past, the present and the future. Injury 2005; 36(Suppl 4):S2–5.

39. Giannoudis PV, Einhorn TA, Marsh D. Fracture healing: a harmony of optimal biology and optimal fixation? Injury 2007;38(Suppl 4):S1–2.

40. Giannoudis PV, Tzioupis C. Clinical applications of BMP-7: the UK perspective. Injury 2005;36(Suppl 3):S47–50.

41. Grauer JN, Patel TC, Erulkar JS, et al. 2000 Young investigator research award winner. Evaluation of OP-1 as a graft substitute for intertransverse process lumbar fusion. Spine 2001;26:127–33.

42. Harwood PJ, Giannoudis PV. Application of bone morphogenetic proteins in orthopaedic practice: their efficacy and side effects. Expert Opin Drug Saf 2005;4:75–89.

43. Wozney JM. Bone morphogenetic proteins. Prog Growth Factor Res 1989;1:267–80.

44. Friedlaender GE, Perry CR, Cole JD, et al. Osteogenic protein-1 (bone morphogenetic protein-7) in the treatment of tibial nonunions. J Bone Joint Surg Am 2001;83(Suppl 1):S151–8.

45. Govender S, Csimma C, Genant HK, et al. Recombinant human bone morphogenetic protein-2 for treatment of open tibial fractures: a prospective, controlled, randomized study of four hundred and fifty patients. J Bone Joint Surg Am 2002;84: 2123–34.

46. Quarto R, Mastrogiacomo M, Cancedda R, et al. Repair of large bone defects with the use of autologous bone marrow stromal cells. N Engl J Med 2001;5:385–6.

47. Quarto R, Thomas D, Liang CT. Bone progenitor cell deficits and the age-associated decline in bone repair capacity. Calcif Tissue Int 1995;56(2):123–9.

48. Bianco P, Riminucci M, Kuznetsov S, et al. Multipotential cells in the bone marrow stroma: regulation in the context of organ physiology. Crit Rev Eukaryot Gene Expr 1999;9(2):159–73.

49. Vats A, Tolley NS, Polak JM, et al. Stem cells: sources and applications. Clin Otolaryngol 2002;27(4): 227–32.

50. Keller GM. In vitro differentiation of embryonic stem cells. Curr Opin Cell Biol 1995;7(6):862–9.

51. Pittenger MF, Mackay AM, Beck SC, et al. Multilineage potential of mesenchymal stem cells. Science 1999;284:143–7.

52. Hanada K, Solchaga LA, Caplan AI, et al. BMP-2 induction and TGF-beta 1 modulation of rat periosteal cell chondrogenesis. J Cell Biochem 2001; 81(2):284–94.

53. Perka C, Shultz O, Spizer RS, et al. Segmental bone repair by tissue-engineered periosteal cell transplants with bioresorbable fleece and fibrin scaffolds in rabbits. Biomaterials 2000;21(11): 1145–53.

54. Williams JT, Southerland SS, Souza J, et al. Cells isolated from adult human skeletal muscle capable of differentiating into multiple mesodermal phenotypes. Am Surg 1999;65:22–6.

55. Zuk PA, Zhu M, Mizuno H, et al. Multilineage cells from human adipose tissue: implications for cell-based therapies. Tissue Eng 2001;7:211–28.

56. McKay R. Stem cells in the central nervous system. Science 1997;276:66–71.

57. Gage FH. Mammalian neural stem cells. Science 2000;287:1433–8.

58. Toma JG, Akhavan M, Fernandes KJL, et al. Isolation of multipotent adult stem cells from the dermis of mammalian skin. Nat Cell Biol 2001;3(9):778–84.

59. Bruder SP, Fink DJ, Caplan AL. Mesenchymal stem cells in bone development, bone repair, and skeletal regeneration therapy. J Cell Biochem 1994;56: 283–94.

60. Mankani MH, Krebsbach PH, Santomura K, et al. Pedicled bone flap formation using transplanted bone marrow stromal cells. Arch Surg 2001;136: 263–70.

61. Fuchs JR, Hannouche D, Terada S, et al. Fetal tracheal augmentation with cartilage engineered from bone marrow-derived mesenchymal progenitor cells. J Pediatr Surg 2003;38:984–7.

62. Chen SL, Fang WW, Ye F, et al. Effect on left ventricular function of intracoronary transplantation of autologous bone marrow mesenchymal stem cell in patients with acute myocardial infarction. Am J Cardiol 2004;94:92–5.

63. Price MJ, Chou CC, Frantzen M, et al. Intravenous mesenchymal stem cell therapy early after reperfused acute myocardial infarction improves left ventricular function and alters electrophysiologic properties. Int J Cardiol 2006;111:231–9.

64. Crisan M, Yap S, Casteilla L, et al. A perivascular origin for mesenchymal stem cells in multiple human organs. Cell Stem Cell 2008;3(3):301–3.

65. Takahashi K, Yamanaka S. Induction of pluripotent stem cells from mouse embryonic and adult fibroblast cultures by defined factors. Cell 2006;126: 663–76.

66. Takahashi K, Koji T, Mari O, et al. Induction of pluripotent stem cells from adult human fibroblasts by defined factors. Cell 2007;131:861–72.

67. Carmeliet P. Angiogenesis in health and disease. Nat Med 2003;9:653–60.

68. Coultas L, Chawengsaksophak K, Rossant J. Endothelial cells and VEGF in vascular development. Nature 2005;438:937–45.

69. Ramirez-Bergeron A, Runge K, Dahl HJ, et al. Hypoxia affects mesoderm and enhances hemangioblast specification during early development. Development 2003;130:4393–403.

70. Le Noble F, Moyan D, Pardanaud L, et al. Flow regulates arterial-venous differentiation in the chick embryo yolk sac. Development 2004;131:361–75.

71. Street J, Bao M, deGuzman L, et al. Vascular endothelial growth factor stimulates bone repair by promoting angiogenesis and bone turnover. Proc Natl Acad Sci U S A 2002;99:9656–61.

72. Nakagawa M, Kaneda T, Arakawa T, et al. Vascular endothelial growth factor (VEGF) directly enhances osteoclastic bone resorption and survival of mature osteoclasts. FEBS Lett 2000;473:161–4.

73. Kaigler D, Wang Z, Horger K, et al. VEGF scaffolds enhance angiogenesis and bone regeneration in irradiated osseous defects. J Bone Miner Res 2006;21:735–43.

Cleft Lip and Palate Surgery: An Update of Clinical Outcomes for Primary Repair

Andrew Campbell, DDS, FRCD(C)[a,b],
Bernard J. Costello, DMD, MD, FACS[a,b,c],*,
Ramon L. Ruiz, DMD, MD[d,e,f]

KEYWORDS

• Cleft lip • Cleft palate • Nasal repair • Palatoplasty

The comprehensive management of cleft lip and palate has received significant attention in the surgical literature over the last half century. It is the most common congenital facial malformation in the United States and has a significant developmental, physical, and psychological impact on those with the deformity and their families. In the United States, current estimates place the prevalence of cleft lip and palate or isolated cleft lip at 16.86 per 10,000 live births (approximately 1 in 600).[1] There is significant phenotypic variation in the specific presentation of facial clefts. Care of children and adolescents with orofacial clefts needs an organized team approach to provide optimal results.[2–4] Specialists from multiple areas are needed for successful management from infancy through adolescence. These include oral and maxillofacial surgery, otolaryngology, plastic surgery, genetics and dysmorphology, speech-language pathology, social work, psychology, orthodontics, pediatric dentistry, prosthodontics, audiology, and nursing.[4] The specific goals of surgical care for children born with cleft lip and palate include:

• Normalized esthetic appearance of the lip and nose
• Intact primary and secondary palate
• Normalized speech, language, and hearing
• Nasal airway patency
• Class I occlusion with normal masticatory function
• Good dental and periodontal health
• Normal psychosocial development

These goals are best achieved when surgeons with extensive training and experience in all phases of care are actively involved in the planning and treatment.[5–7] Surgical treatment must be based on the best available clinical research to avoid unfruitful, biased treatment schemes and optimize outcomes. Ideally, randomized prospective controlled trials with comparative data and appropriate outcome measures would guide one's decisions. Outcome studies pertaining to the multiple outcome measures, such as facial appearance, facial growth, occlusion, patient satisfaction, and psychosocial development, are essential. Unfortunately, this level of published

[a] Private Practice Austin, TX, USA
[b] Division of Craniofacial and Cleft Surgery, Department of Oral and Maxillofacial Surgery, University of Pittsburgh School of Dental Medicine, 3471 Fifth Avenue, Suite 1112, Pittsburgh, PA 15213, USA
[c] Pediatric Oral and Maxillofacial Surgery, Children's Hospital of Pittsburgh, Pittsburgh, PA, USA
[d] Department of Pediatric Craniomaxillofacial Surgery, Arnold Palmer Hospital for Children, Orlando, FL 32806, USA
[e] Department of Surgery, University of Central Florida College of Medicine, Orlanda, FL, USA
[f] Arnold Palmer Children's Hospital, 1814 Lucerne Terrace, Suite D, Orlando, FL 32806, USA
* Corresponding author. Division of Craniofacial and Cleft Surgery, Department of Oral and Maxillofacial Surgery, University of Pittsburgh School of Dental Medicine, 3471 Fifth Avenue, Suite 1112, Pittsburgh, PA, 15213.
E-mail address: bjc1@pitt.edu

Oral Maxillofacial Surg Clin N Am 22 (2010) 43–58
doi:10.1016/j.coms.2009.11.003
1042-3699/10/$ – see front matter © 2010 Elsevier Inc. All rights reserved.

evidence is lacking for this patient population.[8] The cleft population as a whole is heterogeneous, making it difficult to standardize groups of patients and to provide valid comparison and outcome data. Individual clefts of the lip or palate are as unique, as are the patients with the deformity. Patients have complete or incomplete clefts that may be isolated to the lip or palate only, can be unilateral or bilateral, wide or narrow, and found in syndromic or nonsyndromic individuals, to mention the most obvious variations. Infants with clefting can present with cardiac, neurologic, renal, and other developmental deficits that can delay treatment and affect outcome, further complicating this patient population. The heterogeneity of the population, the difficulty in coordinating and compiling multi-center data, and the final results of surgical intervention not being seen for approximately 2 decades make high-level outcome research with long-term, reliable results difficult. Few studies currently stand up to the rigorous criteria of level I evidence. The vast majority of publications deal with single-surgeon experience, retrospective cohort studies, and case series. A lack of comparison or control groups in these studies provides little for evidence-based decision making. However, considerable experience can be used to guide some of one's decisions. Thus, dogmatic claims about the best therapies across large populations of patients are often inappropriate, given the lack of valid data. This article provides an update on current primary cleft lip and palate outcome data and its implications in our treatment decisions.

CLEFT LIP REPAIR

Cleft lip and palate is a complicated and 3-dimensional malformation. Distortion of the skin, musculature, mucous membranes, underlying skeletal structures (bones and cartilage), and dentition occurs with varying severity. The goals of unilateral cleft lip repair include the creation of an intact upper lip with appropriate vertical length and symmetry, repair of the underlying muscular structures producing normal function, and primary treatment of the associated nasal deformity (**Fig. 1**). Original lip reconstruction techniques consisted of simple straight-line closures. In the mid-1800s, the first reports of lip repair that diverged from previous simple closures were published by Malgaine[9] and Mirault.[10] The Tennison[11] technique with use of a triangular flap to vertically reposition cupids bow was presented in 1952. Millard[12] changed cleft lip surgery when he published the rotation-advancement flap technique in 1957. In short order, the technique became popular and remains the most common technique used today.[12,13] Numerous modifications to Millard's original description have been published since then. Prominent surgeons around the world modified their own and others' distinctive repairs, including Asensio,[14] Delaire and colleagues,[15,16] and Nakajima and Yoshimura,[20] lending to the diversity that is cleft lip and nose repair.

Recent surveys of active North American cleft surgeons indicate that the Millard rotation advancement or a modification of the technique is used by 84% of respondents; triangular flaps are used by 9%; and Delaire functional cheilorhinoplasty, by 2%.[13] A detailed description of each repair is presented elsewhere and the reader is referred to a prior publication for detailed discussions.[17] Studies providing comparison data for results of the various repairs are lacking. The few available randomized comparison studies investigated nasal and labial esthetics of patients treated with the rotation advancement technique versus a triangular flap technique.[18,19] Overall, these studies found no significant differences in esthetic outcomes and ultimately advocated either technique. The variations in technique for repairing cleft lip and nasal deformities and the uniqueness of each cleft make comparison studies difficult. Surgical results are also influenced by other variables, such as the use of presurgical orthodontic/orthopedic treatment, simultaneous gingivoperiosteoplasty (GPP), and specific timing of surgery—the particular procedure perhaps being only one of many important factors.[20] The surgical repair of the cleft lip, more than any other area of cleft care, remains an art with little compelling evidence to promote one technique over the other. There currently are no adequate controlled studies published that compare different primary techniques of lip repair and their long-term outcomes.

Primary Nasal Reconstruction

The reconstruction of a cleft lip defect also involves correction of the associated nasal deformity. Thompson and Reinders[21] found that residual nasal deformity required approximately twice as many revisions as the lip. In the past 2 decades, much attention has been given to performing cleft nasal reconstruction in a primary fashion, but controversy still exists. In 2008 Sitzman[13] found that 52% of active cleft surgeons in North America performed primary nasal reconstruction routinely, and 22% never used the technique. The typical nasal deformity is characterized by a cleft-side dome depression, splaying of the ala, and eversion of the alar rim exposing the nasal mucosa. The septum is directed to the noncleft

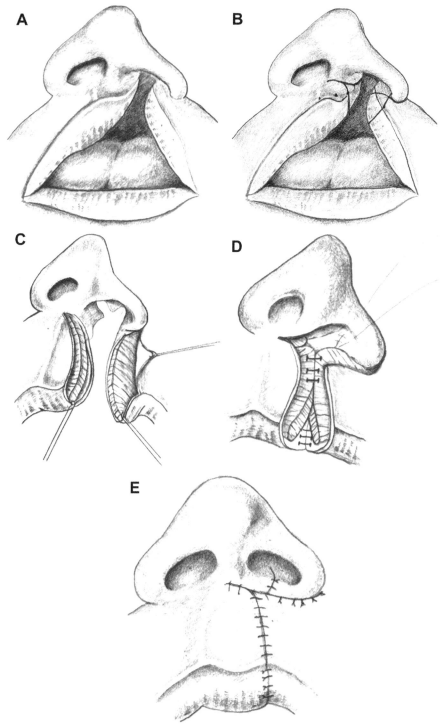

Fig. 1. Complete unilateral cleft lip illustrating the typical deformities of cleft-side alar displacement, deviation of nasal septum, and cleft of the nasal floor (*A*). Markings for typical cleft repair design incorporates the goals of hypoplastic tissue excision and precise approximation of lip vermillion and white roll (*B*). Dissection of all 3 tissue layers (skin, muscle, mucosa) and excision of hypoplastic tissue is completed. Abnormal muscle insertions at the anterior nasal spine and nasal ala are completely freed (*C*). Functional repair of the orbicularis oris muscle with multiple interrupted sutures; the nasal floor and oral mucosa are approximated (*D*). Completed repair with advancement of the cleft side lateral flap and inferior rotation of the medial segment. Vertical scar designed to resemble the philtral column on the unaffected side, with the remaining incisions being hidden in the contours of the nose and lip (*E*). (*From* Fonseca R, Marciani R, Turvey T, editors. Oral and Maxillofacial Surgery, vol. 3. 2nd edition. St Louis (MO): Saunders; 2009. p. 730; with permission.)

side along with the premaxilla and nasal dorsum because of aberrant muscular insertions and activity.[22] Traditionally, surgeons avoided primary nasal correction for fear of growth retardation and further deformity. McComb[23–25] published his primary cleft rhinoplasty technique in 1975, with follow-up studies in 1985 and 1996. In his technique, access to the nasal cartilages is obtained through the cleft lip incisions; this avoids incisions in the nasal lining, which may contribute to later stenosis. Using the existing incisions, wide undermining of the nasal cartilages from the nasal skin is undertaken from the nostril rim to the nasion; the lower lateral cartilages are then supported in proper position with sutures. McComb reported stable long-term correction with the technique, without drooping of the nasal rim. Anastassov and colleagues[26] found increased nasal deviation, increased nasal obstruction, higher rates of sinusitis, and increased requirement for nasal revision surgery in those treated with delayed rhinoplasty. According to these philosophies, the considerable nasal deformity and functional abnormalities resulting from delayed repair can be explained by growth not being "helped" by a proper initial repair, and the deformities worsen with time.[27] Later, Anderl and colleagues[28] reported a similar technique with more extensive mobilization and undermining of the nasal skin and cheek to allow improved medialization of displaced structures without the need for support sutures. The technique proved to have satisfactory results in 80% of 130 patients, with the remaining 31 individuals requiring revision surgery. Anderl and colleagues concluded that growth is not inhibited and that no adverse sequelae resulted from scar tissue secondary to the wide undermining. The technique benefits unilateral and bilateral deformities. Other surgeons remove some of the fibrofatty tissue located between the domes of the lower lateral cartilages and use interdomal suturing during the primary nasal repair. Studies to date regarding primary nasal reconstruction provide level III evidence illustrated by retrospective case review, observational studies, systematic reviews, and experienced surgeon opinion. No randomized controlled studies are available that compare primary versus secondary nasal reconstruction. Despite the poor level of evidence, results from the studies mentioned and similar reports[29–33] indicate that primary nasal reconstruction can be performed to improve overall nasal esthetics and function and possibly to reduce the number of revision surgeries. Large studies are needed to adequately assess the comparative results between different treatment protocols before strong statements can be made regarding the utility of one protocol or procedure over another.

CLEFT LIP MUSCULAR RECONSTRUCTION

Delaire has described the anterior facial muscles as several different groupings of balanced rings. The middle and lower rings are disrupted when cleft of the lip or palate occurs. The resultant disturbance in muscular function within these anatomic muscular units secondarily produces distortions in the subsequent growth of surrounding skeletal and cartilaginous structures that theoretically increase over time.[34,35] Accurate reconstruction of the various muscular layers of the lip is important for normal lip function and prevents further distortion of underlying hard tissue structures.[34–36] According to this theory, treatment of the clefted skin and muscular components improves soft tissue symmetry and, through molding forces, also improves osseous symmetry. The facial musculature adjacent to the cleft deformity has increased collagen content, atrophy, and hypoplasia.[37] Mooney and colleagues[38] have reviewed these concepts and documented that a 3.5-week delay in muscle development occurs in the unilateral cleft lip and that fiber insertions are abnormal and asymmetric. In nonclefted individuals, the perinasal and perioral muscles attach to the caudal-anterior nasal septum, which functions to exert forward growth of the midface. When a facial cleft is present, the abnormal muscular balance results in the midface deviating to the noncleft side. Nasal distortions include widening of the alar base, vertical displacement of the ala, asymmetric nares, lack of supratip break, underprojected tip, deviated nasal septum, and a short and drooping columella.[26] Clefting causes the orbicularis oris to course obliquely along the cleft edges displacing the superficial musculoaponeurotic system (SMAS) inferoposteriorly on the affected side. The zygomaticus muscles pull the SMAS and perioral musculature laterally, posteriorly, and inferiorly, as attachments with the caudal septum are lost on the cleft side.[27] Each of these theoretically contributes to asymmetry.

Joos[36] retrospectively compared 2 groups of patients undergoing cleft lip repair, one with 50 patients receiving musculoperiosteal reconstruction and no presurgical orthopedics and the other with 60 patients receiving the Millard repair and presurgical orthopedic treatment using a pin-retained device. Improvements in skeletal development were noted in the first group, suggesting to the authors that midfacial muscular reconstruction is important and that this cannot be compensated for by orthopedic therapy. These results were echoed by a similar technique described by Markus and Precious.[39] Confounding variables make it difficult to make direct comparisons between the 2 studies. These reports are theoretical and represent Level III evidence. Whether to perform the midfacial dissection in the supraperiosteal or subperiosteal plane is another controversial technical point. Regardless of the depth of dissection, modern techniques rely on restoration of the perinasal and perioral muscular anatomy in at attempt to create balanced facial growth. When such a correction does not occur, the secondary deformities that plagued earlier repairs are the result.[40] These concepts have been generally self-reported by those who advocate them and using mostly Level III data. However, considerable positive experience with these techniques warrants additional investigation to determine the possible improved results purported by the advocates of these techniques and philosophies.

PRESURGICAL ORTHOPEDICS

Some of the more significant challenges commonly discussed in the literature on cleft lip and nasal repair are the optimal results of nasal reconstruction and repair of the wide unilateral or bilateral cleft lip. Wide and extensive cleft deformities are associated with more significant nasolabial deformity.[41] In an attempt to improve results in these difficult cases, surgeons and orthodontists have developed presurgical methods to approximate the soft tissues and osseous structures. One of the best known devices was introduced by Latham in 1975 and subsequently used in the Millard-Latham protocol. This pin-retained active device widened lateral segments while approximating the alveolar arches and, in bilateral cases, retracted the protruding premaxilla.[42] Long-term follow-up of patients treated with these pin-retained orthopedic devices has revealed significant negative effect on maxillary growth making their use limited.[43–45]

The modern era of presurgical nasoalveolar molding (PNAM) was introduced by Grayson and colleagues[46] in 1993, using a passive intraoral device with the addition of nasal prongs. It is theorized that neonatal nasal cartilages have plasticity and can be actively molded and repositioned to the benefit of long-term esthetics. Overall goals of PNAM have been described as improved nasal appearance that persists, fewer secondary nasal surgeries, columellar elongation, minimizing the need for alveolar bone grafting, limited maxillary growth disturbance, and economics.[47] Controversy exists as to whether these benefits are truly achieved and maintained over time. Lack of adequate long-term controlled studies prevents evidence-based recommendations on use of

PNAM. Bennum and colleagues[48] report improved nasal symmetry lasting into childhood when PNAM is used, compared with children excluded from orthopedic treatment. Conversely, subsequent publications note that the initial improvement in nasal symmetry noted with PNAM before unilateral repair has shown significant relapse in the first year after surgery.[49,50] Nasal asymmetry is known to worsen with growth in cleft patients, especially at the prepubertal growth spurt; therefore, a controlled study with follow-up into adulthood is required.

Many surgeons using PNAM also perform GPP and report reduction in the need for secondary bone grafting and minimal growth inhibition. Results show that at least 40% of patients having GPP require secondary bone grafting to obtain alveolar continuity and allow tooth eruption.[51] Secondary maxillary bone grafting procedures have a success of 96%, making the 40% failure rate of GPP unreasonably high. GPP has been abandoned at some centers because of the frequent lack of adequate bone formation and its detriment to growth and the final overall result.[52] Experiences with similar primary bone grafting techniques in the 1960s had poor growth results, leading to recommendations against the procedure.[53,54]

Additional stated benefits of PNAM are improved feeding efficiency and growth.[55] A randomized 2-arm long-term multicenter trial providing rare level I evidence is being carried out in the Netherlands (Dutchcleft) and is providing interesting results regarding presurgical orthopedics using passive plates without active nasal molding. Results have shown that there were no sustained effects on maxillary arch dimensions in the primary dentition; initial improvements in language skills and facial esthetics were no longer realized by age 6 years; no benefits were noted in feeding or weight gain; greater satisfaction with treatment results was not shown by mothers; and ultimately, the cost-effectiveness of presurgical orthopedic treatment should be questioned.[56–60] Similar to other studies, Dutchcleft lacks follow-up into adulthood; future results of this well-performed study are anxiously awaited. A randomized controlled trial of 50 nonsyndromic infants with cleft palate by Masarei and colleagues[61] found no benefit in feeding efficiency or body growth when presurgical orthopedics were used. The published or stated benefits of PNAM have largely been unproven and are based mainly on self-reported level III evidence. Incorporating these devices into cleft care bears a significant financial cost and parental burden. Currently, they are without proven benefit and show poor results in well done comparative studies. The clinical use of PNAM is not strongly supported by the literature.

TIMING OF CLEFT LIP REPAIR

Cleft lip/nasal repair represents the initial surgical endeavor in the care of an individual with cleft lip and palate. Each cleft team advocates a slightly different timing for lip reconstruction, with actual correction being performed from the neonatal period to 6 months or later. Intrauterine repair of the cleft lip deformity has been contemplated, but it is not viable considering the life-threatening position in which it places the mother and fetus. Antenatal and neonatal repair have prompted interest based on experimental findings indicating that wounds in the fetus heal without scar tissue early in gestation.[62,63] Despite theoretical and experimental benefits, neonatal repair has not seen improvement in esthetic outcomes over repair at 3 months.[64,65] In fact, problems with excessive scarring and less esthetic outcomes have resulted. Proponents of traditional repair at 10 to 12 weeks argue that this timeline provides for improved esthetic results, because the lip musculature is more developed and allows for proper reconstruction, decreased risk of anesthesia-related complications, and time for the parents to accept the malformation. Early cleft lip repair has not been shown to improve maternal bonding or have other psychosocial benefits.[66,67] Surgery was traditionally delayed for several weeks based on the "rule of tens." These guidelines included the infant weighing a minimum of 10 pounds, having a hemoglobin level of 10 g/mL, and reaching an age of 10 weeks and were based on minimizing anesthetic morbidity and mortality. Current anesthesia and pharmacologic methods make earlier surgery safe, but without a significant benefit to neonatal repair; most teams choose to wait the traditional 3 months. There is currently no compelling evidence for a repair performed at an earlier time.

SUMMARY: CLEFT LIP

Cleft lip repair has many aspects that require consideration; surgeons have the responsibility of making decisions using the best available data to optimize results. A critical appraisal of the literature reveals deficient level I evidence. Decisions need to be made using published cohort studies, comparison data, case series, and reviews by experts in the field. Based on the best available evidence, some statements can be made

regarding primary cleft lip repair. Repair is still appropriate when performed at age 3 months or older. Earlier repair can be safely performed but offers no benefits in esthetics or maternal bonding. The use of presurgical orthopedics and GPP has many advocates but hypothesized benefits remain largely unsupported, and results of the available level I evidence indicate no significant improvements in outcome. Significant financial and parental resources are required when presurgical orthopedics is undertaken, making the cost-benefit ratio unreasonable. There is little debate over the need to perform accurate perinasal/perioral muscular reconstruction and nasal reconstruction at the time of primary lip repair. Insufficient data exist to advocate one type of repair over another; if the principles of muscular and nasal repair are followed, one can perform the rotation-advancement, Delaire cheilorhinoplasty, or triangular technique and obtain excellent results.

CLEFT PALATE

Le Monnier, a French dentist, reported the first successful cleft palate repair in Paris in 1766.[68,69] Subsequently, many surgical techniques for cleft palate closure have been described. There is still active debate over which technique produces superior results. A lack of clinical data from prospective trials forces clinical decisions to be made from retrospective studies, cohort studies, and surgeon experience. Because of the inherent bias and uncontrolled nature of this level of evidence, clinicians need to be aware of the shortcomings and incorporate the information appropriately into practice. It may be prudent to consider repair of the hard and soft palates as separate entities, because the outcome measures for each are different. The primary objective of soft palate closure is the development of normalized speech.[70] Outcome measures for hard palate closure should include maxillary growth, facial profile, dental occlusion, and fistula formation.[71] An overall detrimental effect of surgery on growth has been shown, and this should be minimized by considering the timing of the repair.[72] Bernard von Langenbeck described a palatoplasty technique in 1861, which is the oldest such procedure used today. The von Langenbeck palatoplasty involves bipedicled mucoperiosteal flaps with medialization of nasal and oral side mucosa for closure. The technique leaves minimal hard palate exposed but does not lengthen the velum and can impair access for repair of the nasal lining and velar musculature. Subsequently, multiple palate repair techniques incorporated a push-back component designed to lengthen the palate and decrease the incidence of velopharyngeal insufficiency (VPI).[76] These include variations of the V-Y pushback described separately by Veau,[73] Kilner[74], and Wardill.[75] Mucoperiosteal flaps are raised based on the greater palatine vasculature, then retropositioned via a V-Y technique, resulting in lengthening of the velum at the expense of denuded anterior hard palate. Poor growth outcomes and anterior fistula formation has limited the use of this technique.

The Bardach 2-flap palatoplasty was described in 1967 and further refined with excellent anatomic and functional results.[77,78] In the Bardach repair, 2 mucoperiosteal flaps based on the greater palatine vessels are raised; as the flaps are not pedicled anteriorly, visibility is optimal for closure of the nasal layer and velar musculature (**Fig. 2**). The technique also limits hard palate bone exposure, because the flaps are rotated downward at the expense of palatal depth. These cleft palate surgical procedures are now collectively termed the 2-flap palatoplasties. In 1978, Leonard Furlow[79] introduced a novel technique of repairing palatal clefts using double-opposing z-plasties of

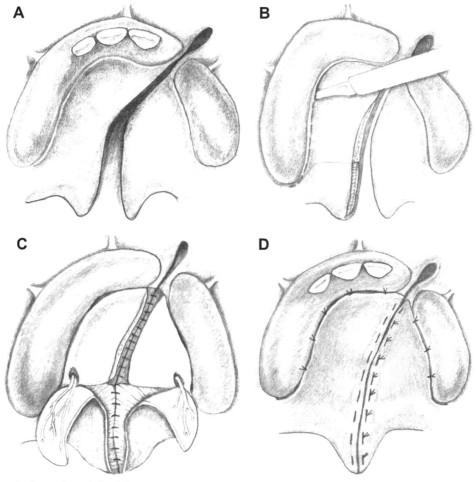

Fig. 2. Typical complete cleft of the primary and secondary palates (*A*). In the Bardach palatoplasty, incisions are designed along the cleft edges and at the junction of the alveolus and hard palate, bilaterally. Two large full-thickness mucoperiosteal flaps are raised on the hard palate; the soft palate is dissected into 3 layers (nasal mucosa, soft palate muscle, oral mucosa). Incisions end at the area of the incisive foramen anteriorly (*B*). Layered palatal closure proceeds with approximation of the nasal mucosa followed by release of the levator palatini muscles from the posterior hard palate. The newly released levator muscles are then posteriorly repositioned and repaired to create a dynamic sling that allows for velar closure (*C*). Closure of the oral mucosal flaps completes the repair; first, the midline is sutured, followed by the lateral releases. Rarely, the lateral releases are left to heal by secondary intention. The cleft anterior to the incisive foramen is left untouched and will be repaired in the mixed dentition stage of development (*D*). (*From* Fonseca R, Marciani R, Turvey T, editors. Oral and Maxillofacial Surgery, vol. 3. 2nd edition. St Louis (MO): Saunders; 2009. p. 730; with permission.)

the oral and nasal layers, with anatomic orientation of the soft palate musculature. Furlow has reported superior results using this procedure as compared with his experience with the 2-flap palatoplasty.[80] Many centers adopted the Furlow palatoplasty and have reported better outcomes.[81–84] These reports consist mostly of experience from a single center or surgeon and limited retrospective comparisons of techniques. They do not provide powerful enough data to make definitive statements. Currently, only some Level II and mostly Level III evidence is available to help make clinical decisions regarding repair techniques. Successful cleft palate repair requires adequate muscular reconstruction of the velum to create a dynamic and functional soft palate. The 2-flap and Furlow palatoplasties reconstruct the velar musculature (ie, levator veli palatini and palatopharyngeus) into a dynamic sling but do so in different ways.

TWO-FLAP PALATOPLASTY

In these techniques, hard palate repair is performed in a 2-layered fashion, with mucoperiosteal flaps for oral side closure and nasal mucosa with or without vomer flaps to reduce tension and fistula formation. The amount of denuded hard palate should be minimized, because this has been shown to inhibit maxillary growth in all dimensions. Ross[72,85–90] found improved maxillary incisor position when von Langenbeck repair is performed instead of push-back procedures, and similar results were reported by Friede.[91] This is probably due to the reduced scarring present with more limited procedures during the early part of the maxillary growth process.

In the 2-flap technique an intravelar veloplasty (IVV) is performed with dissection of the levator palatini muscle (and palatopharyngeus), releasing its abnormal attachment to the posterior hard palate followed by retropositioning of the muscular posteriorly. Ultimately, the muscle fiber direction is reoriented from a sagittal direction to a transverse one. The idea of IVV was first proposed by Kriens[92] in 1969 and has since been incorporated into many techniques. Comparative data on IVV are lacking and conflicting, most probably because of variability in how surgeons perform the muscular dissection and repositioning. In a prospective study, Marsh and colleagues[93] found no significant difference in speech outcome or incidence of VPI among patients who had their clefts repaired with IVV versus those who did not. However, the IVV group showed a tendency toward less VPI. In contrast, Sommerlad[94,95] reported improved outcomes with his version of

IVV. Andrades and colleagues[96] reported lower reoperation rates for VPI and better speech outcomes when IVV was performed than when IVV was omitted. Similarly, Hassan and Askar[97] did a prospective cohort study of nonsyndromic patients with cleft palate, comparing those who received IVV with those who had a 2-layered closure. Improved velopharyngeal and eustachian tube function was found in the IVV group. Currently, the consensus among surgeons seems to suggest that soft palate function is improved when IVV is performed. The available literature also supports the procedure. Reasonable Level II and III evidence is available to guide decisions in this area, and considerable experience seems to indicate that using an IVV in some manner is important to long-term speech results. Level I evidence is still lacking to a great extent in this particular area of cleft palate repair and outcome measurements.

DOUBLE-OPPOSING Z-PLASTY

Closure of a cleft using the Furlow technique involves hard palate closure in a similar manner to that described in the 2-flap palatoplasty, with the goal of a tension-free 2-layered closure. The soft palate is closed in a unique manner that allows theoretical lengthening of the soft palate and reconstruction of the musculature into an anatomically appropriate position (**Fig. 3**). The technique uses opposing, mirror-imaged z-plasties, one on each side of the oral mucosa and the other on each side of the nasal mucosa. The posteriorly based flaps on the nasal and oral surfaces contain mucosa and muscle; the anteriorly based flaps contain only mucosa. The posteriorly based oral myomucosal flap is designed on the patients left side; the incision is made along the cleft edge just shy of the midline hard palate junction, extending toward the hamular notch. The flap containing muscle and mucosa is then raised with a posterior base, leaving the nasal side mucosa intact. On the patient's right side, an oral side mucosa-only flap is developed based anteriorly; the incision is along the cleft edge and extends from the uvular area to the hamular notch, leaving the musculature attached to the nasal mucosa. The nasal side z-plasties are a mirror image of the oral side. On the patient's right, an incision is made just shy of the midline hard palate junction to the hamular notch, making a posteriorly based myomucosal flap. On the left, an incision is made through nasal mucosa from uvula to hamular notch, thus creating an anteriorly based mucosal flap. Dissection proceeds bilaterally into the space of Ernst, and the tensor palatini tendons are released to allow

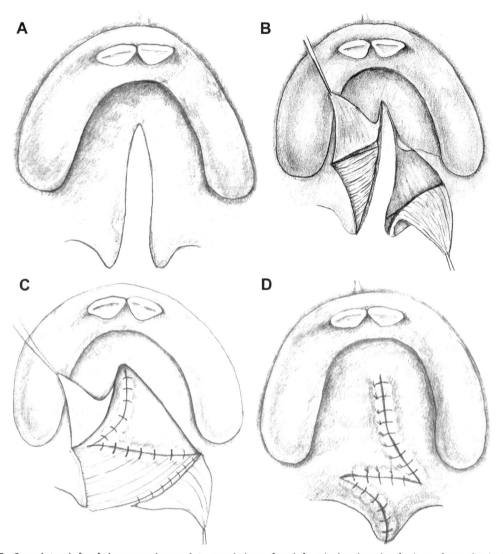

Fig. 3. Complete cleft of the secondary palate consisting of a defect in hard and soft tissue from the incisive foramen to the uvula (*A*). A Furlow double-opposing z-plasty requires the creation of oral side and nasal side z-plasties. Note that both musculomucosal flaps are based posteriorly (*B*). The nasal flaps are transposed for lengthening the soft palate and creating a dynamic levator palatini sling to enhance velar closure. Closure of the nasal mucosa anterior to the hard/soft palate junction is performed in the standard manner (*C*). The oral side flaps are transposed, placing the musculomucosal flap posteriorly; closure proceeds with interrupted sutures (*D*). (*From* Fonseca R, Marciani R, Turvey T, editors. Oral and Maxillofacial Surgery, vol. 3. 2nd edition, St Louis (MO): Saunders; 2009. p. 730; with permission.)

adequate mobilization of all flaps. The flaps are re-positioned and closed accordingly. This repair has many similarities to the IVV, without having to dissect the muscle off the mucosal flaps as is performed in a 2-flap palatoplasty. This effectively reduces the volume of the closure port for the velum, making it easier for the palate to achieve closure. Documentation of "lengthening" of the palate is not present in the literature, but observation during the repair reveals a 3-dimensional

narrowing of the space that the velum must close during speech.

One criticism of this technique relates to the higher fistula rates found by many studies when compared with 2-flap techniques. Fistula rates reported in the literature are infamous for reporting bias, for differing definitions and classifications of fistulae, and for faulty study design. This makes meaningful comparisons nearly impossible, and several investigators have recommended strategies to decrease fistula rates—particularly with the Furlow technique. The placement of acellular dermis between the oral and nasal flaps is recommended by some, and this has shown a significant reduction in fistula rates comparable to 2-flap closures.[98–100] Some recent reviews of fistula formation after 2-flap palatoplasty revealed the fairly low rates of 3.4% and 3.2%, respectively.[101,102] Helling[100] reported a fistula rate of 3.2% when acellular dermis was used in conjunction with the Furlow technique.

The outcome data for the Furlow palatoplasty technique compared with the 2-flap techniques have generally been favorable. Multiple investigators have reported improved speech results and low rates of VPI with Furlow versus von Langenbeck.[83,86,103–105] These studies consist of single-surgeon and single-center experience before and after adoption of the Furlow technique. Although compelling, these data represent Level III evidence and have not had the statistical power to convincingly provide a wave of change in the surgical community. Despite flaws in the study designs, the reduction in reported rates of VPI is impressive. Randall and colleagues[106] confirmed a decrease in VPI from 68% to 25% after instituting the Furlow technique. Williams amd colleagues[104] report a VPI rate of 13% with the Furlow and 25% with von Langenbeck palatoplasties. A small number of uncontrolled studies have reported no significant difference in speech or VPI outcomes between the Furlow and Veau-Wardill-Kilner or von Langenbeck techniques.[107,108] A current and impressive study being conducted at the University of Florida and Sao Paolo, Brazil seeks to compare outcomes of the Furlow and von Langenbeck palatoplasties. The results are unpublished but preliminary findings have suggested only minor differences in outcome, with the exception that the Furlow group has a higher fistula rate and the von Langenbeck, increased amounts of hypernasality as only one element of a comprehensive speech evaluation.[109] The available published data has been weak Level II or Level III, and, as such, has been difficult to use when deciding between repair techniques. Consequently, the data at this time is not convincing enough to advocate the Furlow over the 2-flap palatoplasties. As evidenced by the available literature, good results can be obtained with 2-flap or double-opposing z-plasty techniques.

GROWTH

Growth outcome is a major area of study in cleft lip and palate care and an important long-term outcome variable. Outcomes traditionally measured include degree of maxillary horizontal and vertical retrusion, transverse arch restriction, and occlusion. It is generally accepted that the surgical repair (and resultant scarring) of the palate and lip and other interventions in cleft correction contribute greatly to midface growth restriction. Ross[72,85–90] has demonstrated, however, that the final facial form is a result of treatment effects, inherent growth potential, and features specific to each deformity. He also concluded that surgeons performing the same repairs can have significantly different growth outcomes. With such an integrated mechanism complicated by the myriad of surgical variables, growth inhibition continues to be an area of controversy. Among dozens of studies, a minority based their results on a series of consecutively treated patients (eg, longitudinal). Many of these have reported maxillary growth deficiency in adolescents with a decreased sella-nasion-subspinale angle (an average of 4.5°) compared with noncleft controls.[110–112] To improve growth outcomes, centers have attempted delayed hard palate closure with conflicting results, increased fistula rates, and poor speech outcomes in the short term. A major stated advantage of 2-stage repairs is the narrowing of the hard palate cleft after primary veloplasty.[40] The reduced defect size allows for closure later in the growth curve, with smaller flaps and, presumably, less of a negative effect on future growth. Excellent growth results have been reported with this technique.[113,114]

One-stage palate repair remains the most common protocol in North America. Scarring of the hard palatal tissues is associated with maxillary growth inhibition.[115] Techniques that minimize the degree of palatal scarring are considered beneficial to overall maxillary growth. The push-back palatoplasties leave areas of the anterior hard palate denuded to heal by secondary intention with resultant scarring. Multiple studies have reported greater growth impairment secondary to these techniques versus the von Langenbeck palatoplasty, with some centers abandoning the push-back for that reason.[72,84–91] When a palatoplasty has been performed, there is the possibility of a residual palatal fistula developing at or posterior to the incisive foramen region. Oronasal communications anterior to the foramen are purposely left open, with plans for repair at the time of alveolar/maxillary bone grafting. A decision needs to be made on whether to repair symptomatic residual fistulae early or wait until more growth has occurred. The best data to aid in the decision making comes from a thorough speech examination, performed when the child is cooperative and linguistically developed enough to do one—often at about 3 years of age. Fistulae large enough to interfere with proper language development or cause significant oronasal regurgitation need to be repaired. Repair of insignificant fistulae at an early age will probably restrict maxillary growth further and should be delayed.

Whatever the cause of hypoplastic maxillae, a significant cohort of treated cleft lip and palate patients require maxillary advancement surgery. The frequency with which LeFort I surgery is required in the cleft population has a wide range, depending on the subgroup treated. A retrospective cohort study of a heterogeneous cleft population by Good and colleagues[116] found an overall need for maxillary advancement of 20.9%. When subgroups were considered, they found a range of 0.0% to 47.7%; no patient with isolated clefting of the lip or secondary palate required LeFort I advancement, but 47.7% of those with cleft lip and palate required an osteotomy. Posnick[117] states that rates of maxillary advancement range from 25% to 75% in a cleft population, depending on the criteria applied. The evidence available on this topic is level III in nature and often does not control for cleft type or the surgical variables. To reduce the need for maxillary advancement, consistent team care with a minimum number of surgical procedures and timely orthodontic intervention has been advocated.[118] With roughly one-quarter of the cleft population requiring this additional surgical intervention, growth needs to remain an area of active investigation. More importantly, the concepts of how to potentially alter the current protocols based on the available Level III evidence remains a mystery. Given the multiple variables assessed in the long-term outcome of patients with clefts, larger studies are necessary to strongly advocate for one protocol over another.

TIMING OF PALATE REPAIR

As has been stated earlier, the major goal of cleft palate repair is the development of normalized speech for the affected individual, while limiting the amount of maxillary growth restriction. For normalized speech to develop, an intact and appropriately functioning palate needs to be present at the time a child begins speech production.[119] It is well known that surgery on the hard palate has a negative effect on maxillary growth. To prevent this, some authors advocated delayed hard palate closure.[120,121] In 1944, Schweckendiek[122] advocated early primary repair of the soft palate and delay of hard palate closure until after puberty. Later reports found merit in his technique with less maxillary growth restriction to the extent that up to 90% of patients had normal to near normal midface morphology.[89,122,123] Bardach and colleagues visited Schweckendiek's unit and documented high rates of VPI and compensatory misarticulations among patients treated with this protocol.[124] Additional studies, many with critiques from speech pathologists, confirmed these results when patients were treated with similar protocols.[123–126] Cleft palate centers in North America have mostly abandoned delayed hard palate closure; however, many European units favor these protocols.

Despite the lack of statistical power and the shortcomings of the available literature, some current studies suggest that cleft palate repair performed before age 14 months is associated with better speech when compared with repairs performed later.[127] Dorf and Curtin[128,129] found that children with palatal repair after age 12 months had a 90% likelihood of compensatory articulations (CAs) compared with less than 5% of children with repair before 12 months of age. Chapman and Hardin[130] also found a 90% rate of CAs in their study of children receiving late surgery. Chapman and colleagues[127] recently performed a multicenter prospective study examining 40 children, comparing timing of palatal surgery and lexical status with outcome. They found patients operated on with a mean age of 11 months and less lexical ability had better speech than those with a mean age of 15 months and more lexical ability. Kirschner and colleagues[131] performed modified Furlow palatoplasties on 2 groups of patients, one between 3 and 7 months of age and the second aged 7 months or older. They found no significant differences in speech scores, VPI, or rate of secondary pharyngoplasty and stated that there is no benefit to performing palatoplasty before age 7 months. Chapman's work represents some of the best evidence regarding timing of palate closure, corresponding to high quality level II data. However, most studies in this area consist of level III case series and single-surgeon experience. Consensus from the available data dictates that primary palatal surgery should most often be performed between about 7 and 15 months of age to appropriately balance growth and speech development.

SUMMARY: CLEFT PALATE

Over the past century, improved outcomes have been realized with cleft palate repair, primarily through improved understanding of anatomy, superior techniques, better training, and emphasis on interdisciplinary care. There are limitations in the currently available literature and a high level of heterogeneity exists in the cleft population. There is also variability in how different surgeons perform the same operation. Despite the inherent difficulties in studying this population, there is enough evidence to guide surgeons in repairing the cleft palate deformity. However, it is inappropriate to be dogmatic regarding cleft repair techniques. Consensus has been reached for many general concepts, but the debate continues over several key technical considerations. It is probably beneficial to minimize denuded palatal bone to prevent scar formation and subsequent growth inhibition. Soft palate closure requires the anatomic reconstruction of the levator palatini muscle into a functional sling. Ideally, the levator muscle should overlap at the midline in a significantly retropositioned fashion. The creation of this dynamic sling can be performed with a 2-flap palatoplasty with intravelar veloplasty or Furlow double-opposing z-plasty palatoplasty, with similar results. Using acellular dermis interpositional grafts has been shown to reduce fistula rates—particularly with the Furlow technique. To optimize speech, the traditional timing in North America for cleft palate repair is before about 18 months of age. Recent research suggests that repair before 15 months of age but not earlier than 7 months may benefit speech without endangering growth. When evaluating the currently available literature, controversy still exists over many concepts. There is no current evidence that strongly supports one palate repair technique over another, and continued study is necessary to refine the choices made for repair technique modifications, timing, and other aspects of care.

REFERENCES

1. Canfield MA, Honein MA, et al. National estimates and race/ethnic-specific variation of selected birth defects in the United States. Bir Defects Res A Clin Mol Teratol 2006;76(11):747–56.
2. Kaufman FL. Managing the cleft lip and palate. Pediatr Clin NA 1991;38(5):1127–47.
3. Strauss RP. The organization and delivery of craniofacial health services: state of the art. Cleft Palate Craniofac J 1999;36(3):189–95.
4. Parameters for evaluation and treatment of patients with cleft lip/palate or other craniofacial anomalies. American Cleft Palate-Craniofacial Assoc. March, 1993. Cleft Palate Craniofac J 1993;30(Suppl): S1–16.
5. Adams GR. The effects of physical attractiveness on the socialization process. In: Lucker GW, Ribbibs KA, McNamara JA, editors. Psychological aspects of facial form from craniofacial growth series, monograph no. 11. Ann Arbor (MI): University of Michigan Press; 1981. p. 25–47.
6. Kapp K. Self concept of the cleft lip and or palate child. Cleft Palate J 1979;16:171.
7. Kapp-Simon KA. Psychological interventions for the adolescent with cleft lip and palate. Cleft Palate Craniofac J 1995;32:104–8.
8. Shaw WC, Asher-McDade C, Brattstrom V, et al. A six-center international study of treatment outcome in patients with clefts of the lip and palate. Part 5. General discussion and conclusions. Cleft Palate Craniofac J 1992;29:413–8.
9. Malgaine J. Du bec-de-lievre. J Chir (Paris) 1844;2: 1–6.
10. Mirault G. Lettre sur l'operation du bec-de-lievre. J Chir (Paris) 1844;2:257.
11. Tennison CW. The repair of the unilateral cleft lip by the stencil method. Plast Reconstr Surg 1952;9(2): 115–20.
12. Millard DR. A primary camouflage in the unilateral hairlip. In: Transactions of the International Congress of Plastic Surgeons. Baltimore (MD): Williams and Wilkins; 1957. p. 160.
13. Sitzman TJ, Girotto JA, Marcus JR. Current Surgical practices in cleft care: unilateral cleft lip repair. Plast Reconstr Surg 2008;121(5):261e–70e.
14. Asensio O. A variation of the rotation advancement operation for the repair of wide unilateral cleft lips. Plast reconstr surg 1974;53(2):167–73.
15. Delaire J, Precious DS, Gordeef A. The advantage of wide subperiosteal exposure in primary surgical correction of labial maxillary clefts. Scand J Plast Reconstr Surg Hand Surg 1988;22:147.
16. Markus AF, Delaire J. Functional primary closure of cleft lip. Br J Oral Maxillofac Surg 1993;31:281.
17. Costello BJ, Ruiz R, et al. Repair of the unilateral cleft lip: a comparison of surgical techniques. In: Fonseca R, Marciani R, Turvey T, editors. Oral and Maxillofacial Surgery, vol. 3. 2nd edition. St. Louis (MO): Saunders; 2009. p. 735–58.
18. Chowdri NA, Darzi MA, Ashraf MM. A comparative study of surgical results with rotation-advancement and triangular flap techniques in unilateral cleft lip. Br J Plast Surg 1990;43(5):551–6.
19. Holtmann B, Wray RC. A randomized comparison of triangular and rotation-advancement unilateral cleft lip repairs. Plast Reconstr Surg 1983;71(2): 172–9.
20. Nakajima T, Yoshimura Y. Early repair of unilateral cleft lip employing a small triangular flap method and primary nasal correction. Br J Plast Surg 1993;46:616.
21. Thompson HG, Reinders FX. A long-term appraisal of the unilateral complete lip repair: one surgeon's experience. Plast Reconstr Surg 1995;96:549–56.
22. Schendel SA. Unilateral cleft lip repair-state of the art. Cleft Palate craniofac J 2000;37(4):335–41.
23. McComb H. Treatment of the unilateral cleft lip nose. Plast Reconstr Surg 1975;55:596–601.

24. McComb H. Primary correction of unilateral cleft lip nasal deformity. Plast Reconstr Surg 1985;75: 791–7.

25. McComb H, Coghlan BA. Primary repair of the unilateral cleft nose: completion of a longitudinal study. Cleft Palate Craniofac J 1996;33:23–30.

26. Anastassov GE, Joos U, Zoellner B. Evaluation of the results of delayed rhinoplasty in cleft lip and palate patients: functional and aesthetic implications and factors that affect successful nasal repair. Br J Oral Maxillofac Surg 1998;36:416.

27. Anastassov GE, Joos U. Comprehensive management of cleft lip and palate deformities. J Oral Maxillofac Surg 2001;59:1062–75.

28. Anderl H, Hussl H, Ninkovic M. Primary simultaneous lip and nose repair in the unilateral cleft lip and palate. Plast Reconstr Surg 2008;121(3): 959–70.

29. Brusse C, Van Der Werff JF, Stevens HP, et al. Symmetry and mobility assessment of unilateral complete cleft lip nose corrected with or without primary nasal correction. Cleft Palate craniofac J 1999;36:361.

30. Wolfe A. A pastiche for the cleft lip nose. Plat Reconstr Surg 2004;114:1.

31. Salyer K. Excellence in cleft lip and palate treatment. J Craniofac Surg 2001;12:2.

32. Byrd HS, Salomon J. Primary correction of the unilateral cleft nasal deformity. Plast reconstr Surg 2000;1066:1276.

33. Akuja R. Primary definitive nasal correction in patients presenting for late unilateral cleft lip repair. Plat reconstr Surg 2002;1101:17.

34. Delaire J. La cheilo-rhinoplastic primaire pour fente labio-maxillaire congenitale unilaterale. Essai de schematisation d'une technique. Rev Stomatol Chir Maxillofac 1975;76:193–216.

35. Delaire J. Theoretical principles and technique of functional closure of the lip and nasal aperture. J Maxillofac Surg 1978b;6:109.

36. Joos U. Skeletal growth after muscular reconstruction for cleft lip, alveolus and palate. Br J Oral Maxillofac Surg 1995;53:1025–30.

37. Schendel SA, Pearl RM, De'Armond SJ. Pathophysiology of cleft lip muscle. Plast Reconstr Surg 1989;83:777–84.

38. Mooney MP, Siegel MP, Kimes KR, et al. Development of the orbicularis oris muscle in normal cleft lip and palate human fetuses using three-dimensional computer reconstruction. Plast Reconstr Surg 1988;81:336–45.

39. Markus AF, Precious DS. Effect of primary surgery for cleft lip and palate on midfacial growth. Br J Oral Maxillofac Surg 1997;35:6–10.

40. Markus AF, Delaire J, Smith WP. Facial balance in cleft lip and palate II. Cleft lip and palate deformities. Br J Oral Maxillofac Surg 1992b;30: 296–304.

41. Grayson BH, Maull D. Nasoalveolar molding for infants born with clefts of the lip, alveolus, and palate. Clin Plast Surg 2004;31:148.

42. Georgaide N, Latham R. Maxillary arch alignment in the bilateral cleft lip and palate infant, using pinned coaxial screw appliance. Plast Reconstr Surg 1975;56:52.

43. Berkowitz SB, Mejia M, Bystrik AA. Comparison of the effects of the Latham-Millard procedure with those of a conservative treatment approach for dental occlusion and facial aesthetics in unilateral and bilateral complete cleft lip and palate: part 1: dental occlusion. Plast Reconstr Surg 2004; 113(1):1–18.

44. Posnick JC, Ruiz RL. Management of secondary orofacial cleft deformities. In: Goldwyn RM, Cohen MN, editors. The unfavorable result in plastic surgery: avoidance and treatment. 3rd edition. Philadelphia: Lippincott Williams and Wilkins; 2000. p. 349.

45. Ross RB, MacNamara MC. Effect of presurgical infant orthopedics on facial esthetics in complete bilateral cleft lip and palate. Cleft Palate Craniofac J 1994;31:68–73.

46. Grayson B, Cutting C, Wood R. Preoperative columella lengthening in bilateral cleft lip and palate. Plast Reconstr Surg 1993;92:1422–3.

47. Grayson B, Cutting C. Presurgical nasoalveolar orthopedic molding in primary correction of the nose, lip, and alveolus of infants born with unilateral and bilateral clefts. Cleft Palate Craniofac J 2001;35:193–8.

48. Bennum R, Perandones C, Sepliasrsky V, et al. Nonsurgical correction of nasal deformity in unilateral complete cleft lip: a 6-year follow-up. Plast Reconstr Surg 1999;104:616–30.

49. Pai B, Ko E, Huang C, et al. Symmetry of the nose after presurgical nasoalveolar molding in infants with unilateral cleft lip and palate: a preliminary study. Cleft Palate Craniofac J 2005;42:658–63.

50. Liou E, Subramanian M, Chen P, et al. The progressive changes of nasal symmetry and growth after nasoalveolar molding: a three-year follow-up study. Plast Reconstr Surg 2004;114:858–64.

51. Santiago P, Grayson B, Cutting C, et al. Reduced need for alveolar bone grafting by presurgical orthopedics and gingivoperiosteoplasty. Cleft Palate Craniofac J 1998;1:35.

52. Salyer KE, Genecov ER, Genecov DG. Unilateral cleft lip-nose repair: a 33 year experience. J Craniofac Surg 2003;14(4):549–58.

53. Pruzansky S. Presurgical orthopedics and bone grafting for infants with cleft lip and palate: a dissent. Cleft Palate J 1964;1:164.

54. Robertson NR, Jolleys A. Effects of early bone grafting in complete clefts of the lip and palate. Plast Reconstr Surg 1968;42:414–21.

55. Goldberg WB, Ferguson FS, Miles RJ. Successful use of a feeding obturator for an infant with cleft palate. Spec Care Dentist 1988;8:86–9.

56. Bongaarts CA, van't Hof MA, Prahl-Andersen B, et al. Infant orthopedics has no effect on Maxillary arch dimensions in the deciduous dentition of children with complete unilateral cleft lip and palate (Dutchcleft). Cleft Palate Craniofac J 2006;43(6): 665–72.

57. Bongaarts CA, Prahl-Andersen B, Bronkhorst EM, et al. Effect of infant orthopedics on facial appearance of toddlers with complete unilateral cleft lip and palate (Dutchcleft). Cleft palate craniofac J 2008;45(4):407–13.

58. Prahl C, Prahl-Anderson B, Van't Hof MA, et al. Presurgical orthopedics and satisfaction in motherhood: a randomized clinical trial (Dutchcleft). Cleft Palate Craniofac J 2008;45(3):284–8.

59. Prahl C, Kuijpers-Jagtman AM, Van't Hof MA, et al. Infant orthopedics in UCLP: effect on feeding, weight, and length: a randomized clinical trial (Dutchcleft). Cleft Palate Craniofac J 2005;42(2):171–7.

60. Konst EM, Rietveld T, Peters HFM, et al. Language skills of young children with unilateral cleft lip and palate following infant orthopedics: a randomized clinical trial. Cleft Palate Craniofac J 2003;40(4): 356–62.

61. Masarei AG, Wade A, Mars M, et al. A randomized control trial investigating the effects of presurgical orthopedics on feeding in infants with cleft lip and/or palate. Cleft Palate Craniofac J 2007; 44(2):182–93.

62. Hallock GG. In utero cleft lip repair in A/J mice. Plast Reconstr Surg 1985;75(6):785–90.

63. Longaker MT, Stern M, Lorenz P, et al. A model for fetal cleft lip repair in lambs. Plast Reconstr Surg 1992;90(5):750–6.

64. Mcheik JN, Sfalli P, Bondonny JM, et al. Early repair for infants with cleft lip and nose. Int J Pediatr Otorhinolaryngol 2006;70(10):1785–90.

65. Goodacre TE, Hentges F, Moss TL, et al. Does repairing a cleft lip neonatally have any effect on the longer-term attractiveness of the repair? Cleft Palate Craniofac J 2004;41(6):603–8.

66. Slade P, Emerson DJ, Freedlander E. A longitudinal comparison of the psychological impact on mothers of neonatal and 3 month repair of cleft lip. Br J Plast Surg 1999;52(1):1–5.

67. Field TM, Vega-Lahr N. Early interactions between infants with craniofacial anomalies and their mothers. Infant Behav Dev 1984;7:527.

68. Rogers BO. Hairlip repair in colonial America: a review of 18th century and earlier surgical techniques. Plast Reconstr Surg 1964;34:142.

69. LeMesurier AB. Method of cutting and suturing lip in complete unilateral cleft lip. Plast Reconstr Surg 1949;4:1.

70. Khosla RK, Mabry K, Castiglione CL. Clinical outcomes of the Furlow Z-plasty for primary cleft palate repair. Cleft Palate Craniofac J 2008;45(5): 501.

71. LaRossa D. The state of the art in cleft palate surgery. Cleft Palate Craniofac J 2000;37(3):225.

72. Ross B. Treatment variables affecting facial growth in complete unilateral cleft lip and palate. Part 7: an overview of treatment and facial growth. Cleft Palate J 1987;24:71–7.

73. Veau V. Division palantine. Paris: Masson; 1931.

74. Kilner TP. Cleft lip and palate repair technique. St. Thomas Hosp Rep 1937;2:127.

75. Wardill WFM. The technique of operation for cleft palate. Br J Surg 1937;25:117.

76. Pantaloni M, Hollier L. Cleft Palate and velopharyngeal incompetence. In: Selected readings in Plastic Surgery, 9. Dallas (TX): University of Texas Southwestern; 2001. p. 1–36.

77. Bardach J. Two-flap palatoplasty: Bardach's technique. Oper Tech Plast Reconstr Surg 1995;2:211.

78. Salyer KE, Sng KW, Sperry EE. Two-flap palatoplasty: 20-year experience and evolution of a surgical technique. Plast Reconstr Surg 2006;118:193.

79. Furlow LT. Cleft palate repair: preliminary report on lengthening and muscle transposition by Z-plasty. Paper presented at the annual meeting of Southeastern society of plastic and reconstructive surgeons, Boca Raton, FL, May 16, 1978.

80. Furlow LT. Cleft palate repair by double opposing z-plasty. Oper tech plast recon surg 1995;2:223.

81. Bardach J, Morris HL, LaRossa D, et al. The Furlow double reversing Z-plasty for cleft palate repair: The first 10 years of experience. In: Bardach J, Morris HL, editors. Multidisciplinary management of the cleft lip and palate. Philadelphia: Saunders; 1990. p. 883.

82. Grobbelar AO, Hudson DA, Fernandes DB, et al. Speech results after repair of the cleft soft palate. Plast Reconstr Surg 1985;95:1150.

83. Kirschner RE, Wang P, Jawad AF, et al. Cleft palate repair by modified Furlow double opposing Z-plasty: the Childrens Hospital of Philadelphia experience. Plast Reconstr Surg 1998;104:1999.

84. Pigott RW, Albery EH, Hathorn IS, et al. A comparison of three methods of repairing the hard palate. Cleft Palate Craniofac J 2002;39:383.

85. Ross RB. Treatment variables affecting facial growth in complete unilateral cleft lip and palate. Part 1: treatment affecting growth. Cleft Palate J 1987;24:5.

86. Ross RB. Treatment variables affecting facial growth in complete unilateral cleft lip and palate. Part 2: presurgical orthopedics. Cleft Palate J 1987;24:24.

87. Ross RB. Treatment variables affecting facial growth in complete unilateral cleft lip and palate. Part 3: alveolus Repair and bone grafting. Cleft Palate J 1987;42:33.

88. Ross RB. Treatment variables affecting facial growth in complete unilateral cleft lip and palate. Part 4: repair of the cleft lip. Cleft Palate J 1987;42:45.

89. Ross RB. Treatment variables affecting facial growth in complete unilateral cleft lip and palate. Part 5: timing of palate repair. Cleft Palate J 1987;42:54.

90. Ross RB. Treatment variables affecting facial growth in complete unilateral cleft lip and palate. Part 6: techniques of palate repair. Cleft Palate J 1987;42:64.

91. Friede H, Enemark H, Semb G, et al. Craniofacial and occlusal charactistics in unilateral cleft lip and palate patients from four Scandinavian centers. Scand J Plast Reconstr Surg Hand Surg 1991;25:269.

92. Kriens O. An anatomical approach to veloplasty. Plast Reconstr Surg 1969;43:29.

93. Marsh JL, Grames LM, Holtman B. Intravelar veloplasty: a prospective study. Cleft Palate J 1989; 26:46.

94. Sommerlad BC. The use of the operating microscope in cleft palate repair. Presented at the 9th International Congress on Cleft Palate and Related Craniofacial Anomalies, Goteborg, Sweden, 2001.

95. Sommerlad BC, Mehendale FV, Birch MJ, et al. Palate re-repair revisited. Cleft Palate Craniofac J 2002;39:295.

96. Andrades P, Espinosa-de-los-Monteros A, Shell DH, et al. The importance of radical intravelar veloplasty during two-flap palatoplasty. Plast Reconstr Surg 2008;122:1121.

97. Hassan ME, Askar S. Does palatal muscle reconstruction affect the functional outcome of cleft palate surgery? Plast Reconstr Surg 2007;119(6): 1859–65.

98. Noorchashm N, Duda JR, Ford M, et al. Conversion Furlow palatoplasty: salvage of speech after straight-line palatoplasty and incomplete intravelar veloplasty. Ann Plast Surg 2006;56:505.

99. Seagle MB. Palatal fistula repair using acellular dermal matrix: the University of Florida Experience. Ann Plast Surg 2006;56:50.

100. Helling ER, Dev VR, Garza J, et al. Low fistula rate in palatal clefts closed with the Furlow technique using decellularized dermis. PRS 2006;117(7): 2361–5.

101. Wilhelmi BJ, Appelt EA, Hill L, et al. Palatal fistulas: rare with the two-flap palatoplasty repair. Plast Reconstr Surg 2001;107(2):315–8.

102. Schendel S, Lorenz HP, Dagenais D, et al. A single surgeon's experience with the Delaire palatoplasty. Plast Reconstr Surg 1999;104(7):1993–7.

103. Yu CC, Chen PK, Chen YR. Comparison of speech results after Furlow palatoplasty and von Langenbeck palatoplasty in incomplete cleft of the secondary palate. Chang Gung Med J 2001;24:628.

104. Williams WN, Seagle MB, Nackashi AJ, et al. A methodology report of a randomized prospective trial to assess velopharyngeal function for speech following palatal surgery. Control Clin Trials 1998;19:297.

105. Gunther E, Wisser JR, Cohen MA, et al. Palatoplasty: Furlow's double reversing z-plasty versus intravelar veloplasty. CPCJ 1998;35(6):546–9.

106. Randall P, La Rossa D, Solomon M, et al. Experience with the Furlow double reversing z-plasty for cleft palate repair. Plast Reconst Surg 1986;77:569.

107. Brothers DB, Dalston RW, Peterson HD, et al. Comparison of the Furlow double opposing z-plasty with the Wardill-Kilner procedure for isolated clefts of the soft palate. Plast Reconstr Surg 1995; 95(6):969–77.

108. Spauwen PH, Goorhuis-Brouwer SM, Schutte HK. Cleft palate repair: Furlow versus von Langenbeck. J Craniomaxillofac Surg 1992;20(1):18–20.

109. Seagle MB. Abstract presentation. American Cleft Palate-Craniofacial Association 63rd Annual Meeting, 2006.

110. Fudalej P, Obloj B, Miller-Drabikowska D, et al. Midfacial growth in a consecutive series of preadolescent children with complete unilateral cleft lip and palate following a one-stage simultaneous repair. Cleft Palate Craniofac J 2008;45(6):667–73.

111. Ozturk Y, Cura N. Examination of craniofacial morphology in children with unilateral cleft lip and palate. Cleft Palate Craniofac J 1996;33:32–6.

112. Savaci N, Hosnuter M, TosunZ DA. Maxillofacial morphology in children with complete unilateral cleft lip and palate treated by one-stage simultaneous repair. Plast Reconstr Surg 2005;115:1509–17.

113. Lilja J, Mars M, Elander A, et al. Analysis of dental arch relationships in Swedish unilateral cleft lip and palate subjects: 20-year longitudinal consecutive series treated with delayed hard palate closure. Cleft Palate Craniofac J 2006;43:606.

114. Molsted K, Brattstrom V, Prahl-Anderson B, et al. The Eurocleft study: intercenter study of treatment outcome in patients with complete cleft lip and palate. Part 3: dental arch relationships. Cleft Palate Craniofac J 2005;42:78.

115. Kim T, IshikawaH CS, et al. Constriction of the maxillary dental arch by mucoperiosteal denudation of the palate. Cleft Palate Craniofac J 2002;39:425.

116. Good PH, Mulliken JB, Padwa BL. Frequency of LeFort I osteotomy after repaired cleft lip and palate or cleft palate. Cleft Palate Craniofac J 2007;44(4):396–401.

117. Posnick J. Orthognathic surgery in cleft patients treated by early bone grafting. Plast Reconstr Surg 1991;87:840 [discussion: 840–2].

118. Oberoi S, Chigurupati R, Vargervik K. Morphologic and management characteristics of individuals with unilateral cleft lip and palate who require maxillary advancement. Cleft Palate Craniofac J 2008;45(1):42–9.

119. Peterson-Falzon SJ, Hardin-Jones MA, Karnell MP. Cleft Palate Speech. 3rd edition. St. Louis (MO): Mosby; 2001.

120. Ortiz-Monasterion F, Serrano A, Barrera G, et al. A study of untreated adult cleft palate patients. Plast reconstr Surg 1966;38:36.

121. Gillies HD, Fry WK. A new principle in the surgical treatment of congenital cleft palate and its mechanical counterpart. Br Med J 1921;1:325.

122. Schweckendiek W. Primary veloplasty: long-term results without maxillary deformity. A twenty-five year report. Cleft Pal J 1978;15:268–74.

123. Bardach J, Morris H, Olin WH. Late results of primary veloplasty: the Marburg project. Plast Reconst Surg 1984;73:207–15.

124. Fara M, Brousilova M. Experiences with early closure of the velum and later closure of the hard palate. Plast Reconstr Surg 1969;44:134.

125. Cosman B, Falk AS. Delayed hard palate repair and speech deficiencies: a cautionary report. Cleft Palate J 1980;17:27.

126. Holland S, Gabbay JS, Heller JB, et al. Delayed closure of the hard palate leads to speech problems and deleterious maxillary growth. Plast Reconstr Surg 2007;119:1302.

127. Chapman KL, Hardin-Jones MA, Goldstein JA, et al. Timing of palatal surgery and speech outcome. Cleft Palate Craniofac J 2008;45(3):297.

128. Dorf DS, Curtin JW. Early cleft palate repair and speech outcome. Plast reconstr Surg 1982;70:74–9.

129. Dorf DS, Curtin JW. Early cleft palate repair and speech outcome: a ten-year experience. In: Bardach J, Morris HL, editors. Multidisciplinary management of cleft lip and palate. Philadelphia: WB Saunders; 1990. p. 341–8.

130. Chapman KL, Hardin MA. Phonetic and phonological skills of two-year-olds with cleft palate. Cleft Palate Craniofac J 1992;29:435–43.

131. Kirschner RE, Randall P, Wang P, et al. Cleft palate repair at 3–7 months of age. Plast Reconstruct Surg 2000;105(6):2127–32.

Orbital Surgery: State of the Art

Jason Liss, MD[a,e], S. Tonya Stefko, MD, FACS[b,c,e],
William L. Chung, DDS, MD[d,*]

KEYWORDS

- Orbital • Fracture • Floor • Roof • Medial wall
- Surgery • Management

ORBITAL FLOOR FRACTURES

The floor of the orbit is commonly fractured in children and adults. The floor fracture may be isolated or occur as a component of a panfacial injury. The most frequently encountered combination of fractures is the orbital floor and medial orbital wall, but floor fractures also occur as part of zygomatico-maxillary complex fractures, naso-orbital-ethmoid fractures, LeFort fractures, and frontal sinus and orbital roof fractures. Detailed imaging using multi-planar computed tomography (CT) is essential for understanding the injury completely. Advances in imaging have revolutionized the thought processes and treatment planning; reconstructed sagittal views and three-dimensional rendering with mirror imaging techniques are new areas that provide the surgeon with new insight heretofore unavailable. The reader is referred to the articles by Branstetter and Bell elsewhere in this issue for a more detailed discussion of these new technologies and their use for orbital surgery.

Indications for Repair

Initially many orbital floor fractures may be treated with observation. Indications for repair include enophthalmos or hypoglobus of greater than 2 mm, diplopia at or near central gaze, apparent extraocular muscle entrapment in the fracture, and fractures larger than a critical size (1 or 2 cm).[1,2] Others have pointed out that the size of the fracture is not a critical determinant in the development of enophthalmos, as the periorbita may still be intact and the effective orbital volume not significantly increased.[1,2] The finding on CT of a rounded or inferiorly displaced inferior rectus muscle has been noted to be a predictor of enophthalmos caused by periorbital injury, and an indicator for surgical repair.

Timing of Repair

The theoretic advantage of delaying surgical repair for several weeks or months is to give symptoms of diplopia or disturbances in extraocular motility an opportunity to improve. However, many studies have reported suboptimal results regarding the correction of enophthalmos or diplopia with delayed repair. Almost all of the reports mentioned are retrospective in design and use self-reported data, with the inherent biases that are unavoidable in such circumstances. Level II and III evidence is important and helps guide treatment planning when higher-level evidence is lacking, but critical analysis is necessary when applying these data to particular clinical situations. Dogmatic statements about particular techniques being superior to others are not academically sound (ie, lacking superior evidence, although surgeons make decisions based on the best available data).

[a] Oculoplastic Surgery, University of Pittsburgh Medical Center, 203 Lothrop Street, Pittsburgh, PA 15213, USA
[b] Department of Ophthalmology, University of Pittsburgh Medical Center, 203 Lothrop Street, Pittsburgh, PA 15213, USA
[c] Oculoplastic, Esthetic, and Reconstructive Surgery, University of Pittsburgh Medical Center, 203 Lothrop Street, Pittsburgh, PA 15213, USA
[d] Department of Oral & Maxillofacial Surgery, University of Pittsburgh Medical Center, 3459 5th Avenue, Suite 202 South, Pittsburgh, PA 15213, USA
[e] UPMC Eye Center, 203 Lothrop Street, Pittsburgh, PA 15213, USA
* Corresponding author.
E-mail address: chungwl@upmc.edu

Oral Maxillofacial Surg Clin N Am 22 (2010) 59–71
doi:10.1016/j.coms.2009.11.006

Hawes and Dortzbach[3] found residual diplopia in 38% of patients who had surgery 2 months after injury and in 7% of those operated on within 2 months. Yilmaz and colleagues[4] found that in the 9 fractures they repaired more than 4 weeks after injury, they had 3 results with diplopia and 4 with enophthalmos, compared with just 1 diplopia in 17 early repairs. Some believe that it is more difficult to achieve an anatomic repair with delayed surgery because of early orbital fibrosis and scarring.[5] Others believe that ongoing damage to orbital tissue leads to orbital fat atrophy and extraocular muscle dysfunction.[4,6–10] Harris[6] suggests that if soft-tissue displacement is disproportionate to the bony defect on radiographic imaging, there is a high risk for soft-tissue ischemia and surgery should be undertaken as soon as possible. Thus, if a fracture is determined to require surgery, the surgeon may consider performing the repair within the first 2 to 3 weeks, if not within the first several days, after injury.

Surgical Incisions

Initially, orbital floor fractures were accessed by an intraoral transantral approach, and then later by a lower eyelid subciliary incision. Nam and colleagues[10] performed 405 subciliary incisions with Frost suture removal on postoperative day 3 and subsequent vigorous lower lid massage and reported no cases of lid retraction or ectropion. However, some report a high incidence of eyelid retraction and ectropion with the subciliary incision. The transconjunctival incision provides the obvious advantage of a lack of an external scar. Appling and colleagues[11] found 12% transient ectropion and 28% permanent increased scleral show in subciliary incisions compared with no ectropion and 3% increased scleral show with transconjunctival incisions. Villareal and colleagues[12] and Patel and colleagues[13] also report highly favorable results using a transconjunctival incision. Lane and colleagues[14] documented 1 case of lid retraction in 85 transconjunctival incisions. Schmal and colleagues[15] performed 209 transconjunctival incisions for floor repairs, and found no cases of ectropion or lid retraction, and 2 unsatisfactory scars from his 181 lateral canthotomies. These reports represent lower-level evidence, but are the best available literature for use in careful decision making. Based on these reports, the transconjunctival incision, with or without a lateral canthotomy, has become favored over the subciliary incision.

Orbital Implants

The subject of greatest debate regarding the repair of orbital fractures surrounds the choice of implant. Classically, autogenous bone was the material of choice for repairing facial fractures because of its resistance to infection, low risk of rejection, and perceived incorporation into new bone growth.[16–20] Certain injuries and fracture patterns may be well suited for such grafts (**Fig. 1**A–H). However, its use for internal orbital fractures has declined, primarily because of concerns regarding the potential for donor-site morbidity, unpredictable resorption, and difficulty molding the material to the desired shape of the orbital wall(s).[1,16,17,21] Autogenous conchal or nasal cartilage has also been used because of its ease of harvest and potentially decreased donor-site morbidity compared with bone. However, cartilage is not commonly used for floor fractures because of difficulty in custom-molding, its tendency to warp, lack of tensile strength, and the patient's possible need for nasal cartilage for other future surgical procedures.[22]

Numerous alloplastic materials have been described and studied for use in orbital floor fracture repair (**Table 1**). Alloplastic materials can be thought of as either nonporous or porous. Nonporous silicone rubber (Silastic sheets) was studied by Morrison and colleagues[23] in a 20-year period, and found to have an overall complication rate of 13%, including 6.8% infection and migration and worsening diplopia. Late migration is a frequently documented problem with this material, which might be caused by poor fixation rather than the material itself.[17] Initially Teflon had been reported with good results,[24] but recent case reports of late complications have led to a decrease in its use.

Nylon sheets (SupraFOIL) (**Fig. 2**) were similarly felt to have complications of hemorrhage into the implant capsule,[25] but recent studies have suggested that prior complications may have been caused by poor implant fixation. Park and colleagues[26] studied 181 patients whose injuries were repaired with nylon sheets of varying thickness using a transconjunctival approach with a single-screw fixation of the implant. They reported 1 case of orbital hemorrhage and 1 late infection. Su and Harris[27] showed no complications in 19 repairs of combined floor and medial wall fractures using an implant 0.3-mm thick with prepunched holes to encourage fibrovascular ingrowth to aid in stabilization.

Titanium mesh is the most popular alloplastic nonporous material for repair of most facial fractures (**Fig. 3**A–C). It is strong, malleable, visible on radiography, and fairly infection resistant.[17] However, some of its disadvantages include difficulty sliding the implant into desired spaces because of its sharp edges, difficulty in its removal

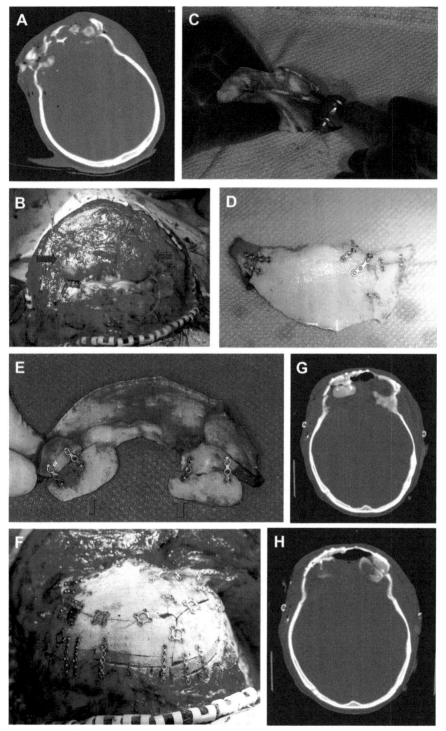

Fig. 1. (*A*) Axial CT scan of comminuted frontal sinus and orbital roof fractures secondary to gunshot wound. (*B*) Exposed, unroofed orbits (*arrows*) by frontal craniotomy. (*C*) Split-thickness frontal (sinus) bone graft in sagittal plane. (*D*) Inner table frontal sinus used to recreate orbital roofs (*arrows*). (*E, F*) Anterior table and frontal bone reconstruction. (*G, H*) Postoperative axial CT scans of reconstructed orbital roofs and frontal sinus.

Table 1
Characteristics of common alloplastic orbital implants

Implant	Porous	Nonporous	Rigid	Soft	Absorbable	Osteoconductive
Silicon (Silastic)		X	X			
Nylon (Supramid, SupraFoil)		X	X			
Titanium		X	X			X
Vitallium		X	X			X
Porous Polyethylene (Medpor)	X		X			X
PTFE (Teflon)	X		X			+/−
PGLA	X		X	X		

Abbreviations: PTFE, polytetrafluoroethylene; PGLA, polyglycolic-polylactide.

(when necessary) because of fibrovascular ingrowth, and a concern that it may cause adhesions to orbital tissue.[17,21]

Porous polyethylene is a porous alloplastic material that has been used widely and reported to have excellent clinical results. It is available in sheets 0.85-mm and 1.5-mm thick, is malleable yet strong, and allows for fibrous ingrowth. One study[28] of 37 patients reported correction of hypoglobus in all documented cases, resolution of diplopia in 15 of 27 cases (with improvement in 7 more), and correction of enophthalmos in 9 of 18 cases. This study also reported only 1 case of infection. In the study by Nam and colleagues[10] of 214 floors repaired with porous polyethylene 12 cases with complications (5.6%) were found, including 7 cases of enophthalmos. Romano and colleagues[29] had only 1 case of infection in 128 implants of porous polyethylene. Documented infection rates were low, and most surgeons typically soak the implant in antibiotic before insertion as standard practice.

An implant that has recently gained much attention and use is titanium-embedded porous polyethylene (**Fig. 4**A–B). It has the malleability, strength, memory, and radiopacity of titanium, with the potential for fibrous ingrowth of porous polyethylene. It is also coated on 1 side to prevent inflammation and adhesion of orbital tissue. Garibaldi and colleagues[30] studied 100 patients (83 orbital floor fractures) who received Medpor Titan implants, 70% of which were fixated with a single screw. One case each of orbital hemorrhage and vertical overcorrection attributed to the thickness of the implant were reported, and no case of either extrusions or infection was reported.

With respect to various implant choices, comparative well-designed trials are lacking and the available literature assesses only the outcome of the materials individually with level III evidence. Considerable reported experience outlines important differences in outcome. As with all evidenced-based decision making, the surgeon must not blindly follow prospective evidence only, but integrate the best available knowledge with individual experience and patient factors to make the best choices possible.

After the surgeon decides the best implant material for reconstruction, placing it precisely becomes the primary objective. Before inserting the implant over the floor fracture, it is ideal to expose and directly visualize the stable posterior shelf of the orbital floor. The surgeon should conceptually understand that the orbital floor slopes superiorly toward the most posterior portion of the orbit, so that the posterior shelf is superior to the orbital rim (**Fig. 5**). Keeping this in mind prevents placement of the implant directly into the posterior maxillary sinus. A useful technique for locating the stable posterior shelf is to run a periosteal elevator along the posterior wall of the maxillary sinus until it curves anteriorly to join the undersurface of the posterior orbital floor.[1] Alternatively, endoscopic approaches, image guidance, and active navigation techniques may be used to assist in placement of a material and

Fig. 2. SupraFOIL alloplastic orbital implant.

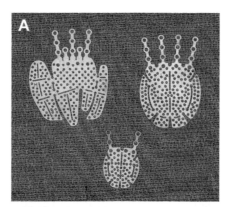

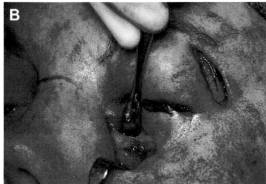

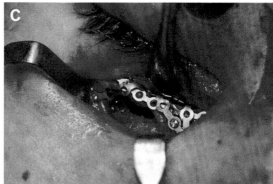

Fig. 3. (*A*) Titanium orbital floor implant. (*B*) Orbital rim and floor fractures exposed. (*C*) Titanium orbital rim and floor implants fixated through lower eyelid crease incision.

optimize the reconstruction. These concepts are discussed by McCain and Bell in other articles in this issue.

Fixation Methods and Wound Closure

After the implant is positioned over the floor defect, alternatives exist regarding the fixation of the implant and closure of the incision. Implant fixation methods include titanium microscrews,[26] cyanoacrylate,[31,32] fibrin glue,[6] and even insertion of a tab of the implant under any stable bone anteriorly.[2] The need for fixation primarily depends on the type of implant. Park and colleagues[26] suggest that implant fixation may be instrumental in significantly reducing the incidence of hemorrhage within the implant capsule in nonporous implants, a problem that resulted in decreased use of

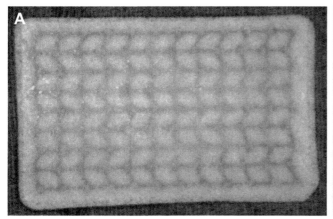

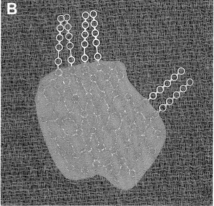

Fig. 4. (*A*) Titan Mesh orbital floor implant. (*B*) Titan Mesh orbital implant with medial and lateral wings and titanium extensions for fixation onto the orbital rim.

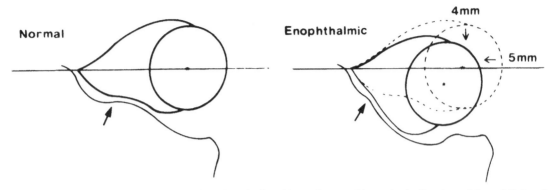

Fig. 5. The posterior ledge of bone must be identified and is used as a guide to the inclination of the orbital walls in reconstruction and as a support for the orbital implant or graft. (*From* Holck DEE, Ng JD. Evaluation and treatment of orbital fractures. Philadelphia: WB Saunders; 2006. p. 146; with permission.)

nonporous alloplastic materials in favor of porous polyethylene.[25,33] Some have reported excellent results without fixation of the implant. Lane and colleagues[14] placed Medpor implants in 85 orbits without fixation or closure of the periosteum, and reported no cases of migration or extrusion. Nam and colleagues[10] did not fixate the porous polyethylene or hydroxyapatite implants in 405 patients, but did close the periosteum, and found no cases of extrusion, migration, or hemorrhage.

Some surgeons advocate closing the periosteum.[2,10,21] Theoretic advantages of closing the periosteum include decreasing the chance of implant migration, and the chance of adhesion or scar formation between orbital contents and the implant material. Lane and colleagues[14] favored foregoing closure of the periosteum to reduce iatrogenic morbidity from incorrect layered closure and tethering of the orbital tissue. These investigators also did not close the conjunctiva in the 85 cases, and had only 1 case of eyelid retraction. The advantage of a sutureless closure of the incision is the lack of potential for corneal irritation from the conjunctival sutures. Although these reports may exhibit some degree of reporting bias and lack a high level of evidence, there are valuable points to consider. As with all technique-sensitive operative endeavors, surgeon skill and experience variability can also be factors that affect outcome when considering outcome data in a particular study.

If postoperative enophthalmos persists because of either nonanatomic repair of a floor fracture or tissue atrophy, several treatment options exist to recreate the orbital floor properly, short of removing the inadequately positioned implant. One option is to insert a porous polyethylene enophthalmos wedge implant to correct the enophthalmos. The implant should be inserted in a subperiosteal plane

posteroinferior to the globe.[34] Another option is to inject retrobulbar hyaluronic acid for volume augmentation.[35] Detailed imaging and modeling can be helpful in understanding the planning of the volume correction and executing the placement of materials to improve less-than-optimal positioning of the globe.

MEDIAL ORBITAL WALL FRACTURES

The medial wall of the orbit is commonly fractured in facial trauma. The reported frequency of an isolated medial wall fracture is variable, ranging from extremely rare[36] to the most commonly isolated orbital wall fracture.[37] As with orbital floor fractures, there is evidence that long-term results are better with earlier surgical intervention.[7,27]

Surgical Approaches

Several approaches to the medial orbital wall have been described. The approach that offers the greatest exposure and access is the coronal incision, and this approach is optimal in cases of extensive facial trauma. However, concerns such as scarring in male pattern baldness, alopecia, frontalis palsy, scalp numbness, and increased surgical time make other more direct approaches desirable in certain situations.

In 1921 Lynch[38] described a semilunar incision between the medial canthal tendon and the nasal dorsum (**Fig. 6**). This incision provides good access but carries the risk of scarring or webbing, and injury to the lacrimal system or canthal tendon.[39] Variations of the Lynch incision are commonly used for approach to the medial wall. Nunery and colleagues[7] repaired 102 combined medial wall and floor fractures using a 1-cm vertical skin incision just anterior to the medial canthal tendon, and found 1 patient with resultant enophthalmos

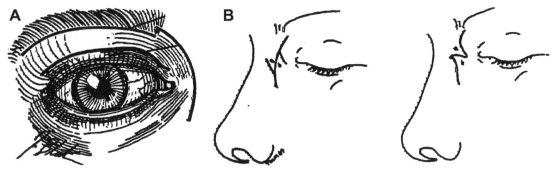

Fig. 6. Lynch incision. (*From* Holck DEE, Ng JD. Evaluation and treatment of orbital fractures. Philadelphia: WB Saunders; 2006. p. 293.)

but no other complications, including unsightly scars. The investigators sutured the skin to the underlying medial canthal tendon and periorbita to avoid webbing of the skin of the medial canthal region. Two other studies[40,41] used either a transcaruncular (**Fig. 7**) or W-shaped incision from the medial brow to the medial canthus, without webbing or unsightly scarring.

The upper eyelid crease incision may be used with better cosmetic results (**Fig. 8**), but access to the posterior and inferior medial wall is limited.[39,42] Lower eyelid incisions provide adequate access to the lower half of the medial orbital wall, with generally good cosmetic results. The transconjunctival incision carries a lower risk of postoperative eyelid malposition.[11,39] However, neither incision provides sufficient access to the superior part of the medial wall.[27,39]

The transcaruncular and precaruncular incisions have recently been described with good results.[27,39,43] These incisions reportedly provide sufficient exposure without notable scarring. Using Desmarres retractors for the eyelids and protecting the globe with a malleable retractor, an incision is made medial to the plica semilunaris, either through the caruncle (transcaruncular) or just lateral to the caruncle (precaruncular), and blunt dissection is carried to the posterior lacrimal crest. The periosteum is first incised and lifted off the posterior lacrimal crest, then posteriorly off the medial wall. The lacrimal sac and the inferior oblique muscle can be elevated with their periosteal attachments as required. After sufficient exposure of all fractures, an implant is positioned, with or without fixation. Su and Harris[27] described the use of Tisseel glue to fixate medial wall implants, whereas others did not fixate the implants and reported no cases of extrusion.[7,39] Meningaud and colleagues[44] described the use of a retrocaruncular incision in conjunction with an endoscope to provide better visualization of the posterior part of the fracture.

A unique approach to medial wall fracture repair has been described by Kim and colleagues.[41] In an

attempt to maximize the advantages of several surgical approaches, a W-shaped skin incision is made from the canthus to the brow (described earlier), followed by an ethmoid osteotomy 5 mm above the medial canthus. Through this incision, the fracture is reduced from the ethmoid sinus with a periosteal elevator, and a balloon is then inflated in the sinus to support the fracture reduction and provide hemostasis. The subperiosteal dissection continues in the orbit to expose the fracture, and an implant is inserted. Of 54 patients, 39 of whom had preoperative diplopia and 16 of whom had enophthalmos, 2 developed postoperative diplopia and 3 retained enophthalmos. No webs or unsatisfactory scars were reported.[41]

Orbital Implants

Implant selection for a medial wall fracture involves the same issues as for a floor fracture,

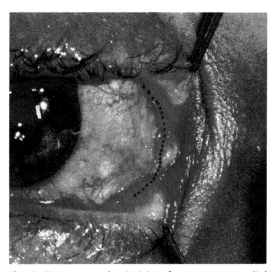

Fig. 7. Transcaruncular incision for access to medial orbital fractures (*From* Holck DEE, Ng JD. Evaluation and treatment of orbital fractures. Philadelphia: WB Saunders; 2006. p. 290; with permission.)

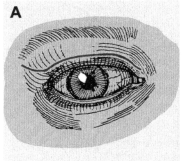 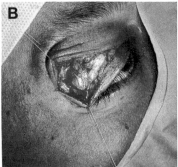 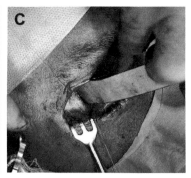

Fig. 8. Upper eyelid crease incision for lateral and superior orbital rim exposure. (*A*) Incision placed in lateral half of upper eyelid crease and extended either direction for exposure as needed. (*B*) Subcutaneous dissection in suborbital fascial plane. (*C*) The periosteum is incised and elevated off the lateral orbital rim, and periorbita is elevated off medial surface. (*From* Holck DEE, Ng JD. Evaluation and treatment of orbital fractures. Philadelphia: WB Saunders; 2006. p. 302; with permission.)

with the exception that a thinner implant may be used for a medial wall fracture because these fractures tend to be smaller and there is less mechanical force pushing on the implant. Nunery and colleagues[7] used 0.4-mm nylon foil, whereas Su and Harris[27] used mostly 0.3-mm nylon implants. Meningaud and colleagues[44] described absorbable polydimethylsiloxane implants for smaller medial wall fractures, but suggested the used of porous polyethylene with imbedded titanium mesh for larger fractures.

Surgical Incision

For combined medial wall and orbital floor fractures, the transconjunctival and transcaruncular (or other medial wall approach) may be used together. Su and Harris[27] fixed 19 patients with combined fractures through a transcaruncular and transconjunctival approach, using primarily 0.3-mm nylon implants. In 12 patients an implant was inserted for each wall fractured, whereas in 7 patients in whom the inferomedial strut was displaced, a third bridging implant was inserted. No infection, implant extrusion, enophthalmos greater than 2 mm, diplopia, vision loss, globe dystopia, or eyelid malposition was reported. As with the previously reported studies, the level of evidence presented in these studies does not allow dogmatic statements about which technique is definitively superior, but it represents the best available literature to guide clinical decisions.

Complications can occur with the transcaruncular incision. One such complication is incision-site edema caused by lack of a surgical plane, a problem that may be improved with the precaruncular incision, described by Moe.[43] Other complications include conjunctival scarring and damage to the inferior oblique muscle, canthal

tendon, or lacrimal system. **Fig. 9** depicts other skin incisions for access to most orbital fractures.

ORBITAL ROOF FRACTURES

Although isolated fractures of the orbital roof or supraorbital rim are uncommon, an estimated 1% to 9% of facial fractures involve the supraorbital rim and the anterior table of the frontal sinus.[45] In adults, orbital roof fractures are often associated with fractures involving the frontal sinus, naso-orbital-ethmoid complex, LeFort fractures, or other portions of the orbit.[46,47] Many of these patients also present with multisystem injuries. In children, orbital roof fractures are often nondisplaced, linear frontobasal fractures.[46,48]

Management of these fractures is dependent on the degree of displacement, and more importantly, any other associated fractures. Nondisplaced roof and supraorbital rim fractures are treated conservatively by observation.[46,48] Associated soft-tissue injuries are repaired while patients are monitored for possible changes in their neurologic status and intracranial pressure (ICP). An isolated blow-in fracture of the orbital roof (**Fig. 10**A–C) should be treated by open reduction and internal fixation if the fracture is causing proptosis, diplopia, or extraocular muscle entrapment.

Surgical Incision

The most direct and cosmetic surgical approach to an isolated orbital roof fracture is the blepharoplasty incision. Subperiosteal dissection along the orbital roof exposes all stable bone around the fracture. Care should be taken when elevating the periosteum beneath the trochlea of the superior oblique muscle, and the lacrimal gland, to avoid damage to these structures. If elevated properly, neither structure needs to be reattached

SKIN INCISIONS FOR ORBITAL FRACTURES

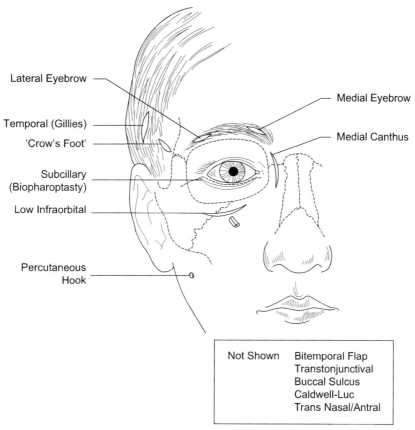

Lateral Eyebrow

Medial Eyebrow

Temporal (Gillies)

Medial Canthus

'Crow's Foot'

Subcillary
(Biopharoptasty)

Low Infraorbital

Percutaneous
Hook

Not Shown	Bitemporal Flap
	Transtonjunctival
	Buccal Sulcus
	Caldwell-Luc
	Trans Nasal/Antral

Fig. 9. Skin incisions for orbital fractures (*From* Rowe NL, Williams JL. Maxillofacial injuries. Edinburgh (UK): Churchill Livingstone; 1994. p. 524; with permission.)

to its bony origin but rather can be allowed to settle back on its periosteum to its origin.[49]

Roof fractures are generally plated with titanium mesh with either microscrew (1.00 mm) or miniscrew (1.3 mm) fixation.[46] Autogenous bone can be used, but concerns about its unpredictable

resorption and difficulty molding the graft to the desired contour limit its effectiveness in this setting.

Orbital blow-up fractures (**Fig. 11**A–C) can be observed unless they cause ocular signs or symptoms. In these cases, if the injury is isolated, it can

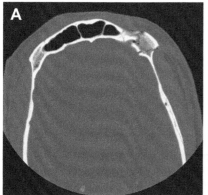
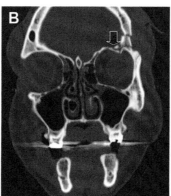
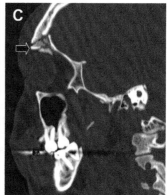

Fig. 10. (*A, B, C*) Axial, coronal, and sagittal CT scans of orbital blow-in fracture. Note displacement of bony roof into the orbit (*arrows*).

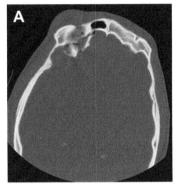
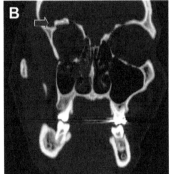
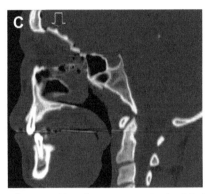

Fig. 11. (*A, B, C*). Axial, coronal, and sagittal CT scans of orbital blow-up fracture. Note large segment of orbital roof displaced superiorly (*arrows*).

be repaired by the same approach as blow-in injuries. If a blepharoplasty incision does not provide sufficient exposure or there are other associated injuries, then a coronal incision may be required for adequate access to the roof or management of any other associated injuries.

When the supraorbital rim and roof are fractured and there are no other injuries, the rim should be reduced first and then the roof defect can be repaired. If frontal sinus or intracranial injuries exist, the treatment should be dictated by the management of these other injuries in consultation with a neurosurgeon, as indicated. In children, a high level of suspicion should be exercised for a growing skull fracture, which occurs with a linear skull fracture and an associated dural defect combined with a growing brain or increased ICP, potentially leading to a slowly enlarging fracture and exophthalmos.[50]

ENDOSCOPIC AND ADVANCED IMAGING TECHNIQUES FOR ORBITAL FRACTURE REPAIR

An alternative to the transorbital approach for orbital floor or medial wall fractures is the endoscopic technique. Endoscopic repair of orbital fractures can be performed either transnasally (**Fig. 12**) or by a transmaxillary approach. The potential advantages of this approach include the lack of a skin incision that can cause scarring and eyelid malposition, excellent exposure of the posterior shelf of the orbital floor (with subsequent proper positioning of an implant), avoidance of intraorbital retraction of the implant (particularly near the orbital apex), and in certain situations, the lack of need of any foreign material being placed into the orbit.

Strong and colleagues[51] classify orbital floor fractures into 3 groups of typical fracture patterns. The medial trapdoor fracture occurs at the medial

edge of the infraorbital canal and the medial floor is still hinged at the base of the lamina papyracea. In medial blow-out fractures, the medial wall fragment is comminuted and not hinged medially. In lateral blow-out fractures, the floor is fractured medial and lateral to the infraorbital canal. Strong and colleagues note that lateral blow-out fractures are more difficult by the endoscopic approach because they place the maxillary division of the trigeminal nerve (V_2) at greater risk of injury, and concludes that complex, 2-walled fractures are not amenable to endoscopic repair.

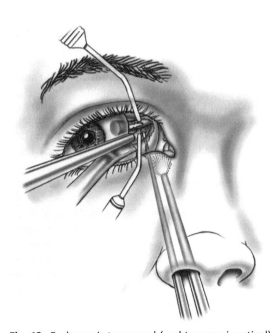

Fig. 12. Endoscopic transnasal (and transconjunctival) approach to optic canal. Biportal access allows for 2-point confirmation of essential anatomic structures. (*From* Holck DEE, Ng JD. Evaluation and Treatment of Orbital Fractures. Philadelphia: WB Saunders, 2006, p. 396; with permission.)

In Strong and colleague's transmaxillary endoscopic technique,[51] a Caldwell-Luc incision is made followed by subperiosteal dissection up the anterior wall of the maxilla. A 1- to 2-cm maxillary antrostomy is made and a notch is created to seat the endoscope and provide tactile feedback to the assistant holding the scope. The sinus ostium and V_2 are identified. The orbital floor anatomy is visualized, and a pulse test consisting of applying pressure to the globe while visualizing the prolapse of orbital contents through the fracture, is performed. Trapdoor fractures are reduced without an implant by carefully reducing the orbital contents with a malleable retractor and reducing the hinged fragment back into apposition with the lateral part of the orbital floor. For medial blow-out fractures, the entire fracture is exposed with a 5- to 7-mm margin of exposed bone on the sinus side, and a 3- to 5-mm margin on the orbital side. A porous polyethylene 0.85-mm implant sheet can be placed into the orbit, extending 1 to 2 mm over the posterior, anterior, and lateral shelves of stable bone.

In addition to the advantages already stated, Strong and colleagues[51] note the opportunity to operate early on eyes with hyphemas and other intraocular disease because of the lack of retraction on the globe itself. Strong and colleagues also propose that orbital floors can be explored to assess the need for surgical repair after a fracture in the zygomaticomaxillary complex is reduced and rigidly fixated. Potential disadvantages of endoscopic repair include injury to V_2, enopthalmos, diplopia, and optic nerve damage.

In a series of 10 patients with orbital floor fractures, Strong[52] successfully repaired 9 of the fractures endoscopically, and reported 3 cases of postoperative diplopia, which resolved after just 1 month. Nahlieli and colleagues[53] repaired 10 patients with this same approach, using titanium mesh on the sinus side of the fracture, with screw fixation, and noted no complications and similar advantages.

Jeon and colleagues[54] describe repair of medial and orbital floor fractures with an endonasal endoscopic approach, using a feeding tube inflated balloon for floor support, and a silastic sheet with Merocel packing retained for 4 weeks for medial wall support. These investigators reported 2 cases of resultant diplopia in 11 isolated floor fractures, 1 case of enophthalmos in 17 medial wall fractures, and 4 cases of diplopia in the 12 combined floor and medial wall fractures. They conclude that this technique should be considered a safe alternative for isolated floor or medial wall fractures, but should perhaps not be considered for combined fractures or if there is an orbital rim fracture.

Computer software and modern image-guidance technology can be used to create a template of the desired orbital floor implant, based on the patient's contralateral, unfractured orbit. Metzger and colleagues[55] have reported a small series using computer-assisted design of orbital implants and have shown an excellent degree of similarity between the repaired orbit and the uninvolved orbit postoperatively. This technology can be particularly useful with repairing more extensive orbitozygomatic fractures.

SUMMARY

Orbital fractures occur in isolation or as a component of other facial fractures. As with any other operation, the surgeon has a multitude of decisions and options in the overall management of these fractures. These complex decisions include the timing of repair, methods of incision (and closure), surgical approaches, and specific implant material. A substantial amount of effort and time has been devoted in the scientific literature to these topics. Comparative studies with strong data and a high level of evidence are lacking, but the available literature allows the astute surgeon to incorporate the available experience into his or her practice with careful decision making. The ultimate treatment of any orbital fracture must take into account the specific circumstances surrounding the patient's fracture, and more importantly, the surgeon's experience and comfort level regarding the management of these injuries.

REFERENCES

1. Cole P, Boyd V, Banerji S, et al. Comprehensive management of orbital fractures. Plast Reconstr Surg 2007;120(7 Suppl 2):57S–63S.
2. Lelli GJ Jr, Milite J, Maher E. Orbital floor fractures: evaluation, indications, approach, and pearls from an ophthalmologist's perspective. Facial Plast Surg 2007;23(3):190–9.
3. Hawes MJ, Dortzbach RK. Surgery on orbital floor fractures. Influence of time of repair and fracture size. Ophthalmology 1983;90(9):1066–70.
4. Yilmaz M, Vayvada H, Aydin E, et al. Repair of fractures of the orbital floor with porous polyethylene implants. Br J Oral Maxillofac Surg 2007;45(8):640–4.
5. Ng SG, Madill SA, Inkster CF, et al. Medpor porous polyethylene implants in orbital blowout fracture repair. Eye 2001;15(Pt 5):578–82.
6. Harris GJ. Orbital blow-out fractures: surgical timing and technique. Eye 2006;20(10):1207–12.

7. Nunery WR, Tao JP, Johl S. Nylon foil "wraparound" repair of combined orbital floor and medial wall fractures. Ophthal Plast Reconstr Surg 2008;24(4):271–5.

8. Hosal BM, Beatty RL. Diplopia and enopthalmos after surgical repair of blowout fracture. Orbit 2002;21(1):27–33.

9. Biesman BS, Hornblass A, Lisman R, et al. Diplopia after surgical repair of orbital floor fractures. Ophthal Plast Reconstr Surg 1996;12(1):9–16.

10. Nam SB, Bae YC, Moon JS, et al. Analysis of the postoperative outcome in 405 cases of orbital fracture using 2 synthetic orbital implants. Ann Plast Surg 2006;56(3):263–7.

11. Appling WD, Patrinely JR, Salzer TA. Transconjunctival approach vs subciliary skin-muscle flap approach for orbital fracture repair. Arch Otolaryngol Head Neck Surg 1993;119(9):1000–7.

12. Villarreal PM, Monje F, Morillo AJ, et al. Porous polyethylene implants in orbital floor reconstruction. Plast Reconstr Surg 2002;109(3):877–85 [discussion: 886–7].

13. Patel PC, Sobota BT, Patel NM, et al. Comparison of transconjunctival versus subciliary approaches for orbital fractures: a review of 60 cases. J Craniomaxillofac Trauma 1998;4(1):17–21.

14. Lane KA, Bilyk JR, Taub D, et al. "Sutureless" repair of orbital floor and rim fractures. Ophthalmology 2009;116(1):135–8.

15. Schmal F, Basel T, Grenzebach UH, et al. Preseptal transconjunctival approach for orbital floor fracture repair: ophthalmologic results in 209 patients. Acta Otolaryngol 2006;126(4):381–9.

16. Al-Sukhun J, Lindqvist C. A comparative study of 2 implants used to repair inferior orbital wall bony defects: autogenous bone graft versus bioresorbable poly-L/DL-Lactide [P(L/DL)LA 70-30] plate. J Oral Maxillofac Surg 2006;64(7):1038–48.

17. Ellis E, Tan Y. Assessment of internal orbital reconstruction for pure blowout fractures: cranial bone grafts versus titanium mesh. J Oral Maxillofac Surg 2003;61(4):442–53.

18. Wolfe SA, Ghurani R, Podda S, et al. An examination of posttraumatic, postsurgical orbital deformities: conclusions drawn for improvement of primary treatment. Plast Reconstr Surg 2008;122(6):1870–81.

19. Jaquiery C, Aeppli C, Cornelius P, et al. Reconstruction of orbital wall defects: critical review of 72 patients. Int J Oral Maxillofac Surg 2007;36(3):193–9.

20. Kontio R. Treatment of orbital fractures: the case for reconstruction with autogenous bone. J Oral Maxillofac Surg 2004;62(7):863–8.

21. Lin IC, Liao SL, Lin LL. Porous polyethylene implants in orbital floor reconstruction. J Formos Med Assoc 2007;106(1):51–7.

22. Lai A, Gliklich RE, Rubin PA. Repair of orbital blow-out fractures with nasoseptal cartilage. Laryngoscope 1998;108(5):645–50.

23. Morrison AD, Sanderson RC, Moos KF. The use of silastic as an orbital implant for reconstruction of orbital wall defects: review of 311 cases treated over 20 years. J Oral Maxillofac Surg 1995;53(4):412–7.

24. Polley JW, Ringler SL. The use of Teflon in orbital floor reconstruction following blunt facial trauma: a 20 year experience. Plast Reconstr Surg 1987;79(1):39–43.

25. Custer PL, Lind A, Trinkaus KM. Complications of supramid orbital implants. Ophthal Plast Reconstr Surg 2003;19(1):62–7.

26. Park DJ, Garibaldi DC, Iliff NT, et al. Smooth nylon foil (SupraFOIL) orbital implants in orbital fractures: a case series of 181 patients. Ophthal Plast Reconstr Surg 2008;24(4):266–70.

27. Su GW, Harris GJ. Combined inferior and medial surgical approaches and overlapping thin implants for orbital floor and medial wall fractures. Ophthal Plast Reconstr Surg 2006;22(6):420–3.

28. Rubin PA, Bilyk JR, Manson PN. Orbital reconstruction using porous polyethylene sheets. Ophthalmology 1994;101(10):1697–708.

29. Romano JJ, Iliff NT, Manson PN. Use of Medpor porous polyethylene implants in 140 patients with facial fractures. J Craniofac Surg 1993;4(3):142–7.

30. Garibaldi DC, Iliff NT, Grant MP, et al. Use of porous polyethylene with embedded titanium in orbital reconstruction: a review of 106 patients. Ophthal Plast Reconstr Surg 2007;23(6):439–44.

31. Seiff SR. Cyanoacrylate fixed silicone sheet in medial blowout fracture repair. Ophthalmology 2000;107(8):1459–63.

32. Tse DT. Cyanoacrylate tissue adhesive in securing orbital implants. Ophthalmic Surg 1986;17(9):577–80.

33. Jordan DR, St Onge P, Anderson RL, et al. Complications associated with alloplastic implants used in orbital fracture repair. Ophthalmology 1992;99(10):1600–8.

34. Kempster R, Beigi B, Galloway GD. Use of enophthalmic implants in the repair of orbital floor fractures. Orbit 2005;24(4):219–25.

35. Tay E, Olver J. Intraorbital hyaluronic acid for enophthalmos. Ophthalmology 2008;155(6):1101–1101.e2.

36. Jank S, Schuchter B, Emshoff R, et al. Clinical signs of orbital wall fractures as a function of anatomic location. Oral Surg Oral Med Oral Pathol Oral Radiol Endod 2003;96(2):149–53.

37. Burm JS, Chung CH, Oh SJ. Pure orbital blowout fractures: new concepts and importance of medial orbital blowout fractures. Plast Reconstr Surg 1999;103(7):1839–49.

38. Lynch RC. The technique of a radical sinus operation which has given me the best results. Laryngoscope 1921;31:1–5.

39. Edgin WA, Morgan-Marshall A, Fitzsimmons TD. Transcaruncular approach to medial orbital wall fractures. J Oral Maxillofac Surg 2007;65(11):2345–9.

40. Kim S, Helen L, Chung SH, et al. Repair of medial orbital wall fractures: transcaruncular approach. Orbit 2005;24(1):1–9.

41. Kim KS, Kim ES, Hwang HJ, et al. Combined transcutaneous transethmoidal/transorbital approach for the treatment of medial orbital blowout fractures. Plast Reconstr Surg 2006;117(6):1947–55.

42. Katowitz JA, Welsh MG, Bersani TA. Lid crease approach for medial wall fracture repair. Ophthalmic Surg 1987;18(4):288–90.

43. Moe KS. The precaruncular approach to the medial orbit. Arch Facial Plast Surg 2003;5(6):483–7.

44. Meningaud JP, Pitak-Arnnop P, Bertrand JC. Endoscopic-assisted repair of medial orbital wall fractures using a retrocaruncular approach. J Oral Maxillofac Surg 2007;65(5):1039–43.

45. Mohadjer Y, Hartstein ME. Endoscopic orbital fracture repair. Otolaryngol Clin North Am 2006;39(5):1049–57.

46. Haug RH, Van Sickels JE, Jenkins WS. Demographics and treatment options for orbital roof fractures. Oral Surg Oral Med Oral Pathol Oral Radiol Endod 2002;93(3):238–46.

47. Sullivan WG. Displaced orbital roof fractures: presentation and treatment. Plast Reconstr Surg 1991;87(4):657–61.

48. Greenwald MJ, Boston D, Pensler JM, et al. Orbital roof fractures in childhood. Ophthalmology 1989;96(4):491–6 [discussion: 496–7].

49. Haug RH. Management of the trochlea of the superior oblique muscle in repair of orbital roof fractures. J Oral Maxillofac Surg 2000;58(6):602–6.

50. Mohindra S, Mukherjee KK, Chhabra R, et al. Orbital roof growing fractures: a report of four cases and literature review. Br J Neurosurg 2006;20(6):420–3.

51. Strong EB, Kim KK, Diaz RC. Endoscopic approach to orbital blowout fracture repair. Otolaryngol Head Neck Surg 2004;131(5):683–95.

52. Strong EB. Endoscopic repair of orbital blow-out fractures. Facial Plast Surg 2004;20(3):223–30.

53. Nahlieli O, Bar-Droma E, Zagury A, et al. Endoscopic intraoral plating of orbital floor fractures. J Oral Maxillofac Surg 2007;65(9):1751–7.

54. Jeon SY, Kwon JH, Kim JP, et al. Individual preformed titanium meshes for orbital fractures. Oral Surg Oral Med Oral Pathol Oral Radiol Endod 2006;102(4):442–7.

55. Metzger MC, Schon R, Weyer N, et al. Anatomical 3-dimensional pre-bent titanium implant for orbital floor fractures. Ophthalmology 2006;113(10):1863–8.

Technology in Microvascular Surgery

Alessandro Cusano, DDS, MD,
Rui Fernandes, DMD, MD, FACS*

KEYWORDS

• Free-tissue transfer • Microvascular surgery

With the refinement of microvascular technique, free-tissue transfer has emerged as the standard of care in head and neck reconstruction. Success rates in the 90% to 99% range[1–4] and significant reductions in operative time have reduced "flap take" from being the marker of reconstructive success to being an expectation. Interest has shifted to improvement of technique, with surgeons placing increasing importance on factors such as donor site morbidity, quality of tissue harvested, and esthetic and functional outcomes.

Much of the recent success can be attributed to technological advances; directly, through improvement in instrumentation and technique, and indirectly, through enhanced understanding of flap physiology and anatomy. This article reviews some of the recent advances and how they have affected microvascular surgery from preoperative, operative, and postoperative standpoints. To gain a deeper appreciation of recent achievements, the first section examines microvascular surgery from a historical perspective.

THE HISTORY OF MICROVASCULAR SURGERY AND FREE-TISSUE TRANSFER

The emergence of microvascular surgery as a distinct surgical discipline can be regarded as a culmination of achievement in vascular surgery. John Benjamin Murphy, an American surgeon, is credited with performing the first vascular anastomosis in 1896, when he successfully repaired a femoral artery that had been severed in a gunshot wound.[5] Although a monumental achievement, illustrating that vascular repair was indeed

possible, his success was limited by patency rates that were less than ideal.

Alexis Carrel, a French surgeon, improved on Murphy's work, reporting a reliable and reproducible method of vascular anastomosis in his description in 1902 of the "triangulation of vessel technique."[6] Using this technique, he and Guthrie, an American vascular surgeon, went on to devise methods for whole-organ transplantation[7]; in 1912, in recognition of his work, Carrel was awarded the Nobel Prize in Medicine and Physiology.

The concept of microscopic vascular surgery was not introduced until 1960, when Jacobson and Suarez, recognizing the need for improvement in small-vessel surgery, pioneered the use of the operating microscope[8]:

The great success in vascular surgery during the last decade is most remarkable in surgery of large vessels. It is less striking in the intermediate sizes, and virtually stops in the small vessels. This communication briefly describes a new technique, called microvascular surgery, which promises the same success with small vessel surgery as that obtained in large vessels.

The significance of this achievement was immediately recognized by Bunke, who envisioned its usefulness in tissue replantation and transplantation. With his 1965 report on experimental digital amputation and replantation he demonstrated that these procedures were indeed possible in the animal model.[9] A year later he reported a rabbit ear replant, which was the first successful

Section of Head Neck Surgery, Division of Oral Maxillofacial Surgery, Divison of Surgical Oncology, Department of Surgery, University of Florida College of Medicine – Jacksonville, 653-1 West 8th Street, Jacksonville, FL 32209, USA
* Corresponding author.
E-mail address: rui.fernandes@jax.ufl.edu

Oral Maxillofacial Surg Clin N Am 22 (2010) 73–90
doi:10.1016/j.coms.2009.11.001
1042-3699/10/$ – see front matter © 2010 Published by Elsevier Inc.

reattachment of an amputated body part using blood vessels of submillimeter size.[10] With these 2 landmark publications, the value of microvascular surgery was quickly becoming evident. In 1968, Komatsu and Tamai were the first to report successful replantation of a human thumb,[11] and in 1972, Bunke and MacLean followed with their report of the first successful microvascular free-tissue transplant using omentum for coverage of a scalp defect.[12]

It was more than a decade, however, before these achievements garnered any significant enthusiasm in the head and neck community. In head and neck reconstruction, surgeons continued to struggle with the inherent limitations of random-pattern skin flaps. These random-pattern flaps were raised without regard for a known blood supply, and because of this, they were restricted to rigid length/width ratios to ensure viability.

It was not until McGregor's description of the forehead flap in 1963[13] and Bakamjian's deltopectoral flap in 1965[14] that it was realized that it was possible to transfer significantly larger areas of cutaneous tissue without strict adherence to dogmatic ratios, as long as the flaps were oriented along the axis of a vascular pathway. This finding is what McGregor and Morgan later referred to as an axial-pattern blood supply,[15] and it was the impetus for what, over the next several decades, evolved into a comprehensive understanding of the vascular anatomy of flaps.

The 1970s saw the resurgence of the musculocutaneous flap. Although use of such flaps had been reported several decades earlier, it was Orticochea in 1972,[16] and later McCraw and Dibbell in 1977,[17] who illustrated the beneficial effect of incorporating muscle in flaps secondary to its significant contribution to the cutaneous circulation. This improved knowledge of vascular anatomy led to Mathes and Nahai's classification of the vascular anatomy of muscle, and to their description of the clinical implications for musculocutaneous flaps.[18–20]

Numerous reports on musculocutaneous flaps followed; perhaps the most significant was the pedicled pectoralis major flap. Although it was initially described for chest-wall defects,[21] Ariyan was the first to report its use in the head and neck.[22] Its potential was soon recognized, as it enabled single-stage transfer of large areas of well-vascularized skin for virtually any defect of the aerodigestive tract, face, and skull base. This development revolutionized head and neck surgery, and is arguably the main reason why the usefulness of free-tissue transfer was not immediately recognized from a head and neck perspective.

The understanding of vascular anatomy of the integument continued to progress when Ponten, with his series of 23 superflaps of the lower leg, demonstrated that the inclusion of the deep fascia in a skin flap gave an advantage to its reliability.[23] This produced the concept of the fasciocutaneous flap, and led Cormack and Lamberty to devise a classification system based on the various patterns of vascularization.[24] About the same time, large series of fasciocutaneous free flaps were being reported from China. Yang's 1981 report on 60 forearm free-skin transplantations with only 1 failure[25] was immediately followed by an equally impressive series of forearm flaps by Song.[26] A couple of years later, Song described a new free flap from the thigh based on the concept of the septocutaneous artery.[27] These 2 fasciocutaneous flaps, known today as the radial forearm flap and the anterolateral thigh flap, remain the flaps of choice for soft-tissue reconstruction in the head and neck.

Osseous defects, however, continued to present significant challenges for the head and neck surgeon, particularly the composite defect of the anterior mandible. The development of the mandibular reconstruction plate in the mid-1970s[28] was a partial solution to the problem, enabling the reestablishment of mandibular contour and, in the process, dispensing with the infamous Andy Gump deformity. Wound breakdown and plate exposure were inevitable, however, without a reliable means of restoring the tissue deficit. The pectoralis major flap, because of its bulk and reliability, was well suited for this purpose, but it did not address the issue of missing bone.

Until the introduction of the osteocutaneous free flap, various osteocutaneous and osteomyocutaneous pedicled flaps had been described, but outcomes were marginal at best.[29–32] Failure was frequent secondary to a tenuous vascular supply and a lack of maneuverability of the osseous component. Osteocutaneous free-tissue transfer was the answer, and for this Taylor deserves much of the credit.[33,34]

Taylor reported the first free vascularized bone graft, when in 1975 he described the use of a vascularized segment of fibula for reconstruction of a traumatic tibial defect.[33] It was Taylor again, in 1978, who described the first vascularized iliac crest transfer using it, along with vascularized groin skin, for single-stage repair of compound defects of the lower extremity.[34] One year later, he and Sanders independently recognized the deep inferior epigastric artery as the principal blood supply to the iliac crest,[35,36] giving rise to what is known as the deep circumflex iliac artery

(DCIA) flap; and it was Taylor again, in 1982, who first reported use of the DCIA flap for reconstruction of mandibular defects.[37]

Reports of other osteocutaneous free flaps soon followed. Soutar was first to describe the osteocutaneous radial forearm flap in 1983.[38] Gilbert and Teot are credited with the free scapular flap in 1982,[39] although it was Silverberg and colleagues[40] in 1985 and Swartz and colleagues[41] in 1986 who popularized its use for maxillomandibular reconstruction. In 1989, Hidalgo's revolutionary application of the free fibula flap for reconstruction of the near-total mandibular defect[42] established free-tissue transfer as an accepted and reliable tool in head and neck reconstruction.

Microvascular surgeons now had at their disposal all that they needed to reconstruct virtually any defect in the head and neck. Soft-tissue defects were addressed with either the radial forearm free flap or the anterolateral thigh flap, and composite defects were reconstructed with the vascularized fibula, scapula, or iliac crest. As experience with these flaps grew and success rates increased to the 90% to 99% range, "flap take" was no longer sufficient to constitute a successful outcome. Surgeons were now more interested in maximizing tissue quality, minimizing donor-site morbidity, and improving function and esthetics.

In search of the ideal flap, surgeons sought once again to further their understanding of vascular anatomy. The concept that skin overlying certain muscles could be transferred reliably as musculocutaneous flaps had been well documented. In 1989, Koshima recognized that these muscles served only as passive carriers, and that if the musculocutaneous perforating vessels could be dissected free of the muscle, a skin flap devoid of muscle could be raised, preserving donor site function.[43,44] This was an exciting discovery, as these so-called perforator flaps combined the reliable blood supply of the musculocutaneous flap with the reduced bulk and donor site morbidity of the skin flap. In essence, the same skin territories could be transferred as before, but in a more elegant manner.[45]

The perforator flap, and its descendant, the free-style free flap, represent the latest genre of reconstructive tissue transfer. Surgeons can now uniquely tailor flaps to specific defects by selecting tissue that maximizes function and esthetics and minimizes donor site morbidity. This evolution, however, has not occurred overnight. Rather, it represents the culmination of decades of discovery and rediscovery in flap surgery and anatomy.[46]

Endemic with any new development is technological advance, and microvascular surgery is no exception. The next section investigates some of the current technology in microvascular surgery, focusing on imaging assessment, anastomotic technique, and flap monitoring as selective examples in the preoperative, operative, and postoperative settings, respectively.

TECHNOLOGY IN MICROVASCULAR SURGERY
Preoperative: Imaging Assessment

The reconstructive process, regardless of the reconstructive modality selected, begins with a preoperative assessment of the defect. If one subscribes to the principle of replacing like with like, then the nature of the defect, to a certain degree, dictates flap selection. Ultimate flap choice, however, depends on several factors, not the least of which is whether or not the flap is feasible from a vascular perspective.

In conventional free-flap surgery, this point holds true for the radial forearm free flap and fibula free flap. With these flaps, uneventful sacrifice of 1 principal blood supplier to the respective extremity depends on whether the in situ vessels can pick up the slack. In these cases, preoperative donor site evaluation is crucial in preventing a catastrophic outcome. Although the Allen test is often all that is required for safe harvest of the radial forearm free flap, most would agree that harvest of the fibula necessitates some form of preoperative imaging.

In perforator flap surgery, and certainly in free-style free flap surgery, preoperative donor site evaluation also plays an integral role. The identification of perforating vessels preoperatively, as opposed to relying on intraoperative identification, facilitates skin-paddle design. It may also help to prevent raising a flap with no substantial perforator, forcing the surgeon to change design considerably or abort the harvest altogether.

Preoperative assessment of the recipient site is also of paramount importance. With the reconstructive surgeon becoming more adept at free-tissue transfer, the challenges are becoming more complex. Complicated, three-dimensional defects of the facial skeleton, once primarily addressed with prostheses, are now being addressed with free flaps. Similarly, reconstruction of defects in the irradiated vessel-depleted neck is not uncommon. In either case, thorough preoperative planning is critical to success, and often necessitates the use of various imaging modalities.

Donor Site Assessment

In conventional free-flap surgery, harvest of either the radial forearm free flap or the fibula free flap places the respective extremity at risk for ischemic complications. The Allen test is often all that is required for safe harvest of the radial forearm free flap. Safe harvest of the fibula, however, is often the subject of much debate. Most would agree that some form of routine preoperative imaging of the lower extremity vasculature is warranted when harvest of the fibula is anticipated. However, there are those who would argue against it, suggesting that it is unnecessary.[47]

The argument against was perhaps more valid when the only reliable means of imaging the vasculature of a lower extremity was with conventional angiography (**Fig. 1**). Although still the gold standard, conventional angiography is an invasive procedure requiring intra-arterial cannulation, and as a result, it carries substantial risk for the patient.[48] The newer, noninvasive imaging modalities have removed much of the inherent risk, significantly tipping the risk/benefit ratio in favor of preoperative imaging. The more commonly used noninvasive vascular imaging modalities include color duplex ultrasonography (CD-US),

magnetic resonance angiography (MRA), and computed tomographic angiography (CTA).

CD-US

US typically refers to gray-scale ultrasound. Gray-scale US provides extensive information regarding the topography and morphology of blood vessels, but not function.[49] Continuous-wave Doppler sonography, on the other hand, provides information regarding the function of the vascular system, because there is a change in the frequency of the emitted sound waves when the distance between the sound source (ie, the US transducer) and the reflecting object (ie, the red blood cell) changes.[49] The combination of gray-scale US and Doppler sonography is referred to as duplex US, and provides an integral assessment of all 3 measures: topography, morphology, and function.[49]

Color duplex US is perhaps the most informative of the US techniques (**Fig. 2**). In color duplex US all stationary soft tissues are imaged in different gray-scale values. Flowing blood, in contrast, is demonstrated in blue or red, depending on the direction of flow in relation to the transducer.[49] Although color duplex US has been proposed as a noninvasive alternative to conventional angiography, its

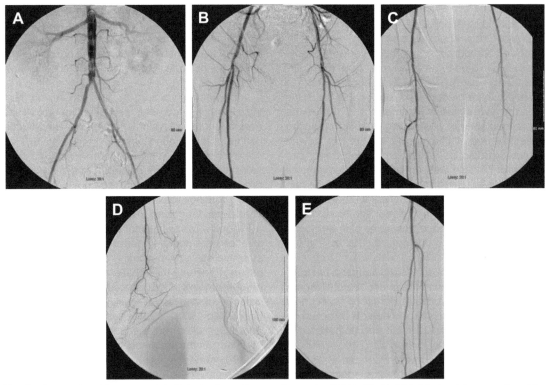

Fig. 1. Conventional intra-arterial digital subtraction angiography (DSA). (*A–D*) DSA bilateral lower extremities from renal arteries to runoff. (*E*) Left lower extremity with clear depiction of the trifurcation and 3-vessel runoff.

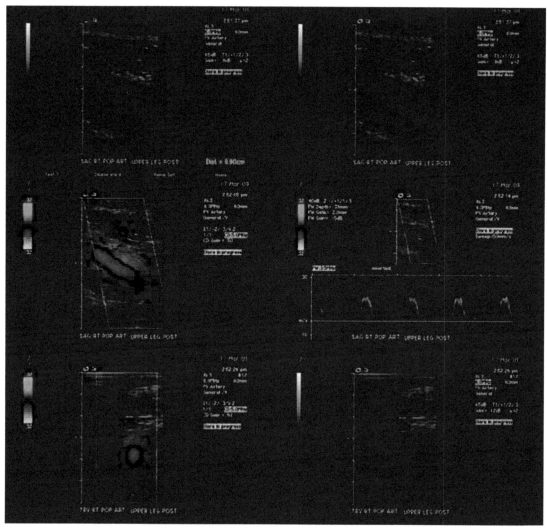

Fig. 2. Arterial CD-US of the right lower extremity in a 70-year-old man with a history of a right popliteal artery aneurysm. Transverse and longitudinal images of the right popliteal artery are displayed. Mild aneurysmal dilatation of the artery can be seen. Directional flow is readily appreciated by the contrasting red and blue colors.

inability to image the entire vascular tree in an acceptable examination time, and the degree of technical expertise it requires, limit its use in many centers.[49]

MRA

Magnetic resonance imaging (MRI) uses a powerful external magnetic field to first align the nuclear magnetization of hydrogen atoms in the body. Then with the application of radiofrequency pulses it sequentially changes their magnetization, systematically altering the net magnetization vector. The net magnetization vector is then detected by a receiver coil, thereby inducing a voltage and producing the MR signal.[50]

MRA uses MRI techniques to visualize the vascular system selectively. Contrast-enhanced MRA is perhaps the most common method of MRA image acquisition, and involves intravenous administration of a contrast medium, typically via the antecubital vein. The images are then acquired during the first pass of the agent through the vascular system. Correct timing of image acquisition relative to contrast injection is therefore critical, such that arterial opacification is ensured and venous contamination is avoided, resulting in high-quality images (**Fig. 3**).[51]

Gadolinium is 1 of the more commonly used contrast agents in MRA. Because it is highly paramagnetic, it markedly reduces the T1 relaxation time of water in blood; as a result, when used in conjunction with a T1-weighted sequence, it effects high-quality contrast separation between vessel and surrounding tissue.[51] Gadolinium has the

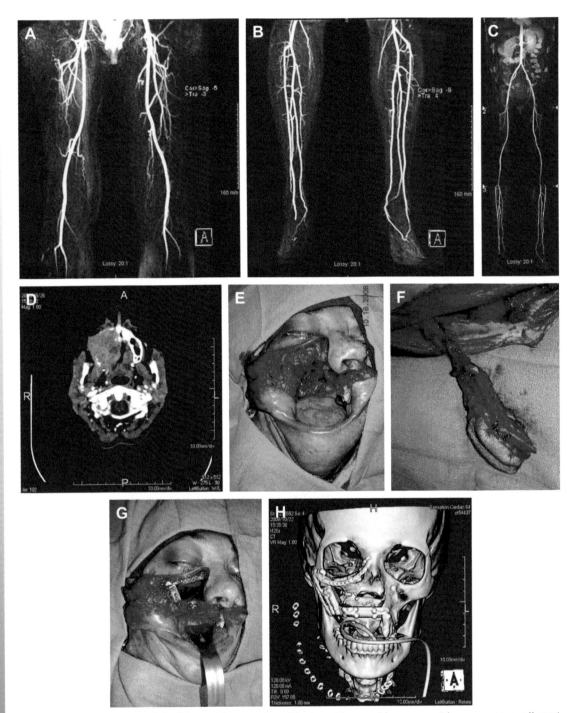

Fig. 3. Preoperative MRA of the bilateral lower extremities in a 48-year-old woman with a squamous cell carcinoma of the right maxilla. (*A*) Thigh level image. (*B*) Lower leg level image. (*C*) Composed body shot. Good 3-vessel runoff is seen bilaterally. The patient went on to have uneventful resection and reconstruction with an osteocutaneous free fibula flap. (*D*) Preoperative CT demonstrating tumor in the right maxilla. (*E*) Postablative defect. (*F*) Osteocutaneous free fibula flap before pedicle ligation. (*G*) Flap inset. (*H*) Postoperative volume-rendered three-dimensional CT reconstruction.

added advantage of being non–iodine-based, with minimal risk of nephropathy or hypersensitivity.[51]

Many reports in the literature advocate use of MRA for imaging the vasculature of lower extremities, citing sensitivities and specificities that rival if not surpass conventional angiography.[51] Not unlike CD-US, however, MRA is also a time-consuming process. In addition, there is a group of patients for whom these studies are contraindicated: patients with implantable defibrillators, permanent pacemakers, or intracranial aneurysm clips are not suitable candidates.[52] Claustrophobia is also a major issue, preventing approximately 10% of patients from completing the examination.[52]

CTA

CT images are graphical representations of the radiographic density of a tissue at different points in space.[53] A radiograph source fires a beam of radiographs that passes through the patient before being picked up by a detector. The detectors compare the intensities of the transmitted radiographs against the source intensities and, using advanced mathematical algorithms, construct a matrix of tissue densities from which the images are generated.[53]

The present generation of CT scanners, multidetector CT scanners (or spiral CT scanners), is the epitome of technological development, with incremental improvements in several technologies. Seven generations ago, the first CT scanner used only a thin pencil beam of radiographs and only 2 detectors. The 2 detectors were slowly translated across the field of view, before being rotated by a single degree. The process was repeated 180 times, for a total arc of rotation equal to 180°.[53]

Modern CT scanners, in contrast, use a fanlike radiograph beam that encompasses the entire patient and that continuously rotates about the patient. Up to 16 detectors are set in several parallel linear arrays, which are then arranged to form a broad arc within the gantry. The detectors remain constantly active while the patient is slid continuously through the gantry under the rotating radiograph beam.[53] This technique has significantly shortened scan times, having the added benefit of more efficient use of injected contrast media.[53]

CTA uses CT technology to visualize the vascular system preferentially. Like MRA, it requires the use of a contrast medium, typically administered via the antecubital vein. After a predetermined delay to select for arterial phase, scanning is initiated (**Fig. 4**).[53]

With the latest generation of multidetector row CT scanners, CTA has overcome many of the limitations of the other vascular imaging modalities. Complete noninvasive, angiographic visualization of the entire peripheral vascular tree from abdominal aorta to distal lower extremities can be completed in a single scan lasting less than a minute.[53] Unlike with MRA, patients with implantable defibrillators, permanent pacemakers, or intracranial aneurysm clips are not excluded; and claustrophobia is almost not an issue. Furthermore, that CTA is less expensive, less user-dependent, and more widely available than the other modalities, justifies its use in peripheral vascular assessment.[54] Radiation exposure and the use of potentially nephrotoxic contrast agents deserve consideration; however, the shortened scan times with the new generation of scanners reduce the level of risk.

Recipient Site Assessment

Recipient site assessment is integral to the reconstructive process, from the perspective of the defect to be reconstructed and the recipient vessels on which to perform the anastomosis. With respect to defect assessment, those defects that warrant considerable investigation are, more often than not, composite in nature with a substantial osseous component. CT is therefore the preferred imaging modality; with volume-rendered three-dimensional reconstructed imaging a three-dimensional stereolithographic model can be manufactured, greatly facilitating the reconstructive process (**Fig. 5**).

Preoperative imaging of recipient vessels for anastomosis is also often advantageous, especially in the irradiated vessel-depleted neck (**Fig. 6**). Like CT, CTA can use volume-rendered three-dimensional imaging to provide a detailed three-dimensional representation of the vascular system. The image generated can then provide the diagnostician with a clear and concise depiction of available recipient vessels in an otherwise complex environment.

Stereolithography

Stereolithography uses digital image data acquired from CT or MRI to produce a physical model. Specific software is required to reformat the data, generating a three-dimensional image with a series of internal and external reference points. Based on these reference points, the stereolithographic apparatus then uses a laser beam to selectively polymerize and solidify an ultraviolet (UV)-sensitive photopolymerizing resin, generating the three-dimensional model. The model is then placed in a UV radiation bath for postcuring, which covalently cross-links the resin, rendering it

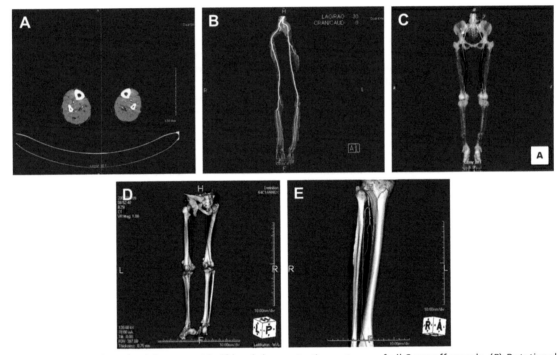

Fig. 4. CTA. (*A*) Selected axial cut at midcalf level demonstrating patency of all 3 runoff vessels. (*B*) Rotational three-dimensional image of bilateral lower extremities (BLE) in the same patient, demonstrating good 3-vessel runoff bilaterally. (*C*) Rotational three-dimensional image of BLE in a patient with poor visualization of all vessels beyond mid leg, precluding use of a free fibula flap. (*D*) Volume-rendered rotational three-dimensional image of BLE in another patient, allowing assessment of the vascular tree in relation to the surrounding bone. Poor 3-vessel runoff is again seen. (*E*) Volume-rendered rotational three-dimensional image of right lower extremity, demonstrating good 3-vessel runoff and clear visualization of the peroneal artery along the entire length of the fibula.

resistant to heat deformation and allowing it to be sterilized for intraoperative use.[55]

Stereolithography, by providing an enhanced understanding of the complex three-dimensional anatomic relationships, gives the surgeon the practical advantage of preoperative simulation surgery, which may then facilitate the ultimate reconstruction, particularly for complex structural defects of the facial skeleton (**Fig. 7**).

Three-dimensional spiral CTA

In the same way stereolithography uses volume-rendered three-dimensional reconstructed CT imaging to manufacture a three-dimensional model of the facial skeleton, three-dimensional spiral CTA uses the same process to generate a three-dimensional image of the vascular system.

For imaging of the head and neck vasculature, an intravenous contrast agent is administered rapidly by a power injector, followed by contrast-enhanced scanning in the arterial phase approximately 6 seconds after bolus tracking in the common carotid artery.[54] Spiral CT scans are then obtained in the usual fashion, preferably using

1-mm slices. The CT data sets are then reformatted into a set of volume-rendered, rotational, three-dimensional images, allowing visualization of the cervical vasculature from multiple viewpoints (**Fig. 8**).[54]

The appeal of three-dimensional spiral CTA is the simplicity of its interpretation. Full diagnostic information is retained in the original set of axial images, but by compiling the entire data set into a single three-dimensional image, visual comprehension of the area of interest is enhanced.[54] In the same single image, CTA also allows the assessment of the vasculature in relation to the surrounding tissues, which may further benefit preoperative planning.

Intraoperative: Anastomotic Technique

The fundamentals of vascular surgery were established by Alexis Carrel in 1902 when he described the "triangulation of vessel technique" for vascular anastomosis.[7] The placement of 3 stay sutures 120° apart essentially triangulates the vessel, thereby facilitating equidistant placement of

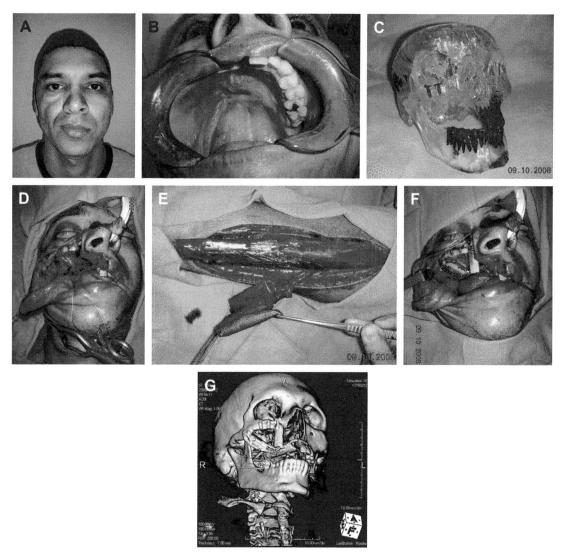

Fig. 5. A 32-year-old man referred for reconstructive evaluation several years after resection of an odontogenic myxoma of the right maxilla. He presented with complaints of right midfacial deficit (*A*), persistent oronasal fistula (*B*), and dissatisfaction with obturator. A three-dimensional stereolithographic model was obtained to facilitate assessment of the defect and planning of the reconstruction (*C*). He went on to have uneventful reconstruction with an osteocutaneous free fibula flap (*D–F*). (*G*) Postoperative volume-rendered three-dimensional CT reconstruction.

additional sutures in the intervening segments. This technique has withstood the test of time, and continues to have application in vascular and microvascular surgery.

In their original description of microvascular surgery, Jacobson and Suarez reported that an average 3-mm-diameter arterial anastomosis required from 25 to 30 stitches, and that for an endarterectomy incision of less than 2 cm, 62 stitches were used.[8] This seems absurd in comparison with today's standards in which a typical arterial anastomosis contains only 8 stitches at best. Nevertheless, it is enlightening

to take a look back at the origin of surgical technique and to view its evolution to modern-day applications.

Microvascular anastomosis continues to be the most critical determinant of successful free-tissue transfer, with technical errors occurring during anastomosis accounting for most free-flap failures. Simple interrupted suture placement remains the gold standard, although other methods have been described, with the aim of simplifying anastomotic technique, reducing operative time, and increasing patency rates. The most widely accepted of these is the microvascular

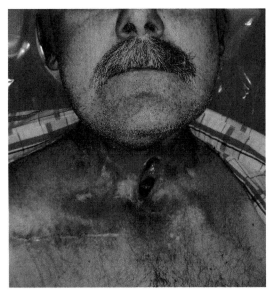

Fig. 6. A 47-year-old man with a history of laryngeal cancer status post total laryngectomy and adjuvant radiotherapy with pharyngocutaneous and tracheoesophageal fistulae. Proper assessment of the cervical vasculature is critical in these patients if reconstruction with free-tissue transfer is anticipated.

anastomotic Coupler system (Synovis Micro Companies Alliances Inc, Birmingham, AL, USA).

Microvascular anastomotic Coupler system

The prototype microvascular anastomotic device was developed by Nakayama in 1962 and consisted of 2 metallic rings with 12 interlocking pins and holes. The vessel ends were passed through the rings, everted onto the pins, and then mechanically approximated.[56] The Nakayama device was later modified by Ostrup and Berggren in 1987,[57] and their version in turn evolved into the present-day device.

Commercially available since 1990, the present-day coupler consists of 2 high-density polyethylene rings each with 6 stainless-steel pins that interlock with holes on the opposite ring.[58] Rings with internal diameters ranging from 1.0 to 4.0 mm at 0.5-mm intervals are available, permitting use of the device over a wide range of vessel sizes (**Fig. 9**).

The present-day device functions in a similar manner as the original Nakayama device. A measuring gauge is used to determine the correctly sized coupler, which is then loaded onto the applicator. The vessel ends are then passed through the rings, everted onto the pins, and with a clockwise turn of the applicator handle, brought into approximation. A hemostat is then used to compress the opposing rings further,

and with an additional clockwise turn of the applicator handle the completed anastomosis is ejected (**Fig. 10**).

Theoretically, the patency rates of coupled anastomoses should compare favorably with those that are hand-sewn. By achieving intima-to-intima contact of the vessel ends without the presence of intraluminal foreign material (ie, suture), the coupler device should theoretically reduce the risk of thrombosis. In addition, the rigidity of the plastic rings has been suggested to stent open the anastomosis, increasing luminal diameter in a region that might otherwise be slightly constricted.[59] Furthermore, viewing the lumen of both vessels in their entirety before their apposition provides the surgeon with the added confidence that a successful anastomosis will be achieved. Nevertheless, with success rates of free-tissue transfer now in the high 90% range irrespective of anastomotic method used, it might be questioned whether the theoretic advantage has translated into any clinically significant benefit. In terms of patency, the question is valid. However, if time is considered as an additional outcome variable, the argument might differ.

The biggest advantage of using the coupler device rather than the traditional hand-sewn method is the reduction in time taken to complete the anastomosis. Anastomoses performed with the coupler device are consistently completed in less than 7 minutes,[58] which is unattainable with traditional methods. Another advantage of the coupler is its ability to manage size discrepancy.[58] By selecting a coupler with a ring size equal to the diameter of the smaller vessel, and then pleating the wall of the larger vessel evenly over the pins, an anastomosis free of leakage is created, which may not have occurred had it been hand-sewn.

The microvascular anastomotic Coupler system continues to be most commonly used for veins, and it has been approved for use in an end-to-end and end-to-side fashion. Its use for arterial anastomoses remains controversial. It has been suggested that the inherent thickness of the arterial wall renders it impliable for eversion onto the pins, complicating the procedure and significantly reducing luminal diameter if indeed an intact anastomosis can be achieved.[58]

Recently, however, Chernichenko and colleagues[60] reported a retrospective review of 127 free-tissue transfers in which a coupler device was used for the arterial and venous anastomoses. Their flap survival rate was 97.6% and they reported only 4 complications related to arterial insufficiency. With these results they concluded that for arterial anastomoses use of a coupler is a safe alternative to the traditional hand-sewn method.

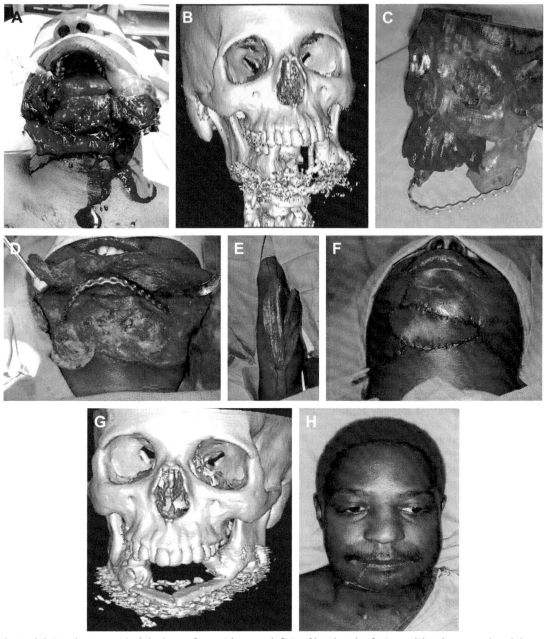

Fig. 7. (*A*) Gunshot wound of the lower face with gross deficit of hard and soft tissue. (*B*) Volume-rendered three-dimensional CT image of the defect. (*C*) Preoperative contouring of reconstruction plate to fit the stereolithographic model. (*D–F*) Uneventful reconstruction with osteocutaneous free fibula flap. (*G*) Volume-rendered three-dimensional CT image of the reconstruction. (*H*) Postoperative clinical photograph.

Although the numbers in this study are significant, this is level III evidence, with its inherent shortcomings.

In summary, the microvascular anastomotic Coupler system has proved to be an invaluable tool, particularly for use in venous anastomosis. Its main advantage is the significant decrease in time taken to complete the anastomosis, thereby reducing ischemia time of the flap. Although its use for arterial anastomosis has also been reported, corroboratory literature is lacking.

Postoperative Flap Monitoring

With the refinement of microvascular technique, success rates of free-tissue transfer have

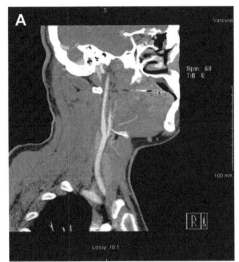
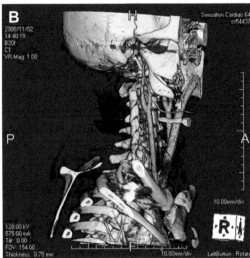

Fig. 8. CTA of the neck. (*A*) Selected sagittal view. (*B*) Volume-rendered rotational three-dimensional image (different patient) enhancing visualization of the cervical vasculature.

increased into the 90% to 99% range; salvage rates, however, have not shared the same level of success.[4] The failure of flap salvage to improve in parallel with flap transfer suggests that the problem is not one of technical expertise, but rather delayed recognition of the failing flap. Early intervention is the key to a successful salvage attempt, emphasizing the need for improved monitoring methodology.

Numerous methods have been described, including intravenous fluorescein,[61] optical spectroscopy,[62] transcutaneous laser Doppler,[63] photoplethysmography,[64] and transcutaneous Po_2 monitoring.[65] All are based on assessment of surface capillary blood flow, and as a result rely on an externalized skin paddle. In this respect,

these techniques are no different from the traditional method of clinical examination, and they have failed to demonstrate any significant benefit in comparison.

Clinical examination is regarded as the gold standard for postoperative monitoring of flap perfusion. It typically entails frequent interval assessment of flap color, capillary refill, turgor, warmth, and bleeding to pinprick. Based on these measures alone, the experienced observer is able to ascertain the status of flap circulation. However, it is rare that an experienced observer performs the assessment. Most of the time, the welfare of the flap is at the mercy of the inexperienced discretion of the support clinicians and staff, who may lack experience and judgment regarding the

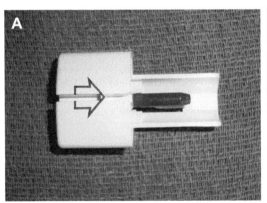
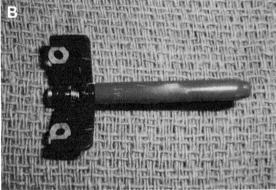

Fig. 9. 1.5-mm microvascular anastomotic Coupler device. (*A*) Coupler as it appears on removal from the manufacturer's packaging. The different-sized couplers are color-coded with a blue shaft denoting a 1.5-mm coupler. (*B*) Coupler removed from plastic housing (for illustration purposes only). The Coupler is seen in its open position, with clear visualization of polyethylene rings and stainless-steel spikes.

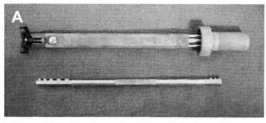

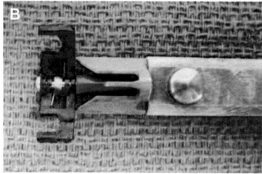

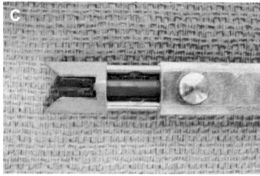

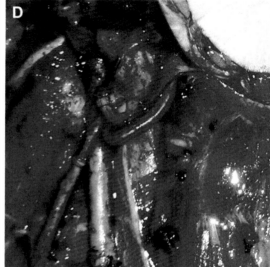

Fig. 10. Coupler instrumentation and technique. (*A*) Measuring gauge and applicator device. (*B*) Loaded applicator in open position (actual Coupler absent). (*C*) Loaded applicator in closed position following clockwise turn of the applicator handle (actual Coupler absent). (*D*) Intraoperative photograph depicting 2 venous anastomoses completed with the microvascular anastomotic Coupler system. A hand-sewn arterial anastomosis is also seen.

subtle changes seen with these flaps in the early postoperative time period.

Observer experience aside, the issue of the buried flap must be considered. The absence of an externalized skin paddle precludes the use of clinical examination or any other method of assessment reliant on surface capillary phenomena. Disa and colleagues[66] proved this to be a real problem. In their retrospective review of 750 free flaps monitored with conventional methods, vascular compromise in non-buried flaps was identified early (generally <48 hours), prompting an urgent return to the operating room, and resulting in flap salvage in 77% of cases. Conversely, in buried flaps, vascular compromise went unrecognized until it manifested as a wound complication (generally

>7 days postoperatively), at which time reexploration was too late, resulting in a flap salvage rate of 0%.

In 1988, Swartz and colleagues[67] devised a method of providing continuous real-time monitoring of flap perfusion that proved to be the solution to the problem of the buried flap.

Cook-Swartz Implantable Doppler probe system

Swartz's original device consisted of a 1.0-mm Doppler probe secured with a small amount of silicone to a polytetrafluoroethylene (Gore-Tex; WL Gore and Associates, Flagstaff, AZ, USA) cuff that was then wrapped around the flap vessel and secured to itself by suture.[67] It has since evolved into the Cook-Swartz implantable Doppler

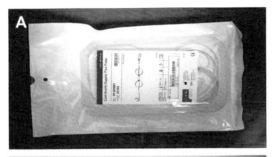

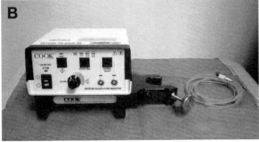

Fig. 11. Implantable Doppler instrumentation and technique. (*A*) Cook-Swartz implantable Doppler probe as it appears in the manufacturer's packaging. (*B*) Cook Doppler blood-flow monitor, pole mount, and extension cable.

flow system (Cook Vascular Inc, Vandergrift, PA, USA), arguably today's standard of care for the buried free flap.

The Cook-Swartz implantable Doppler flow system consists of the Cook-Swartz implantable Doppler probe, an extension cable for the probe, a Doppler blood-flow monitor, an external power supply, and a pole mount (**Fig. 11**). The probe contains a 20-MHz ultrasonic Doppler crystal that is attached to a silicone cuff (8 × 5 mm^2) that gets wrapped around the vessel and secured on itself with a surgical clip. The probe exits the wound as a thin wire (internal segment) that converts itself into a cable (external segment) before connecting to the extension cable that attaches to the monitor. Retention tabs exist at the junction of the internal and external segments to secure the probe externally to the patient's skin (**Fig. 12**). The monitor is portable and can be either battery or power operated. The thin wire (internal segment) is designed to disengage from the silicone cuff with only minimal tension, allowing for safe removal of the device (silicone cuff left in situ) when flap monitoring is complete.

The device was initially designed for use with the venous anastomosis because of the superior sensitivity of monitoring venous blood flow in detecting flap compromise.[67] In his initial work, Swartz found that venous probes detected

a venous problem immediately and detected an arterial problem on average with only a 6-minute delay. Arterial probes, however, detected an arterial occlusion immediately, but for up to 6 hours after venous occlusion continued to record an arterial pulsation. The device was therefore designed to be used on venous anastomosis with the rationale that, whereas the presence of a venous signal confirms venous and arterial flow, the converse is not necessarily true.

Over the years, numerous studies have demonstrated the positive effect the device has had on flap salvage. Kind and colleagues[4] in 1998 reported a 100% salvage rate of 20 ischemic flaps (147 flaps total), De la Torre and colleagues[68] in 2003 reported an 83% salvage rate of 8 ischemic flaps (118 flaps total), and Pryor and colleagues[69] in 2006 reported a 66.7% salvage rate of 3 ischemic flaps (24 flaps total). In each of the studies the number of false-negatives was zero; however, false-positives were encountered 4, 6, and 3 times, respectively. This finding suggests that although it is unlikely that the device fails to recognize a compromised flap when it is compromised, it will on occasion overshoot and indicate that a flap is compromised when it is not. The question then becomes "what is the significance of this overshoot"?

With nonburied flaps, the answer is probably nothing. The presence of an externalized skin paddle in instances of conflicting data allows one to rely on conventional clinical examination to prevent a needless intervention. With buried flaps, however, an overshoot of the device translates into an unnecessary return to the operating room, which places the patient at risk of an additional invasive procedure, and is often regarded as the principal weakness of the device.

Recently, in their retrospective review of 369 free flaps, Guillemaud and colleagues[70] found that of the 7 false-positives that occurred in the presence of an altered Doppler signal, 5 were from probes placed on the venous pedicle. These investigators concluded by stating that use of the probe on the venous pedicle was unreliable in their experience, and that if used on the arterial pedicle, a lower incidence of false-positives would result.

The implantable Doppler has proven to be a valuable tool for the monitoring of free flaps, with significant improvements in rates of salvage. Its use is perhaps most warranted and beneficial with buried flaps, in which case lack of an externalized skin paddle precludes clinical evaluation. It may be argued, however, that its use is equally justified in the nonburied flap, in which its continuous, real-time signal is easily interpreted by the novice

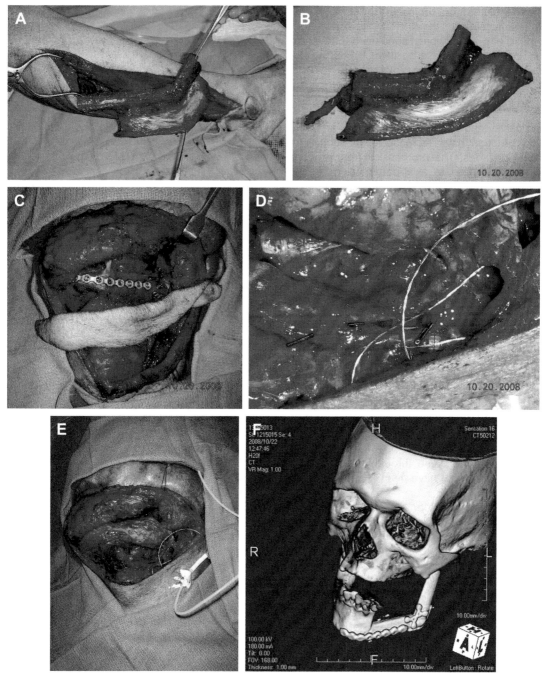

Fig. 12. A 57-year-old man with squamous cell carcinoma of the left mandible treated with segmental mandibular resection, ipsilateral neck dissection, and reconstruction with osteocutaneous free fibula flap. (*A*) Harvested free fibula flap before pedicle ligation. (*B*) Pedicle ligated and fibula osteotomized according to defect dimensions. (*C*) Osseous component of flap inset. (*D*) Hand-sewn arterial anastomosis and coupled venous anastomosis complete with implantable Doppler placed on the venous pedicle. (*E*) Cook-Swartz implantable Doppler probe in position with internal segment, retention tabs, and external segment clearly visualized. (*F*) Postoperative volume-rendered three-dimensional CT image of the reconstruction.

practitioner and is not subject to the delay of interval assessment. Placing the probe on the arterial anastomosis has recently been suggested to decrease the incidence of false-positives, reducing the number of unnecessary reexplorations.

SUMMARY

The quality and sophistication of head and neck reconstruction have increased exponentially in recent decades. The progression from random-pattern skin flaps to axial-pattern skin flaps to musculocutaneous and osteomusculocutaneous composite flaps reflected the need at that time to incorporate more bulk of tissue into the reconstruction. By doing so, surgeons were able to better address the larger, more complex defects while maintaining a robust blood supply to the flap.

The advent of microvascular surgery freed the surgeon from the constraints of locoregional tissue and prompted the exploration of distant tissue as new potential donor sites. The evolution of musculocutaneous flaps to fasciocutaneous flaps to perforator flaps to free-style free flaps reflects a second wave of progression, which in contrast to the first is dominated by the desire to reduce tissue bulk.

With free-style free flaps being essentially skin flaps raised from potentially any site with a Dopplerable perforator, the development has come full circle. The distinction, however, is that the development has come through the knowledge and experience that have been afforded by technological advance.

Technological development has been integral to the refinement of microvascular technique. This article has reviewed several tools that have simplified practice and improved performance. As the complexity and sophistication of this technical surgical art develop, advancement in technology will remain a key to progress in the field.

REFERENCES

1. Schusterman MA, Miller MJ, Reece GP, et al. A single center's experience with 308 free flaps for repair of head and neck cancer defects. Plast Reconstr Surg 1994;93(3):472–8.
2. Kroll SS, Schusterman MA, Reece GP, et al. Choice of flap and incidence of free flap success. Plast Reconstr Surg 1996;98(3):459–63.
3. Hidalgo DA, Disa JJ, Cordeiro PG, et al. A review of 716 consecutive free flaps for oncological surgical defects: refinement in donor-site selection and technique. Plast Reconstr Surg 1998;102(3):722–32.
4. Kind GM, Buntic RF, Buncke GM, et al. The effect of an implantable Doppler probe on the salvage of microvascular tissue transplants. Plast Reconstr Surg 1998;101(5):1268–73.
5. Murphy JB. Resection of arteries and veins injured in continuity – end-to-end suture – experimental and clinical research. Med Rec 1897;51:73–88.
6. Carrel A. [La technique opératoire des anastomoses vasculaires et la transplantation des viscères]. Lyon Med 1902;98:859 [in French].
7. Carrel A. Results of transplantation of blood vessels, organs and limbs. J Am Med Assoc 1908;51:1662.
8. Jacobson JH, Suarez EL. Microvascular surgery. Dis Chest 1962;41:220–4.
9. Buncke HJ, Schulz WP. Experimental digital amputation and replantation. Plast Reconstr Surg 1965;36:62–70.
10. Buncke HJ, Schulz WP. Total ear replantation in the rabbit utilizing microminiature anastomoses. Br J Plast Surg 1966;19(1):15–22.
11. Komatsu S, Tamai S. Successful replantation of a completely cut off thumb. Plast Reconstr Surg 1968;42:374–7.
12. Maclean DH, Buncke HJ. Autotransplant of omentum to a large scalp defect, with microsurgical revascularization. Plast Reconstr Surg 1972;49(3):268–74.
13. McGregor IA. The temporal flap in intraoral cancer: its use in repairing the post-excisional defect. Br J Plast Surg 1963;16:318–35.
14. Bakamjian VY. A two stage method for pharyngoesophageal reconstruction with a primary pectoral skin flap. Plast Reconstr Surg 1965;36:173–84.
15. McGregor IA, Morgan G. Axial and random pattern flaps. Br J Plast Surg 1973;26(3):202–13.
16. Orticochea M. The musculo-cutaneous flap method: an immediate and heroic substitute for the method of delay. Br J Plast Surg 1972;25:106–10.
17. McCraw JB, Dibbell DG. Experimental definition of independent myocutaneous vascular territories. Plast Reconstr Surg 1977;60:212–20.
18. Mathes SJ, Nahai F. Clinical atlas of muscle and musculocutaneous flaps. St. Louis (MO): Mosby; 1979.
19. Mathes SJ, Nahai F. Classification of the vascular anatomy of muscles: experimental and clinical correlation. Plast Reconstr Surg 1981;67:1177–87.
20. Mathes SJ, Nahai F. Clinical applications for muscle and musculocutaneous flaps. St. Louis (MO): Mosby; 1982.
21. Hueston JT, McConchie IH. A compound pectoral flap. Aust N Z J Surg 1968;38(1):61–3.
22. Ariyan S. The pectoralis major myocutaneous flap. A versatile flap for reconstruction in the head and neck. Plast Reconstr Surg 1979;63(1):73–81.
23. Ponten B. The fasciocutaneous flap: its use in soft tissue defects of the lower leg. Br J Plast Surg 1981;34(2):215–20.
24. Cormack GC, Lamberty BGH. A classification of fasciocutaneous flaps according to their patterns of vascularization. Br J Plast Surg 1984;37:80–7.

25. Yang GF, Chen PJ, Gao YZ, et al. Forearm free skin flap transplantation: a report of 56 cases. Chin Med J 1981;61:139–41.

26. Song R, Gao Y, Song Y, et al. The forearm flap. Clin Plast Surg 1982;9(1):21–6.

27. Song YG, Chen GZ, Song YL. The free thigh flap: a new free flap concept based on the septocutaneous artery. Br J Plast Surg 1984;37(2):149–59.

28. Chow JM, Hill JH. Primary mandibular reconstruction using the AO reconstruction plate. Laryngoscope 1986;96(7):768–73.

29. Snyder CC, Bateman JM, Davis CW, et al. Mandibulo-facial restoration with live osteocutaneous flaps. Plast Reconstr Surg 1970;45:14–9.

30. Conley J. Use of composite flaps containing bone for major repairs in the head and neck. Plast Reconstr Surg 1972;49:522–6.

31. Ariyan S. Pectoralis major, sternomastoid, and other musculocutaneous flaps for head and neck reconstruction. Clin Plast Surg 1980;7:89–109.

32. Panje W, Cutting C. Trapezius osteomyocutaneous island flap for reconstruction of anterior floor of mouth and the mandible. Head Neck Surg 1980;3: 66–71.

33. Taylor GI, Miller GD, Ham FJ. The free vascularized bone graft: a clinical extension of microvascular techniques. Plast Reconstr Surg 1975;55(5): 533–44.

34. Taylor GI, Watson N. One stage repair of compound leg defects with free, revascularized flaps of groin skin and iliac bone. Plast Reconstr Surg 1978; 61(4):494–506.

35. Taylor GI, Townsend P, Corlett R. Superiority of the deep circumflex iliac vessels as the supply for free groin flaps. Plast Reconstr Surg 1979;64(5): 595–604.

36. Sanders R, Mayou BJ. A new vascularized bone graft transferred by microvascular anastomoses as a free flap. Br J Plast Surg 1979;66(11):787–8.

37. Taylor GI. Reconstruction of the mandible with free composite iliac bone grafts. Ann Plast Surg 1982; 9(5):361–76.

38. Soutar DS, Schelier L, Tanner N, et al. The radial forearm flap: a versatile method for intraoral reconstruction. Br J Plast Surg 1983;36(1):1–8.

39. Gilbert A, Teot L. The free scapula flap. Plast Reconstr Surg 1982;69(4):601–4.

40. Silverberg B, Banis JC, Acland R. Mandibular reconstruction with microvascular bone transfer. Am J Surg 1985;150(4):440–6.

41. Swartz WM, Banis JC, Newton ED, et al. The osteocutaneous scapula flap for mandibular and maxillary reconstruction. Plast Reconstr Surg 1986;77(4): 530–45.

42. Hidalgo DA. Fibula free flap: a new method of mandibular reconstruction. Plast Reconstr Surg 1989;84(1):71–9.

43. Koshima I, Fukuda H, Utunomiya R, et al. The anterolateral thigh flap: variations in its vascular pedicle. Br J Plast Surg 1989;42(3):260–2.

44. Koshima I, Soeda S. Inferior epigastric artery skin flaps without the rectus abdominis muscle. Br J Plast Surg 1989;42(6):645–8.

45. Cavadas PC, Sanz-Gimenez-Rico JR, Gutierrez-de la Camara A, et al. The medial sural artery perforator free flap. Plast Reconstr Surg 2001;108:1609–15.

46. Morris SF, Miller BF, Taylor GI. Vascular anatomy of the integument. In: Blondeel PN, Morris SF, Hallock GG, et al, editors. Perforator flaps: anatomy, technique, and clinical applications. St Louis (MO): Quality Medical Publishing, Inc; 2006. p. 12–36.

47. Ahmad N, Kordestani R, Panchal J, et al. The role of donor site angiography before mandibular reconstruction utilizing free flap. J Reconstr Microsurg 2007;23(4):199–204.

48. Abu Rahma AF, Robinson PA, Boland JP, et al. Complications of arteriography in a recent series of 707 cases: factors affecting outcome. Ann Vasc Surg 1993;7(2):122–9.

49. Reimer P, Landwehr P. Non-invasive vascular imaging of peripheral vessels. Eur Radiol 1998;8:858–72.

50. Westbrook C. MRI at a glance. Oxford (UK): Blackwell Science Ltd; 2002.

51. Dellegrottaglie S, Sanz J, Macaluso F, et al. Technology insight: magnetic resonance angiography for the evaluation of patients with peripheral artery disease. Nat Clin Pract Cardiovasc Med 2007; 4(12):677–87.

52. Begelman SM, Jaff MR. Noninvasive diagnostic strategies for peripheral arterial disease. Cleve Clin J Med 2006;73(4):S22–9.

53. Pierce G. Basics of computed tomography angiography of the lower extremity vessels. Semin Vasc Surg 2004;17(2):102–9.

54. Thurmuller P, Kesting MR, Holzle F, et al. Volume-rendered three-dimensional spiral computed tomographic angiography as a planning tool for microsurgical reconstruction in patients who have had operations or radiotherapy for oropharyngeal cancer. Br J Oral Maxillofac Surg 2007;45(7):543–7.

55. Powers DB, Edgin WA, Tabatchnick L. Stereolithography: a historical review and indications for use in the management of trauma. J Craniomaxillofac Trauma 1998;4(3):16–23.

56. Nakayama K, Tamiya T, Yamamoto K, et al. A simple new apparatus for small vessel anastomosis (free autograft of the sigmoid included). Surgery 1962; 52:918–31.

57. Ostrup LT, Berggren A. The UNILINK instrument system for fast and safe microvascular anastomosis. Ann Plast Surg 1986;17:521–5.

58. Jeremic G, Shrime M, Irish JC, et al. The microvascular anastomotic device and its role in free tissue transfer. Univ Toronto Med J 2006;84(1):51–4.

59. Ross DA, Chow JY, Shin J, et al. Arterial coupling for microvascular free tissue transfer in head and neck reconstruction. Arch Otolaryngol Head Neck Surg 2005;131:891–5.

60. Chernichenko N, Ross DA, Shin J, et al. Arterial coupling for microvascular free tissue transfer. Otolaryngol Head Neck Surg 2008;138(5):614–8.

61. Graham BH, Walton RL, Elings VB, et al. Surface quantification of injected fluorescein as a predictor of flap viability. Plast Reconstr Surg 1983;71(6):826–33.

62. Payette JR, Kohlenberg E, Leonardi L, et al. Assessment of skin flaps using optically based methods for measuring blood flow and oxygenation. Plast Reconstr Surg 2005;115(2):539–46.

63. Bruce-Chwatt AJ. Free flap monitoring using a microcomputer linked to a laser Doppler flowmeter. Br J Plast Surg 1986;39(2):229–38.

64. Webster MH, Patterson J. The photo-electric plethysmograph as a monitor of microvascular anastomoses. Br J Plast Surg 1976;29(2):182–5.

65. Serafin D, Lesesne CB, Mullen RY, et al. Transcutaneous PO2 monitoring for assessing viability and predicting survival of skin flaps: experimental and clinical correlations. J Microsurg 1981;2(3): 165–78.

66. Disa JJ, Cordiero PG, Hidalgo DA. Efficacy of conventional monitoring techniques in free tissue transfer: an 11-year experience in 750 consecutive cases. Plast Reconstr Surg 1999;104(1):97–101.

67. Swartz WM, Jones NF, Cherup L, et al. Direct monitoring of microvascular anastomoses with the 20-mHz ultrasonic Doppler probe: am experimental and clinical study. Plast Reconstr Surg 1988;81(2):149–61.

68. De la Torre J, Hedden W, Grant JH, et al. Retrospective review of the internal Doppler probe for intra- and postoperative microvascular surveillance. J Reconstr Microsurg 2003;19(5):287–90.

69. Pryor SG, Moore EJ, Kasperbauer JL. Implantable Doppler flow system: experience with 24 microvascular free-flap operations. Otolaryngol Head Neck Surg 2006;135(5):714–8.

70. Guillemaud JP, Seikaly H, Cote D, et al. The implantable Cook-Swartz Doppler probe for postoperative monitoring in head and neck free flap reconstruction. Arch Otolaryngol Head Neck Surg 2008; 134(7):729–34.

Temporary Skeletal Anchorage Devices for Orthodontics

Bernard J. Costello, DMD, MD, FACS[a],*,
Ramon L. Ruiz, DMD, MD[b,c],
Joseph Petrone, DMD, MDS, MPH[d],
Jacqueline Sohn, DMD, MDS[e]

KEYWORDS
- Miniscrews • Orthodontic mechanics
- Skeletal anchorage • Temporary anchorage devices

Orthodontists have always tried to develop ways to move teeth while minimizing the unwanted reciprocal movement of the teeth they pull or push against. This constant battle is more easily won when ideal anchorage is in place to move teeth in an efficient manner. Although dental implants were used as absolute orthodontic anchorage in the past, they had not become popular for a number of reasons including cost; time of sequencing for osseointegration; and their primary use for dental restoration purposes, not orthodontic mechanics. These concepts of skeletal anchorage are not new, but have gained more attention in the literature because of a number of innovations in design and technique. Even as this article is being written, advances in materials and technique are poised to change how these procedures are planned and performed. The reader is encouraged to review the literature regularly because the pace of change is rapid.

The goals of orthodontic therapy include optimizing occlusion, aesthetics, and facial balance. Traditional orthodontic mechanics are efficient at accomplishing these goals for clinical scenarios that require mild to moderate compensation. Those patients who have more significant discrepancies, however, require additional techniques. This is most evident to the oral and maxillofacial surgeon when one examines patients with moderate to severe skeletal discrepancies. Patients with occlusal discrepancies beyond what can be managed with standard orthodontic therapy are usually treated with techniques that include growth modification or orthognathic surgery in combination with comprehensive orthodontic therapy. Presently, patients with mild to moderate discrepancies may benefit from skeletal anchorage devices to compensate further for malocclusions that were not previously correctable using conventional orthodontic mechanics. Additionally, a variety of problems encountered by the orthodontist on a regular basis are now more efficiently treated with skeletal anchorage as an adjunct to traditional mechanics.

This article discusses the recent advances and basic concepts of skeletal anchorage devices of various types and reviews the current literature on their use. A primer on orthodontic mechanics is required to treat patients with skeletal anchorage devices adequately, and the reader is encouraged to review principles of orthodontic

[a] Department of Oral and Maxillofacial Surgery, University of Pittsburgh School of Dental Medicine, 3471 5th Avenue, Suite 1112, Pittsburgh, PA 15213, USA
[b] Craniomaxillofacial Surgery, Pediatric Oral and Maxillofacial Surgery, Arnold Palmer Children's Hospital, Orlando, FL, USA
[c] University of Central Florida College of Medicine, Orlando, FL, USA
[d] Department of Orthodontics, University of Pittsburgh School of Dental Medicine, Pittsburgh, PA, USA
[e] Private practice, Pittsburgh, PA, USA
* Corresponding author.
E-mail address: bjc1@pitt.edu

Oral Maxillofacial Surg Clin N Am 22 (2010) 91–105
doi:10.1016/j.coms.2009.10.011

mechanics in conjunction with this article. Much like the concepts introduced during the beginnings of orthognathic dentofacial teams, treatment that uses skeletal anchorage requires interdisciplinary collaboration and planning with regular interaction, continuing education, and a regular review of the latest relevant literature. Additionally, frequent communication between orthodontist and oral and maxillofacial surgeon is necessary to achieve superior results.

HISTORY OF SKELETAL ANCHORAGE FOR ORTHODONTICS

Recent technical advances have resulted in an increased level of interest in skeletal anchorage for orthodontic treatment, although the concept of using implantable devices for this purpose has been present for more than a half century.[1–5] Only recently have innovations in materials, new outcome data, and improved techniques thrust this concept forward as a more mainstream option for treatment. In the 1940s, Gainsforth and Higley[6] experimented with vitallium screws and wires in the dog ramus used for skeletal anchorage. This initial experiment was not considered a success.[6] Linkow[7] used blade-type implants in the posterior mandible to apply class II elastics for retraction of maxillary incisors. This cross-arch technique was apparently successful, but had the disadvantage of requiring the surgical placement of a blade implant and then allowing adequate healing time for its osseointegration before use as an anchor. Sherman[8] also used dental implants in dogs for anchorage with limited success. In 1979, Smith[9] noted that dental implants could act like ankylosed teeth during orthodontic movement. In 1988, Shapiro and Kokich[10] discussed how dental implants could be used for orthodontic anchorage before their prosthodontic use, and a number of practitioners used this technique from this point forward. In 1995, Block and Hoffman[11] used a hydroxyapatite-coated onplant placed in the midline palatal tissues for use with an orthodontic anchor device. This was moderately successful, but required the orthodontist to rethink anchorage in terms of palatal mechanics instead of what was typically used with brackets and bands. Costa and coworkers[12] used titanium miniscrews borrowed from plating fixation systems for orthodontic anchorage with some success. In 1999, Umemori and colleagues[3] described techniques for using a modified rigid fixation plate for use as orthodontic anchorage. This was a particularly important leap, because the plating system could be easily placed and significant force could be used without loosening of the device that was seen

rather frequently with individual screws. Loosening of the screw mechanic had been a major drawback of screw systems. Sugawara and colleagues and other authors[3,4,13–17] subsequently described a number of interesting compensation techniques for a variety of problems that traditionally would have required orthognathic surgery to treat, such as the anterior open bite and significant class III deformity.

BASIC ORTHODONTIC MECHANICS AND SKELETAL ANCHORAGE

To understand the indications for skeletal anchorage, the practitioner placing the devices must have a baseline understanding of orthodontic mechanics to ensure superior results. Planning for a team approach to a skeletal anchorage case is in many ways similar to planning for orthognathic surgery. Issues that arise in the preoperative, intraoperative, and postoperative phases of treatment concern both the orthodontist and surgeon. As such, frequent communication must occur to ensure the best outcome.

The term "anchorage," within the context of orthodontic treatment, is defined as the resistance to unwanted tooth movement. The forces involved in orthodontic tooth movement obey Newton's third law, which states that for every action, there is an equal and opposite reaction. For every movement of a tooth in the desired direction, the force is distributed to the anchorage segment, potentially affecting the position of those teeth within the anchorage segment. If an orthodontist wishes to move a canine posterior (distally), but only one molar is present, then the molar has a tendency to drift toward the mesial if the molar is used as an anchor for that movement. If more anchorage is provided to that area, however, then the movement can occur with less of the unwanted mesial movement of the molar.

Using conventional mechanics, anchorage can be increased by using intraoral or extraoral techniques. Intraoral techniques commonly use tooth-borne appliances to improve anchorage. This can be achieved by increasing the number of teeth in the anchorage unit. For example, teeth can be tied together with ligature wire to resist unwanted tooth movement in another area. Another way of increasing teeth in the anchorage segment is to use a transpalatal arch. A transpalatal arch can be fabricated to distribute force to another segment of teeth across the arch. Alternatively, elastic bands can be used between the opposing arches to provide additional anchorage. This technique is commonly used to close space after maxillary premolar extraction by retracting the anterior dentition of the maxilla with elastic bands bilaterally and attaching the elastic to the mandibular posterior teeth. These class II elastics also help to minimize the unwanted mesial movement of the maxillary posterior anchorage segments. This technique is based on compliance, and can be ineffective if the patient does not regularly wear the elastics.

Another way to provide maximum anchorage to the posterior teeth is to use a Nance button appliance that holds the posterior molars in position with an acrylic button on the anterior palate. Force can then be applied to the posterior teeth to close premolar space, and the tendency for the molar teeth to move mesial is resisted by the acrylic button on the palate near the incisive foramen. These appliances may irritate the tissue and become uncomfortable. Extraoral appliances, such as a headgear, can also be used to provide additional anchorage, but are often subject to compliance issues and rarely offer more than 6 to 10 hours of force per day. They are also not readily accepted by some patients, particularly adults.

Skeletal appliances (specialized bone screws or plates) provide anchorage that is not tooth-borne because they are attached to the surrounding bone. As a result, unwanted reciprocal tooth movements involving the surrounding teeth are totally avoided. Other advantages of these devices include the following:

- No or minimal reliance on existing dentition
- Less dependent on patient compliance
- Continuous rather than intermittent force may be applied
- Surgical procedures are necessary, but they are simple in most instances
- May be significantly less expensive than other surgical options, such as orthognathic surgery
- Force may be applied very soon or immediately after placement of the device; devices require mechanical stability instead of osseointegration
- Devices are easily removed.

The anchorage applied may be considered direct or indirect. Direct techniques are those that apply force directly from the anchor to the segment or tooth that is to be moved (**Fig. 1**). For example, maxillary plates placed at the zygomatic buttresses may be designed to provide intrusion force to the maxillary molars with the intent of closing an anterior open bite. This is a direct technique because the force is applied from the anchor directly to the molar teeth. Indirect techniques tie the anchor device to the segment of teeth that requires additional anchorage such that more traditional mechanics can be used in the area (**Fig. 2**). Rather than an active, elastic connection between the anchor and the archwire, indirect anchorage involves an inelastic or even rigid connection between the anchor and the orthodontic appliances. For example, if a maxillary anchor is tied by a steel ligature to the anterior teeth to provide more anchorage to that segment, then a coil spring could be used on the archwire to distalize the molar teeth. This represents an indirect technique because the force used is along the archwire by the coil spring, and represents a traditional type of mechanic in orthodontics. The advantage to the indirect technique is that most orthodontists already design their movements of teeth based on traditional mechanics. Providing additional anchorage by a skeletal device simply increases efficiency without necessitating a new appliance design or vectors and movements difficult to achieve in commonly used orthodontic techniques. Either a direct or indirect technique can be used in most situations, and each case requires careful planning to ensure ideal placement of the anchor for these purposes.

Skeletal anchorage devices allow orthodontic movements to be designed that were previously thought to be difficult, if not impossible.

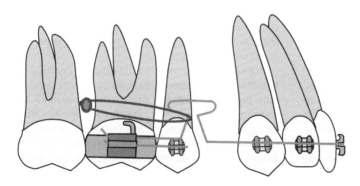

Fig. 1. Direct anchorage is achieved by adding a force from an elastic chain or thread to the loop in an existing orthodontic mechanical system to achieve retraction of the entire anterior segment of teeth. (*Data from* Nanda R. In: Nanda R, editor. Temporary anchorage devices in orthodontics. St Louis: Elsevier; 2008. p. 157.)

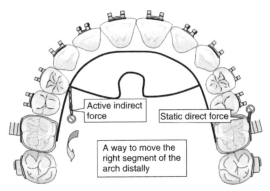

Active indirect force

Static direct force

A way to move the right segment of the arch distally

Fig. 2. An example of indirect anchorage using somewhat complicated palatal mechanics. The left first molar is tied with a ligature wire to a temporary anchor screw providing absolute anchorage. The right segment is planned to move distally, so an elastic chain is threaded from the hook behind the first bicuspid on the transpalatal bar. The final result is distalization of the entire right segment, a vector of force that is traditionally difficult or impossible to achieve with standard mechanics. (*Data from* Anka G. In: Nanda R, editor. Temporary anchorage devices in orthodontics. St Louis: Elsevier; 2008. p. 199.)

Compensation beyond the typical envelope of discrepancy is possible for many clinical indications. Skeletal anchorage devices do not allow faster movement of teeth, or the ability to overcome exceptionally large discrepancies; the devices have limitations. They provide absolute anchorage for orthodontic movement, however, and do so in a number of novel ways. They allow for more efficient movement of teeth and address a number of anchorage problem areas that previously were difficult or impossible to resolve with traditional orthodontic mechanics alone.

DEVICES FOR SKELETAL ANCHORAGE

A number of devices have been used to provide additional anchorage for orthodontic purposes. The early attempts that were successful used dental implants placed with the intention of using them for total skeletal anchorage. These had the significant drawbacks of requiring osteointegration before use and the high cost. They also required aggressive surgery for removal. Although some could be kept in place for prosthetic use, often it was difficult to determine the exact position required at the end of orthodontic treatment when placing them for anchorage purposes before treating the malocclusion. Consequently, the implants were often not in ideal position for the final crown or prosthesis, rendering them either useless or requiring specialized prosthodontic techniques to compensate for poor position.

Various dental implants including miniature dental implants were used in a similar fashion and placed in the retromolar region for anchorage purposes.[8,18] These also required osseointegration before use and surgical removal, and had the same types of drawbacks. Similar devices continue to be used in the palate, either in the midline or parasagittal to the midline. The anatomy in this region does not support full bony integration of an implant in most instances. Midline insertion into the septum may provide initial stability, but may also create problems, such as septal perforation either at the time of placement or at the time of removal. If the implants are placed parasagittal, then a fistula may result when the implant is removed because of the thin bone in this region of the nasal floor and hard palate.

The onplant system, with attachments that penetrate through the palatal tissues for orthodontic anchorage, is an attempt to get around these inadequacies of the endosseous implant approach. These onplants are coated with titanium or hydroxyapatite in the hopes of osseointegration after a small palatal incision is made for a subperiosteal placement. Long-term outcomes of this technique have not been reported, and it has mostly been supplanted by single screws or plates at other locations. As with any palatal implant, the additional drawback of redesigning orthodontic mechanics around a device positioned on the palate requires significant planning by the orthodontist in a manner that is not conventional.

Placement of a bone screw for orthodontic mechanics has been described using a number of different screw devices.[10,14,19,20] Recently, there has been an explosion of these screws commercially available for use. Originally, fixation screws used for craniomaxillofacial surgery were placed and then attached to the orthodontic appliance for use as additional anchorage. Other screw systems used for alternative purposes, such as maxillomandibular fixation, were modified for use as skeletal anchorage. Eventually, screws specifically designed for use in orthodontic skeletal anchorage were manufactured with versatile orthodontic attachments to optimize their use (**Fig. 3**). Both self-tapping and self-drilling systems are currently available.

Screws are typically manufactured in multiple lengths for a number of indications. Short screws can be used, but fail more often because of minimal bone-to-screw interface. Screws that engage cortical bone across the alveolus tend to have more stability, and this technique requires longer screws (8–12 mm). The thread pitch should also be ideal for the type of bone in this area, and

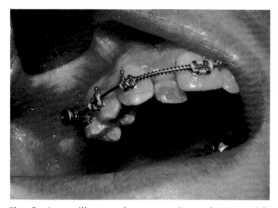

Fig. 3. A maxillary anchor screw is used to provide anchorage to the anterior dentition because of a lack of anchorage in the right posterior maxilla. This allows the orthodontist to distalize the premolars and canine to treat the crowding of the anterior dentition while preserving the dental midline.

typically is approximately 0.6 mm. The attachments come in a variety of designs. The authors prefer an attachment that allows for placement of a ligature, elastomer chain, or wire. Although a number of entities manufacture screws, it is important to consider the quality of the titanium alloy used and the highly engineered aspects of the screw. Poorly made devices are prone to fracture, and as such it is recommended that surgeons use devices with proved use in these indications. Devices should

- Be designed for the purpose of skeletal orthodontic anchorage
- Have a very high quality of manufacturing with standardized quality control
- Have an appropriate pitch thread to ideally engage bone
- Have the appropriate core and external diameter to withstand orthodontic forces in maxillary and mandibular bone
- Be designed well at the runout and shaft-head interface to avoid fracture.

Screws that are smaller than 1.5 mm tend to fail much more often, and are not recommended for indications that require significant force. Additionally, screws with bracket-like head designs offer little advantage to more simple attachments, which tend to be more versatile. Bracket-like attachments require specialized custom bending of the orthodontic wire, and often fail with minimal torque or a force that rotates the screw in the counterclockwise direction, loosening it. The indications, success rates, and limitations of screws used for skeletal anchorage are discussed later.

Plate systems were originally used by Sugawara and others to provide additional three-dimensional stability and increase the success rates over the long-term. Originally these were modified fixation plates used for Le Fort osteotomies and facial trauma repair.[3,4] Eventually, custom-designed plating systems specifically indicated for skeletal orthodontic anchorage were developed.[4,13,21–25] Skeletal anchorage plates have the advantage of increased stability, allowing the use of greater forces. They do not require osseointegration and can be loaded immediately. The plates typically allow for placement of multiple small screws away from the tooth roots, avoiding injury (**Fig. 4**). Skeletal anchorage plates are also easy to remove, but require an additional incision and dissection.

Clinical Indications

Skeletal anchorage devices may be used in many different applications to provide absolute anchorage and optimize the efficiency of tooth movement. The authors prefer plates over screws to provide anchorage using indirect mechanics when possible. Direct anchorage techniques may also be helpful for some indications. Some case examples illustrating the use of skeletal anchorage follow, and new applications are being investigated.

MESIAL OR DISTAL MOVEMENT OF TEETH WITH MAXIMUM ANCHORAGE

The need to move posterior teeth in the mesial direction is difficult because of a lack of anchorage

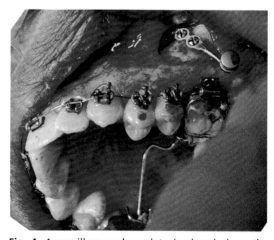

Fig. 4. A maxillary anchor plate is placed along the left maxillary buttress. This allows placement of three or four monocortical screws away from the tooth roots and placement of the orthodontic attachment in an ideal position for intrusion of the maxillary molars.

from the anterior segment.[4,24,25] For example, when an overretained primary first molar is extracted and the succedaneous permanent first bicuspid is missing, the orthodontist may choose to move the remaining posterior tooth or teeth to the mesial to close the space of the primary first molar (**Fig. 5**). This is often difficult because the anterior segment of teeth have a tendency to move to the posterior (distal), causing the incisors to upright and changing the canine position to class II. To maintain the position of the anterior teeth including the class I canine, a skeletal anchor may be placed to provide either indirect anchorage with a rigid attachment to the anterior segment or direct anchorage with and active attachment to the molar segment. This allows for more efficient movement of the posterior molars to close the space, without loosing the position of the canine or disrupting the overbite-overjet relationship of the incisors. To improve a class II relationship, a variety of tooth movements are possible including distalizing the maxillary teeth. By moving the maxillary molars distally, space can be created to reduce the overjet and to achieve a class I canine relationship (**Figs. 6 and 7**).[14,25]

Alternatively, if a patient presents with a class III discrepancy, then the orthodontist may choose to compensate by providing maximum anchorage to the mandibular posterior teeth or to distalize mandibular molar teeth.[26] This allows the mandibular anterior dentition to be retracted and to close the space while providing maximum anchorage to the distal (posterior) segment of teeth. Without

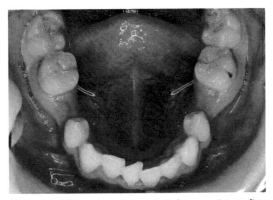

Fig. 5. A patient who has lost their lower primary first molars has good position of the canines (class I), and lacks enough anchorage posteriorly to close the space without the unwanted distal movement of the canines. This is a frequent problem for orthodontists who need to close space with maximum anchorage. Anchorage plates or screws can provide absolute anchorage to close the space efficiently without unwanted tooth movements.

skeletal anchorage, this may be difficult to achieve because the posterior teeth have a tendency to move toward the mesial when using traditional mechanics (**Fig. 8**).

It follows that these techniques can be helpful after extraction of bicuspids if the orthodontist wishes to close the space with maximum anchorage in either segment. Although this is easily done with traditional orthodontic mechanics, in certain instances when anchorage is lacking, or maximum anchorage is desired, then skeletal anchorage appliances can be used to maximize efficiency.

UPRIGHTING OR INTRUDING MOLAR TEETH

One of the more difficult movements in orthodontic treatment is uprighting a molar tooth that has moved mesially into an edentulous space. Most often this occurs in the adult patient who has lost their first molar to caries and the second molar tips to the mesial over a period of time. Subsequent to this event, if a patient presents for orthodontic treatment, it may be very difficult to upright the second molar without extruding the tooth and opening the patient's bite.[14,15,22] With the use of a skeletal anchor, the tooth may be uprighted without the untoward extrusion that often results with conventional orthodontic techniques.

Another difficult problem to remedy is the over-erupted maxillary or mandibular tooth that is in poor position because of an edentulous space in the opposite arch. Intruding teeth in this situation is exceptionally difficult using traditional orthodontic mechanics. The use of a skeletal anchorage device makes intrusion a relatively easy orthodontic movement.[22] This technique may be used in the anterior or posterior dentition. Patients who have a deep class II relationship with excessive overbite can have their anterior maxillary dentition intruded and retropositioned to improve the overbite-overjet relationship. Typically, this is done with an intrusion arch or other traditional mechanics, such as headgear. With skeletal anchorage devices, this is made much more efficient and also requires very little compliance from the patient.

CLOSURE OF ANTERIOR OPEN BITE

There has been a great degree of excitement generated by the initial reports of anterior open bite closure with orthodontic anchorage appliances.[3,4,13,16,22,27–29] Typically, this is performed by placing orthodontic plates or screws in the posterior maxilla, apical to the dentition. Force is then generated to intrude the posterior molars

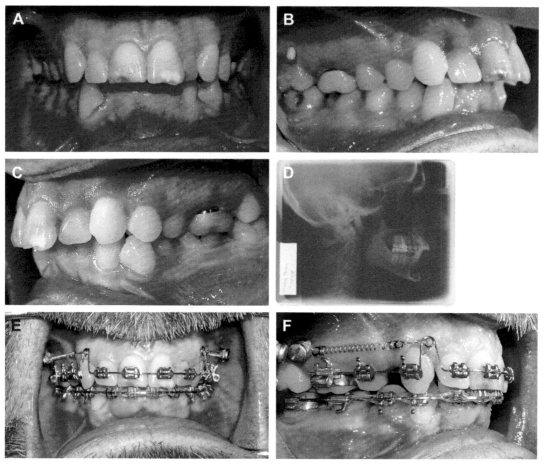

Fig. 6. A patient with a significant class II relationship who is unwilling to undergo orthognathic surgery has upper first premolar extractions, and lower second premolar extractions in preparation for orthodontic therapy. The space in the maxilla is closed with the aid of anchor screws, which allow for closure of the space by bodily moving the anterior centrals, laterals, and canines en mass. (*A–C*) Preoperative occlusion photos. (*D*) Preoperative lateral cephalometric radiograph. (*E, F*) Postoperative occlusion photos after 6 months of orthodontic therapy with closure of the space and improvement of the class II relationship. The force is generated at the optimized vector to allow for efficient movement.

and premolars (as necessary) to close the anterior open bite. A number of case reports have shown this to be successful. Excitement has grown in this area because of the difficulty typically encountered with orthodontic-only closure of the anterior open bite, and the subsequent relapse that often occurs. The alternative is orthognathic repositioning with the presumed improvement in stability. Although the use of skeletal anchorage to close anterior open bite is reported to be stable in case reports and a few case series publications, there are no long-term data on stability of these procedures as there has been for orthognathic surgery.

For this reason, the authors prefer to use this technique for those patients who cannot or will not undergo orthognathic surgery, and for those patients who have minimal open bites. Patients who have already failed orthodontic treatment for

closure of their open bites may be good candidates for this procedure, but retreatment does come with additional risk, such as root resorption. Orthodontists should be careful to not extrude the anterior maxillary teeth, which likely decreases long-term stability of the correction. Intrusion of the posterior maxillary dentition is preferred and has been shown to be effective. Patients should be cautioned regarding the expectations of outcome over the long-term. It is expected that more data will become available to assess the safety, efficacy, and long-term stability of this treatment option.

ORTHOPEDIC GROWTH MODIFICATION

An area of considerable interest is the use of skeletal anchorage to provide forces for orthopedic

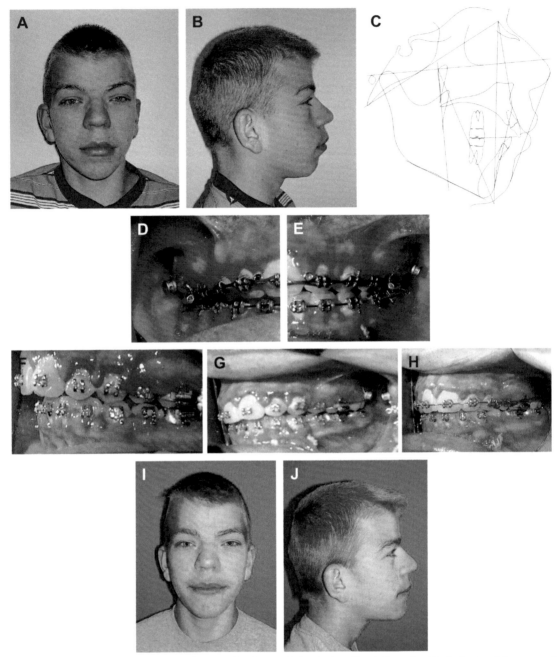

Fig. 7. A patient with Noonan's syndrome who has a skeletal class II relationship. His behavioral issues and bleeding disorder (both associated with this syndrome) make him a poor candidate for orthognathic or other craniofacial procedures. His class II is compensated by distalizing the entire maxillary dentition with two skeletal anchors placed in the posterior maxilla. Over time he develops a class I relationship. At the time of the anchor placement, a genioplasty is performed to balance his facial profile. (*A, B*) Preoperative facial photographs. (*C*) Cephalometric tracing showing a significant class II relationship that would typically be treated with orthognathic surgery. (*D, E*) Photographs of the anchors in place after several weeks with minimal inflammation. (*F–H*) Photographs of the progression of treatment over 9 months as the class II discrepancy improves. (*I, J*) Posttreatment facial photographs.

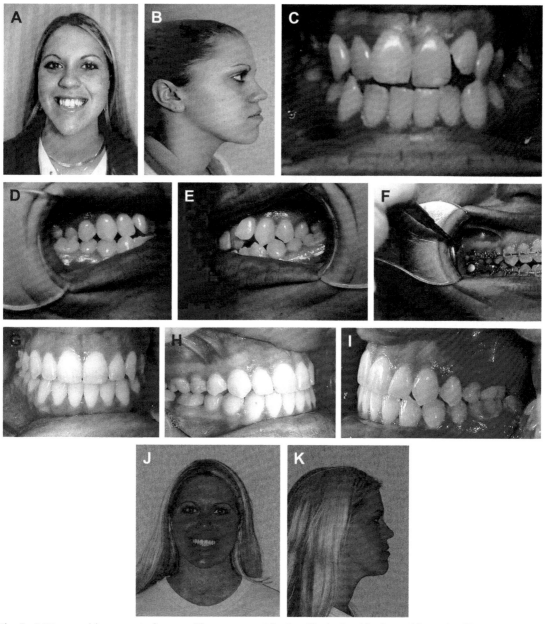

Fig. 8. A 21-year-old woman is shown with an asymmetric class III relationship, but without significant transverse discrepancy. She was unwilling to consider an orthognathic surgery treatment option, so one skeletal anchor plate was placed in the posterior right mandible to bring the entire mandibular dentition to her right. This allowed for distal movement of most of the mandibular arch of teeth, and establishment of a class I canine relationship. (*A–E*) Pretreatment photographs. (*F*) Mandibular anchor plate in place with orthodontic anchorage activated. (*G–K*) Posttreatment photographs.

growth modification in a manner similar to the use of headgear appliances. This has been used by some practioners for children during phase I orthodontic therapy. For patients with a class III skeletal pattern (midface hypoplasia or mandibular prognathism), skeletal anchors can be placed in the mandible and maxilla to provide forward orthopedic force to the maxilla and encourage a more class I relationship.[30] The vector of force is similar to reverse-pull headgear without the need for an external appliance. The mechanics involved are more favorable because of the constant force provided rather than relying on the patient to wear the appliance only for a prescribed time.

Although the concept has been reported in the literature, there is little evidence of its efficacy or safety. Practitioners must be careful to avoid developing tooth structures, and minimize surgical procedures in this growing population so as not to hamper tooth or bone growth. More literature is necessary before the widespread use of this technique.

Surgical Procedures

The application of temporary anchorage devices for orthodontic treatment usually requires only a minor surgical procedure. The exact type of anchor (miniscrew or specialized anchor plate), location, and angle of the device are determined by the orthodontic treatment plan. Preoperative planning requires a careful clinical examination; at least a panoramic radiograph; and clear communication between the orthodontist and surgeon regarding positioning, activation, and removal.

PLACEMENT OF SKELETAL ANCHORAGE PLATES

Bone plates used for anchorage during orthodontic treatment can be placed in a variety of anatomic locations within the maxillary and mandibular arches. These devices typically consist of a bone plate with holes for screw placement and a transmucosal connecting arm that extends from the plate to a specialized working end. The working end of the appliance allows for the attachment of wire, springs, elastics, and other orthodontic constructs.

Within the maxillary arch, the anchor plate is typically placed within one of the vertical buttresses of the midface (eg, zygomaticomaxillary buttress or piriform buttress) where the bone thickness allows for adequate mechanical stability using monocortical screws. Monocortical screws are preferred for fixation of the plate. The mid-anterior maxillary wall is avoided because of the thin cortical bone that is present directly over the maxillary sinuses and the proximity of the infraorbital neurovascular bundle. These considerations are reminiscent of the rationale applied when placing maxillary bone plates within the piriform and zygomatic buttresses during orthognathic surgery and the repair of mid-face fractures.

The procedure is easy to perform for most patients (**Figs. 9** and **10**). First, a vertical incision, approximately 8 to 10 mm in length, is created from the mucogingival junction superiorly into the maxillary vestibule. A small horizontal releasing incision is usually added along the mucogingival line to improve direct visualization and minimize retraction-related trauma to the soft tissues during anchor placement. A periosteal elevator is used to develop a full-thickness mucoperiosteal flap exposing the underlying skeletal buttress. The anchor device is then carefully adapted so that the plate and connecting bar closely follow the contour of the underlying cortical bone of the zygomaticomaxillary or piriform buttress region. Care should be taken to avoid any dead-space or gaps between the bone and the implanted portion of the device. Another critical technical consideration is the location of the connecting bar as it exits the subperiosteal pocket and enters into the oral cavity. The transmucosal position of the connecting bar should be located at approximately the mucogingival junction. Nonkeratinized mucosal tissues should be avoided. When the transmucosal location of the connecting bar is within the unattached tissues of the maxillary vestibule, increased irritation, inflammation, infection, and soft tissue overgrowth may result. Once the anchor has been appropriately contoured and positioned, it is secured using self-drilling or self-tapping monocortical screws. The incision is irrigated and soft tissue closure is carried out using resorbable suture material.

In contrast with the maxilla, the facial cortex of the mandible is composed of dense bone that allows for stable placement of skeletal anchorage devices. Despite the favorable cortical nature of the mandible, however, specific, key anatomic structures including the mental foramen and nerve, and the mandibular canal must be avoided during placement. Placement of anchors in the mandible is most frequently carried out within the symphysis, posterior body, and ramus. In cases where the bone plate is positioned directly over the mandibular canal, monocortical screws should be used to avoid injury to the inferior alveolar neurovascular bundle.

When skeletal anchorage plates are used, the bone plate portion of the device is positioned away from the tooth roots. Even in certain cases, where the bone plate must be placed in closer proximity to the adjacent teeth, the risk of damage to the underlying root structure remains very low. The use of short bone screws that engage only the outer (facial) cortex avoids damage to dental structures and allows for the orthodontic movement of teeth with minimal risk of hardware-related impingement on the roots.

The placement of a skeletal anchorage plate is usually carried out using local anesthesia. The use of local anesthesia in combination with light conscious sedation may be preferable depending on the specific surgical plan, the number of anchors being placed, and patient preference.

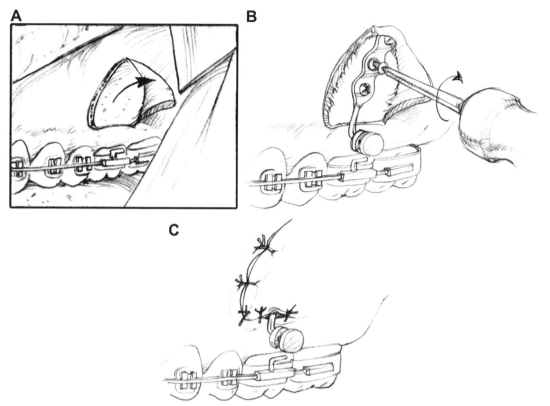

Fig. 9. (*A–C*) Maxillary anchor plate procedure. A small L-shaped incision is used at the mucogingival junction to allow for placement of an anchor plate. Three screws or more are placed with appropriate positioning for the indicated orthodontic mechanics. Closure is achieved with resorbable suture.

PLACEMENT OF MINISCREWS FOR SKELETAL ANCHORAGE

Skeletal anchorage miniscrews are placed near or at the mucogingival junction and engage the cortical and cancellous bone layers. Because the entire anchorage device is dependent on the stability of the single screw, the longest length possible is usually placed. In the maxillary arch, placement can be undertaken at the buttresses (ie, zygomatic or piriform); the hard palate; or within the alveolar process in-between tooth roots. Within the mandible, placement can be undertaken along the alveolar process at the mucogingival junction, the symphysis, and within the retromolar pad region. Because the screws extend into the trabecullar bone, the subsequent orthodontic movement of tooth roots must be anticipated.

The surgical procedure for placement of miniscrews is minimally invasive and does not typically require the elevation of a soft tissue flap. Local anesthesia is used and a simple infiltration is usually adequate for placement of a single bone screw. In areas where a more pronounced tissue depth or thick fibrous tissue is encountered, a small tissue punch or surgical blade may be used to create a small puncture site for introduction. A number of self-drilling screws are available that allow for placement of the anchor screw without the creation of a pilot hole within the outer cortex of the maxilla. When anchor screw placement is undertaken within the mandibular arch, the use of self-drilling screws is generally avoided. The density and thickness of the mandibular cortical plate may cause fracture of the screw when a self-drilling anchor is used. Instead, a pilot hole is made using the surgical handpiece and a self-tapping anchorage screw is placed.

Postoperative Regimen

Postoperative radiographs may be obtained to confirm the position of the skeletal anchorage devices relative to the surrounding anatomic structures. A panoramic radiograph is usually adequate. In cases where miniscrews are placed in between teeth, periapical radiographs may be useful in examining the proximity of adjacent tooth roots.

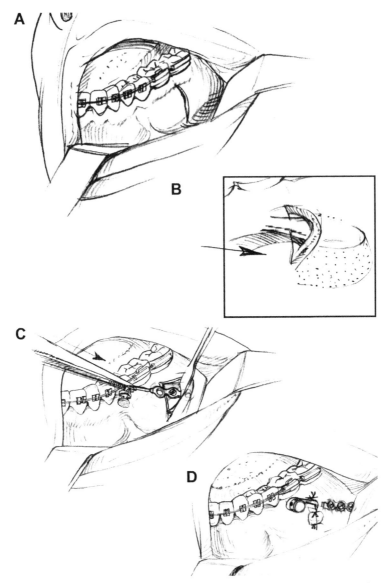

Fig. 10. (*A–D*) Mandibular anchor plate procedure. A small linear or L-shaped incision is used to position the plate in a manner ideal for orthodontic mechanics of the specific case. The incision is placed at or near the mucogingival junction if possible to avoid inflammation. Closure is achieved with resorbable suture.

Because the implants used for skeletal anchorage are transmucosal and involve a portion of hardware that remains exposed to the oral cavity, antibiotic coverage is used during the postoperative phase. Patients are given a 5-day course of oral antibiotics following surgical placement. The most commonly used agents include penicillin, amoxicillin, and clindamycin. In addition, meticulous oral hygiene and chlorhexidine oral rinses during the first week postsurgery dramatically reduce the amount of soft tissue inflammation and risk of infection.

Pain and discomfort following miniscrew placement is generally minimal. Patients undergoing anchor plate placement may require a short course of analgesic coverage because the procedure involves the creation of an incision and greater soft tissue dissection. Patients may also report cheek irritation, which tends to peak at approximately 10 days following surgery before resolving.

Because temporary anchorage devices require primary mechanical stability, and not osseointegration, they may be used for orthodontic treatment immediately following surgical place-ment. Miniscrews may be activated immediately after surgical placement. Manipulation of full orthodontic force using a skeletal anchorage plate is usually delayed for 7 to 10 days following place-ment. This allows for adequate healing at the site of the mucoperiosteal flap and at the soft tissue of the mucogingival junction where the connecting bar is located.

OUTCOMES AND COMPLICATIONS

Although in general the procedures described previously are reported as being very successful, the overall success rate of screw and plate systems warrants a special discussion. There is considerable variation in the reported success of these techniques, and a number of opinions regarding the exact indications for the choice of plates over screws in a given clinical situation. Placement of a screw or plate system is associ-ated with few complications, but the surgeon must be aware of those rare occurrences that can create issues for patients. Problems related to skeletal orthodontic anchorage appliances are typically screw, patient, or operator related.

The overall success rates vary between devices rather dramatically. A number of reports have listed loosening or outright failure of orthodontic anchorage screws to be above 15%.[12,14,19,20,23,31–34] In some indications and anatomic locations, the rate of loos-ening of the screw is higher than 30%. As might be expected, the rate of failure of plates is considerably lower with failure rates below 5%.[4,23,24,27] It is impor-tant to recognize that most of the data published are reported by the individuals who placed and used the devices, and as such the definition of failure may vary. There is an inherent self-reporting bias with such liter-ature. Plate systems offer a greater degree of three-dimensional stability, and a higher integration with the bone structure because of the multiple screws used for fixation. Consequently, the authors tend to use bone plates more often than screws for cases that require longer treatment times or greater forces. Many surgeons and orthodontists believe plates to be more stable, but they often are concerned regarding the additional incision and dissection required for placement despite the minor nature of the procedure.[35] Additionally, although reports of improved outcomes using these techniques appear in the literature, not many prospective studies in the level I evidence category exist.[36] Most studies have significant reporting bias, disparate patient popula-tions, and data analysis flaws.[36,37] Although the avail-able literature is encouraging, any innovation requires scrutiny and comparative study to ultimately deter-mine its use in the treatment armamentarium.

Complications related to the device itself can occur because of device failure (fracture); loos-ening associated with a design flaw; or infection. Most devices are made of titanium alloy that is of a sufficient quality to avoid deformation of the threads, breakage of the screw head or shaft, or fragmentation of the metal during placement with the driver. Manufacturers with experience manufacturing plates and screws rarely encounter issues with material failure because of the exten-sive experience with materials used in rigid internal fixation. If the titanium is not sufficiently strong or the manufacturing process for producing the screw or instrumentation has flaws, then the screw or plate may be more likely to break or fatigue quickly. This can lead to device failure. Screws that are designed with an appropriate pitch thread for the soft bone of the maxilla may also fail because of a lack of contact with cortical bone. This is also true if the run-out of the screw is partic-ularly long because the screw threads do not inter-face with adequate cortical bone for stability. The screw prematurely loosens in this setting. Although infection is rare in this area, it does occur, and the devices should be sterilized before insertion.

Operator-related complications can also occur for a variety of reasons. Small screw systems require very careful placement, and a fine tactile sense is necessary to avoid stripping the bone-screw interface during placement. Overworking the screw material can also lead to failure. Poor stability can also occur because of a poor choice of placement, such as in the mid-maxillary antral sinus wall. Bone is not adequate in this area to support fixation in most patients, and individual screws or plates are prone to failure. Most screws and the working attachments of plates should enter the oral cavity within attached mucosa if possible. Significant inflammation, pain, and even infection may result if moveable mucosa surrounds the screw head or working end of an anchor plate system.

The device must be placed in a location that is helpful for the orthodontic mechanics required by the orthodontist. This should be the case throughout the entire treatment period. For example, if a screw is placed within alveolar bone to allow for distal movement of teeth just anterior to that screw, then the eventual location of those teeth should be anticipated after they are moved. Will the device be in the way of moving teeth? Will it need to be replaced? Is it far enough away from the point of attachment to allow for all of the movement necessary throughout the case? All of these questions should be addressed at the treatment planning stage before surgical placement of the device to avoid the need for additional surgery.

One area requiring special attention is that of root damage from either placement of a screw or the drilling process. Surgeons who are comfortable with the anatomy of these regions typically do not have issues with root damage, but this may still occur because of anatomic variation or other causes. Thankfully, roots have excellent recuperative power that allows for recuperation if a minimal insult occurs. If a device has been placed and the screw is in contact with the root of a viable tooth, then the patient typically experiences discomfort during mastication. Moving the root away from the implant typically relieves this discomfort, or the device can be replaced in a new location.

A number of patient-related complications also can occur. Patients must have good-quality bone to accept the devices and have reasonable hygiene. Quality cortical bone is a necessity for long-term stability of the anchors. Patients who have systemic disorders that affect bone or mucosal healing are not good candidates for these procedures. Likewise, those patients who have undergone radiation therapy in the region or are taking bisphosphonate medications are not good candidates. Those patients who smoke are also prone to mucosal breakdown, infection, and failure of the devices.

SUMMARY

Skeletal anchorage devices allow orthodontic movements that were previously thought to be difficult if not impossible. The devices do not accelerate tooth movement, but do provide the greatest amount of anchorage in a manner that is bone-borne, creating more efficient mechanics for moving teeth while avoiding unwanted (reciprocal) tooth movement in a number of challenging clinical situations. Additionally, unwanted reciprocal tooth movements are minimized or avoided altogether. An additional advantage is the use of mechanics for which the success is not based on compliance factors, such as with headgear or elastic band therapy that requires patient placement and removal. Multiple applications, devices, and technique innovations are evolving. Caution is warranted for some applications because long-term data are not available at this time. It is hoped that additional data will become prevalent and help decide how skeletal anchorage fits in best with the armamentarium of treatment choices for significant skeletal and dental discrepancies.

REFERENCES

1. Park HS, Kim JB. The use of titanium microscrew implant as orthodontic anchorage. Keimyung Med J 1999;18:509–15.
2. Park HS, Bae SM, Kyung HM, et al. Microimplant anchorage for treatment of skeletal class I bialveolar protrusion. J Clin Orthod 2001;35:417–22.
3. Umemori M, Sugawara J, Mitani H, et al. Skeletal anchorage system for open-bite correction. Am J Orthod Dentofacial Orthop 1999;115:166–74.
4. Sugawara J. Dr. Junji Sugawara on the skeletal anchorage system. J Clin Orthod 1999;33:689–96.
5. Bae SM, Park HS, Kyung HM, et al. Clinical application of micro-implant anchorage. J Clin Orthod 2002; 36:298–302.
6. Gainsforth BL, Higley LB. A study of orthodontic anchorage possibilities in basal bone. Am J Orthod 1945;31:406–17.
7. Linkow LI. The endosseous blade implant and its use in orthodontics. J Orthod 1969;18:149–54.
8. Sherman AJ. Bone reaction to orthodontic forces on vitreous carbon dental implants. Am J Orthod 1978; 74:79–87.
9. Smith JR. Bone dynamics associated with the controlled loading of bioglass-coated aluminum endosteal implants. Am J Orthod 1979;76:618–36.
10. Shapiro PA, Kokich VG. Uses of implants in orthodontics. Dent Clin North Am 1988;32:539–50.
11. Block MS, Hoffman DR. A new device of absolute anchorage for orthodontics. Am J Orthod Dentofacial Orthop 1995;107:251–8.
12. Costa A, Raffini M, Melsen B. Microscrew as orthodontic anchorage. Int J Adult Orthodon Orthognath Surg 1998;13:201–9.
13. Sherwood K. Closing anterior open bites by intruding molars with titanium miniplate anchorage. Am J Orthod Dentofacial Orthop 2002;122:593–600.
14. Sung J, Kyung H, Bae S, et al. Microimplants in orthodontics. Daegu (Korea): Dentos; 2006. p. 1–173.
15. Park HS, Kyung HM, Sung JH. A simple method of molar uprighting with micro-implant anchorage. J Clin Orthod 2002;36:592–6.
16. Park HS. Clinical study of the success rate of microscrew implants for orthodontic anchorage. Korean. J Orthod 2003;33:151–6.
17. Woo SS, Jeong ST, Huh YS, et al. A clinical study of the skeletal anchorage system using miniscrews. J Korean Oral Maxillofac Surg 2003;29:102–7.
18. Roberts WE, Smith RK, Zilberman Y, et al. Osseous adaptation to continuous loading of rigid endosseous implants. Am J Orthod 1984;86:95–111.
19. Tseng YC, Hsieh CH, Chen CH, et al. The application of mini-implants for orthodontic anchorage. Int J Oral Maxillofac Surg 2006;35:704–7.
20. Cornelis MA, De Clerck HJ. Maxillary molar distalization with miniplates assessed on digital models:

a prospective clinical trial. Am J Orthod Dentofacial Orthop 2007;132(3):373–7.

21. Jenner JD, Fitzpatrick BN. Skeletal anchorage utilising bone plates. Aust Orthod J 1985;9(2):231–3.

22. Sherwood K. Intrusion of supererupted molars with titanium miniplate anchorage. Angle Orthod 2003; 73(5):597–601.

23. Cornelis MA, Scheffler NR, De Clerck HJ, et al. Systematic review of the experimental use of temporary skeletal anchorage devices in orthodontics. American Journal of Orthodontics & Dentofacial Orthopedics 2007;131(Suppl 4):S52–8.

24. Cornelis MA, De Clerck HJ. Biomechanics of skeletal anchorage. Part 1. Class II extraction treatment. J Clin Orthod 2006;40(4):261–9, quiz 232.

25. De Clerck HJ, Cornelis MA. Biomechanics of skeletal anchorage. Part 2: Class II nonextraction treatment. J Clin Orthod 2006;40(5):290–8, quiz 307.

26. Sugawara J, Daimaruya T, Umemori M. Distal movement of mandibular molars in adult patients with the skeletal anchorage system. Am J Orthod Dentofacial Orthop 2004;125(2):624–9.

27. Sugawara J, Baik UB, Umemori M, et al. Treatment and posttreatment dentoalveolar changes following intrusion of mandibular molars with application of a skeletal anchorage (SAS) for open bite correction. Int J Adult Orthodon Orthognath Surg 2002;17(4): 243–53.

28. Kuroda S, Sakai Y, Tamamura N, et al. Treatment of severe anterior open bite with skeletal anchorage in adults: comparison with orthognathic surgery outcomes. Am J Orthod Dentofacial Orthop 2007; 132(5):599–605.

29. Erverdi N, Keles A, Nanda R. The use of skeletal anchorage in open bite treatment: a cephalometric evaluation. Angle Orthod. 2004;74(3):381–90.

30. Kircelli BH, Pektas ZO, Uckan S. Orthopedic protraction with skeletal anchorage in a patient with maxillary hypoplasia and hypodontia. Angle Orthod 2006; 76(1):156–63.

31. Miyawaki S, Koyama I, Inoue M. Factors associated with the stability of titanium screws placed in the posterior region for orthodontic anchorage. Am J Orthod Dentofacial Orthop 2001;124(4):236–42.

32. Liou EJ, Pai BC, Lin JC. Do miniscrews remain stationary under orthodontic forces? Am J Orthod Dentofacial Orthop 2004;126:42–7.

33. Favero L, Brollo P, Bressan E. Orthodontic anchorage with specific fixtures: related study analysis. Am J Orthod Dentofacial Orthop 2002;122(1).

34. Wilmes B, Rademacher C, Olthoff G, et al. Parameters affecting primary stability of orthodontic mini-implants. J Orofac Orthop 2006;67(3):162–74.

35. Cornelis MA, Scheffler NR, Nyssen-Behets C, et al. Patients' and orthodontists' perceptions of miniplates used for temporary skeletal anchorage: a prospective study. Am J Orthod Dentofacial Orthop 2008;133(1):18–24.

36. Lai EH, Yao CC, Chang JZ, et al. Three-dimensional dental model analysis of treatment outcomes for protrusive maxillary dentition: comparison of headgear, miniscrew, and miniplate skeletal anchorage. Am J Orthod Dentofacial Orthop 2008;134:636–45.

37. Rahimi H. Methodology for orthodontic anchorage study questioned. Am J Orhod Dentofacial Orthop 2009;135:559.

Advances in Head and Neck Imaging

Tao Ouyang, MD[a], Barton F. Branstetter IV, MD[b],*

KEYWORDS

- Computed tomography • Magnetic resonance imaging
- Positron emission tomography
- Radiology in dental and craniomaxillofacial practice

After Wilhelm Roentgen discovered x-rays in 1895, the head and neck region began to be explored in ways that had never been possible before. Suddenly, the osseous structures and the overlying soft tissues could be visualized using various projections using plain film radiography. Fluoroscopy was subsequently introduced, enabling dynamic evaluation of the upper aerodigestive tract and the esophagus with excellent detail.

Linear tomography became available in the 1930s. Subsequently, circular, elliptical, and hypocloidal tomographic tube motions were introduced to evaluate the complex structures of the head and neck, including the facial bones and the temporal bones. Tomography continues to be fundamental in dental imaging with the use of panoramic oral radiographs.

Computed tomography (CT) and magnetic resonance imaging (MRI) were introduced in the 1970s and 1980s and have since become the mainstay of cross-sectional imaging of the human body. With the advent of multislice scanners, which increase resolution and decrease scan time, CT technology has been especially important in changing the landscape of oral and maxillofacial imaging. MRI, with its ability to delineate marrow and soft tissue pathology, especially with the use of gadolinium contrast material, is often complementary to CT. MRI is also vital in the imaging of the temporomandibular joint (TMJ).

Finally, advances have also been made in the field of nuclear medicine. Nuclear medicine had traditionally relied on isotopes, such as those of indium and gallium, for tumor and infection imaging. While the use of such isotopes had been useful, it has been made somewhat obsolete by advances in cross-sectional imaging, especially with the use of intravenous contrast material. However, combination positron emission tomography and CT (PET/CT), introduced in the 1990s, has revolutionized imaging and surveillance of head and neck cancer and has become a vital part of oncological care.

COMPUTED TOMOGRAPHY

When CT was first introduced, it was extremely time-consuming, requiring about 5 minutes per image. It was first used in brain imaging only where a few select slices were imaged. Since then, many advances have been made in CT to enable faster scanning. Helical multidetector CT (MDCT) is the new standard in CT imaging of facial trauma, infections, and neoplasms of the head and neck.

CT uses Hounsfield values as a measure of the attenuation of tissues and assigns shades of gray to different values in generating an image. Depending on the range of values, any particular image can be "windowed" to the anatomy of interest (eg, bone, soft tissues, or brain).

Conventional CT scanners use a single row or multiples (4, 8, 12, 32, and now 64) of solid-state detectors paired with a fan-shaped beam to capture the attenuated x-ray. MDCT depends on pitch, collimation, and reconstruction thickness to make an image. Pitch is the amount of movement of the table through the gantry during one revolution of the detectors. Collimation is the width of the detector

[a] Department of Radiology, Penn State Hershey Medical Center, Hershey, PA, USA
[b] Department of Radiology, University of Pittsburgh Medical Center, 200 Lothrop Street, PUH Room D132, Pittsburgh, PA 15213
* Corresponding author.
E-mail address: Bfb1@pitt.edu

Oral Maxillofacial Surg Clin N Am 22 (2010) 107–115
doi:10.1016/j.coms.2009.10.002

elements. Multiple detectors enable acquisition of several (as many as the number of detectors or "slices") images at once. This increases the speed at which the scan can be completed and enables images made up of thinner slices, thus providing better spatial resolution. Sixteen-slice scanners have been widely available for years, while 64-slice MDCT scanners became available in 2004 and represent significant improvements in image quality and scan time.[1] Decreased scan time is extremely important in the trauma setting as patients are often clinically unstable.

Multislice helical imaging provides excellent detail and is superior to panoramic radiograph in displaying the multiplicity of fragments, degree of dislocation or rotation, and/or skull base involvement in trauma.[2] MDCT also accommodates multiplanar reformats (MPRs). Traditionally, facial CT was often performed in the direct coronal plane. Now all images can be acquired in the axial plane and reformatted into coronal and sagittal planes. Coronal MPRs, rather than direct coronals, are advantageous in the trauma setting because trauma patients, often with cervical spine injuries, are limited in terms of positioning for direct coronal scanning. New postprocessing software for MDCT also makes possible three-dimensional (3D) volume-rendered reconstructions, which can be very useful in surgical planning for trauma and reconstructive imaging of the face.

MPRs can aid in the detection of subtle fractures (**Figs. 1** and **2**). Fractures oriented in the horizontal plane often are occult on the axial images. A study of 35 patients with complex maxillofacial trauma showed that, in 26 cases (74%), MPRs and 3D reconstructions were able to either better detail axial findings or show new injuries not discernible on axial images alone.[3] The same study showed coronal MPRs to be particularly useful in imaging the cribriform plate and the orbital floor and roof. Sagittal MPRs represent an entirely new plane of imaging that would not be otherwise possible. Sagittal MPRs are powerful for visualization of mandibular fractures; in particular, they can offer information about the alignment of the TMJs and the integrity of the inferior alveolar canal.

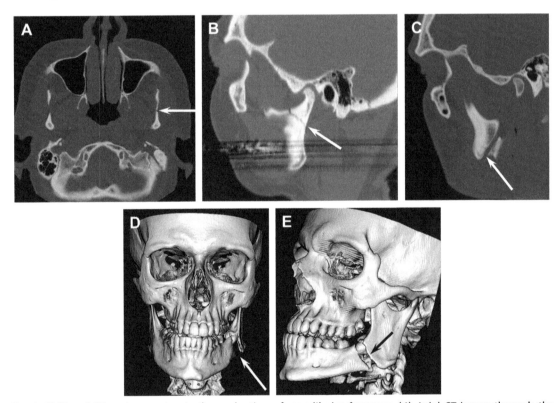

Fig. 1. Utility of CT postprocessing in the evaluation of mandibular fractures. (*A*) Axial CT image through the mandibular ramus depicts a subtle fracture of the left sigmoid notch (*arrow*). The fracture might be easily overlooked in this plane. (*B*) The subcondylar fracture (*arrow*) is much more evident, and better characterized, on sagittal reformatted image. (*C*) Sagittal reformatted image in another patient demonstrates the relationship between the fracture and the inferior alveolar canal (*arrow*). (*D*) Surface-rendered 3D reconstruction in frontal projection provides surgeons with an excellent gestalt of the fracture pattern (*arrow*). (*E*) Surface renderings can be performed in any projection to best depict the fracture (*arrow*).

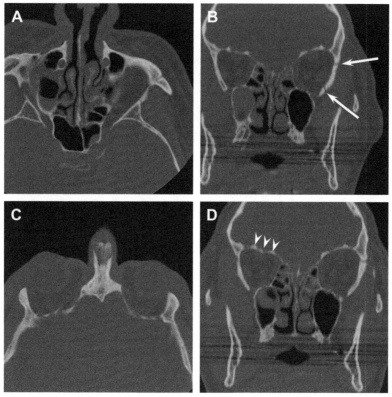

Fig. 2. Utility of CT postprocessing in the evaluation of orbital fractures. (*A*) Axial CT through the orbits does not identify any orbital fractures. (*B*) Coronal reformatted image clearly shows the two fractures (*arrows*) of the left orbital wall. (*C*) Axial CT in another patient demonstrates apparent symmetry between the orbital roofs. (*D*) Coronal reformatted image shows the depressed fracture of the right orbital roof (*arrowheads*).

Because information can be acquired in the helical mode in MDCT, axial reformats can also be rendered. These renderings can be very helpful if the patient positioning was suboptimal, which is often the case in trauma settings. This obviates rescanning the patient, saving radiation dose as well as time.

Panoramic reformats can also be obtained. This is useful in surgical planning for dental implants.[4] Oblique reformatted images can be obtained through the axis of each tooth (**Fig. 3**). This represents a significant advantage over traditional panoramic radiographs for several reasons, not the least of which is higher resolution. Panoramic radiographs, because of the curved cassette used in their acquisition, present a special challenge to digital conversion and storage in a readily available digital archiving system. Traditional films are easily lost, not easily transportable, and require space and manpower to store in libraries. However, the panoramic radiograph is by no means obsolete. Panoramic radiographs are inexpensive and easily accessible. They are also easy to perform in office settings, where they are often obtained. Therefore, the panoramic radiograph

will continue to serve as a useful diagnostic and screening modality for dental disease, although MDCT is superior for evaluation of mandibular fractures and mass lesions.

Faster scan times using MDCT also permit dynamic maneuvers to better evaluate mucosa in the head and neck, in particular the "puffed-cheek technique," to examine closely opposing mucosal surfaces in the oral cavity (**Fig. 4**).[5] Other dynamic maneuvers include modified Valsalva, open-mouth, and phonation maneuvers.[6]

There are several limitations of MDCT as well. Chief among them is radiation risk. Artifacts can also be an issue, especially in the head and neck, where the anatomy is complex and many different tissues types are in close proximity. Beam-hardening artifact, from bone, hardware, or dental amalgam, can obscure images of nearby soft tissues. Motion (eg, from swallowing or phonation) can also cause artifacts, although this is less of an issue with the most current 64-slice scanners, which require less scan time.

Another advance in CT technology that merits discussion is cone-beam CT, which has been

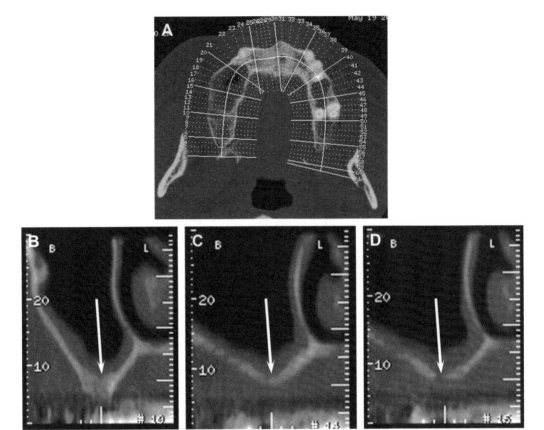

Fig. 3. Utility of CT postprocessing for evaluating the alveolus. (*A*) Scout axial CT image delineates the angles of the reconstructed sagittal oblique images designed to be perpendicular to the alveolar ridge. Each image is numbered so that the exact location can be referenced. The resulting reformatted images show normal thickness of the alveolar ridge (*arrow* in *B*), thinning of the ridge (*arrow* in *C*), or breakthrough into the maxillary sinus (*arrow* in *D*).

commercially available since the beginning of this decade. Cone-beam CT scanners use a cone-shaped beam, rather than a fan-shaped beam of x-rays. The x-ray source and detector make one full rotation around the patient's head and generate "projection data". These data are then processed to generate 3D volumetric data, from which reconstructed images in all three planes can be obtained. Cone-beam CT also has MPR and curved planar capabilities. Its chief advantages are lower radiation dose compared with MDCT,[7] rapid scan time (comparable with that of MDCT systems), availability of display modes unique to maxillofacial imaging, and smaller size and cost than conventional CT units, making it more suitable for use in clinical dental practices.[8,9] Currently, cone-beam CT is best suited to evaluate osseous structures in the craniofacial area (**Fig. 5**). MDCT remains preferable for evaluation of soft tissue processes, including tumors.

MAGNETIC RESONANCE IMAGING

MRI imaging was introduced for clinical use in the 1980s and, because of its inherent multiplanar

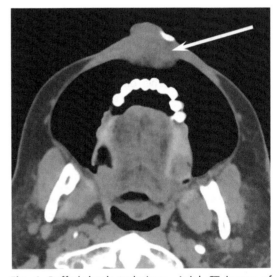

Fig. 4. Puffed-cheek technique. Axial CT image of a patient with squamous cell carcinoma of the lower lip demonstrates the lesion (*arrow*) surrounded by air instead of adjacent to the jaw. Buccal and gingival lesions may be difficult to distinguish and characterize without this technique. Furthermore, bone invasion can be confidently excluded.

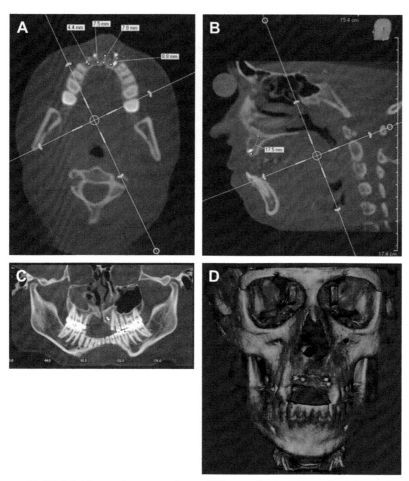

Fig. 5. Cone-beam CT. (*A*) Axial image from cone-beam CT in a patient with repaired dentoalveolar fractures of the anterior maxilla. Although image quality is lower than that for standard CT, and soft tissue is not evaluated, bone structures can still be accurately measured. (*B*) Multiplanar reformatted images are available, just as with standard CT. (*C*) Curved panoramic reformats may be useful for surgeons accustomed to panoramic radiographs. (*D*) Surface renderings do not have the same level of detail available from standard CT, but are usually adequate for surgical planning. (*Courtesy of* BJ Costello.)

capabilities and ability to delineate soft tissue pathology, has become a very powerful tool for imaging of the human body. Although MRI scanning is much more time-consuming and expensive than CT, and while MRI scanners are somewhat less accessible compared with the widespread availability of CT scanners, MRI is proven to have exciting and unique clinical utility in head and neck imaging.

Most clinical scanners available are 1.5 T or less, although 3-T scanners are becoming more widely used. MRI depends on the observation that protons become magnetized when a magnetic field is applied to them and the principle that protons in different environments behave differently when magnetized. These spins are picked up as "signal" and are mathematically process using Fourier transform to generate an image. MRI is much

more flexible than CT, which depends solely on attenuation of x-rays by the tissue of interest. With MRI, sequences can be fine-tuned to take advantage of specific characteristics of tissues and the observation that diseased or inflamed tissues or neoplasms behave differently than normal tissue. MRI is particularly useful for evaluation of suspected osteomyelitis[10] and neoplastic conditions near bone since edema in the bone marrow and soft tissues can be easily detected by specific sequences, in particular inversion recovery sequences (**Fig. 6**).[11] MRI is also the preferred modality for identifying perineural spread of malignancy (**Fig. 7**).[12]

MRI imaging in head and neck infections and neoplasms nearly always requires the use of gadolinium-based intravenous contrast. Primary and secondary neoplasms often demonstrate

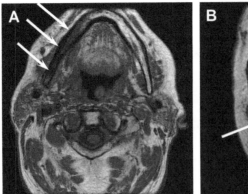
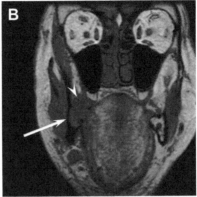

Fig. 6. MRI for bone invasion. (*A*) Axial T1-weighted image shows asymmetric low signal (*arrows*) in the marrow of the right hemimandible. (*B*) Coronal T1-weighted image confirms abnormal low signal in the right hemimandible with cortical thinning (*arrow*) and soft tissue adjacent to the mandible (*arrowhead*). These findings confirm invasion of the mandible by squamous cell carcinoma.

increased "enhancement" because of increased vascular permeability, increased extracellular space, and overall increased blood flow. Dynamic contrast-enhanced gradient-echo MRI imaging may be preferable to conventional contrast-enhanced spin-echo imaging for extent of tumor evaluation.[13]

Finally, MRI can elegantly evaluate TMJ pathology. Because the TMJ is a dynamic joint, sequences are performed in closed- and open-mouthed positions in sagittal and coronal planes. Some investigators advocate dynamic imaging of the joint, in which up to 16 images are generated in various positions, ranging from completely open to completely closed. However, this has not been shown to improve diagnostic accuracy.

In the closed-mouth position, the configuration of the condylar head and the glenoid, the integrity and shape of the intra-articular disc, joint effusion, and marrow edema can be evaluated (**Fig. 8**). In the open-mouth position, the movement of the joint as well as the position of the disc can be evaluated (**Fig. 9**).

MRI does have a few limitations, including relatively high cost and long scan time compared with other modalities. Some patients with extreme claustrophobia cannot tolerate MRI because of the narrowness of the gantry. Gadolinium-based contrast agents, generally considered safe and key in infection/inflammation and tumor imaging, have recently been associated with development of a rare systemic disease called nephrogenic systemic fibrosis in patients with renal insufficiency. Therefore, new guidelines are being established about the safety and dosage of contrast agents to such patients. Lastly, patients with

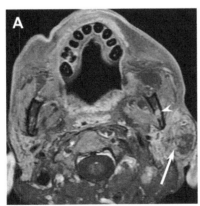
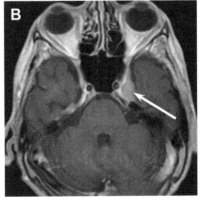

Fig. 7. MRI for perineural spread. (*A*) Axial contrast-enhanced T1-weighted image shows a large enhancing left parotid mass (*arrow*) with abnormal enhancement in the mandibular foramen (*arrowhead*) related to perineural spread along the auriculotemporal nerve to the mandibular nerve. (*B*) More superior image reveals abnormal enhancement in left Meckel cave (*arrow*) from perineural spread of the parotid tumor intracranially.

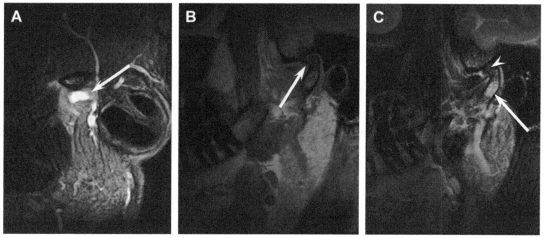

Fig. 8. MRI for TMJ osteoarthropathy. (*A*) Sagittal oblique T2-weighted image shows a high-signal collection (*arrow*), indicating joint effusion. (*B*) Sagittal oblique T1-weighted image reveals a beak-shaped osteophyte on the anterior aspect of the mandibular condyle (*arrow*), as well as narrowing of joint space. (*C*) Sagittal oblique T2-weighted image shows secondary signs of degenerative osteoarthropathy, such as subchondral cysts (*arrowhead*) and bone marrow edema (*arrow*).

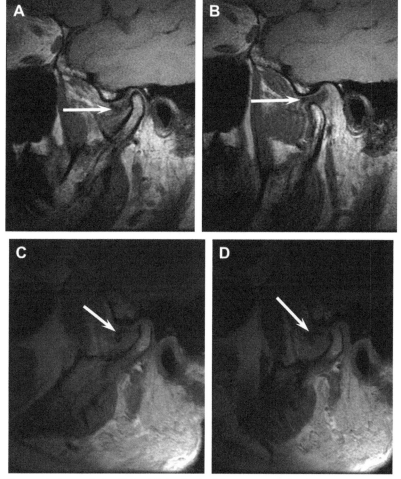

Fig. 9. MRI for disc pathology of the TMJ. (*A*) Sagittal oblique T1-weighted image in closed-mouth position reveals anterior dislocation of the low-signal articular disc (*arrow*). (*B*) Sagittal oblique T1-weighted image in open-mouth position shows recapture of the dislocated disc (*arrow*). (*C*) Sagittal oblique T1-weighted image in closed-mouth position from a different patient also shows anterior dislocation of the articular disc (*arrow*). (*D*) In this second patient, the disc (*arrow*) remains dislocated in the open-mouth position.

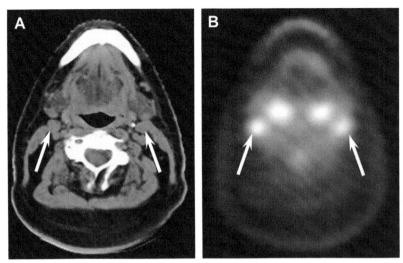

Fig. 10. Combined PET and CT (PET/CT). (*A*) Axial CT image through the upper neck shows normal-sized, symmetric jugulodigastric nodes (*arrows*). (*B*) PET image at the same level demonstrates FDG avidity (*arrows*), indicating metastatic disease.

certain implanted devices, such as pacemakers, some neurostimulators, and metallic fragments near vital structures (eyes, vessels, major organs), cannot undergo MRI scanning because of potential heating, movement, and/or malfunction that the powerful magnetic field might cause.

NUCLEAR MEDICINE

Traditionally, the role of nuclear medicine in head and neck imaging has primarily entailed the use of indium and gallium for infection imaging and radioactive iodine for thyroid imaging. Technetium 99 bone scans are helpful to determine bone metabolic activity and may indicate active growth or infection. Use of gallium and indium for infection has been made essentially obsolete by advances in cross-sectional imaging. However, the development of PET with 18-fluorodeoxyglucose (18FDG), especially when fused with diagnostic CT imaging (PET/CT), has revolutionized oncological imaging as a whole, including head and neck cancer imaging.[14,15] PET imaging is based on the principle that neoplastic processes demonstrate altered glucose metabolism compared with normal tissue. PET is performed by injecting 18FDG intravenously, waiting for approximately 1 hour, and then placing the patient in the scanner. Each positron particle emitted from the patient annihilates into two photons of equal energy in opposite directions. The points of origin of these photons are mathematically determined and mapped to create an image. In general, primary malignancy and metastases show increased 18FDG uptake. CT of the patient is obtained on

the same scanner to allow for fusion of the images and precise anatomic localization of foci of abnormal 18FDG uptake.

PET and, in particular, PET/CT are used for staging and surveillance of a variety of head and neck malignancies, most commonly squamous cell carcinoma. These can also be used for salivary gland tumors and thyroid carcinoma, the latter when thyroglobulin levels are elevated but iodine I 131 scan is negative.[16] It is also standard of care for evaluation and follow-up of lymphoma. Aside from identifying the primary malignancy, which in the head and neck is often clinically evident, PET/CT is particularly useful for finding lymphadenopathy because of the shortcomings of CT alone or MRI alone for such identification. With either CT or MRI, no single imaging feature definitively determines malignancy (**Fig. 10**). On the flip side, PET/CT is useful to exclude malignancy in lesions that are indeterminate by CT but do not have increased 18FDG uptake; this is particularly valuable in post-treatment scans. Finally, using the spatial information provided by fusion technology, PET/CT can help guide biopsies either of the primary lesion or, more likely, in suspected recurrence.[17]

SUMMARY

Imaging plays a key role in dental implantation, management of maxillofacial trauma, facial reconstruction, TMJ pathology, and evaluation and treatment of neoplasms and infections. In addition to traditional conventional radiography, recent advances in CT, MRI, and PET/CT fusion technology have made radiology an even more vital component of patient care in dental and cranio-maxillofacial practice.

REFERENCES

1. McCabe KJ, Rubinstein D. Advances in head and neck imaging. Otolaryngol Clin North Am 2005;38:307–19.
2. Schiknecht B, Graetz K. Radiologic assessment of maxillofacial, mandibular and skullbase trauma. Eur Radiol 2005;3:560–8.
3. Preda L, La Fianza A, DiMaggio EM, et al. Complex maxillofacial trauma: diagnostic contribution of multiplanar and tridimensional spiral CT imaging. Radiol Med 1998;3:178–84.
4. Schwarz MS, Rothman SL, Chafetz N, et al. Computed tomography in dental implantation surgery. Dent Clin North Am 1989;33:555–97.
5. Weissman JL, Carrau RL. "Puffed-cheek" CT improves evaluation of the oral cavity. AJNR Am J Neuroradiol 2001;22:741–4.
6. Henrot P, Blum A, Toussaint B. Dynamic maneuvers in local staging of head and neck malignancies with current imaging techniques: principles and clinical applications. Radiographics 2003;23:1201–13.
7. Schulze D, Heiland M, Thurmann H, et al. Radiation exposure during midfacial imaging using 4- and 16-slice computed tomography, cone beam computed tomography systems and conventional radiography. Dentomaxillofac Radiol 2004;33:83–6.
8. Scarfe WC, Farman AG, Sukovic P. Clinical applications of cone-beam computed tomography in dental practice. Can Dent Assoc 2006;72:75–80.
9. American Academy of Oral and Maxillofacial Radiology executive opinion statement on performing and interpreting diagnostic cone beam computed tomography. Farman AG, editor. Oral and Maxillofacial Radiology 2008;106:561–62.
10. Kaneda T, Minami M, Ozawa K, et al. Magnetic resonance imaging of osteomyelitis in the mandible. Comparative study with other radiologic modalities. Oral Surg Oral Med Oral Pathol Oral Radiol Endod 1995;79:634–40.
11. Lee K, Kaneda T, Mori S, et al. Magnetic resonance imaging of normal and osteomyelitis in the mandible: assessment of short inversion time inversion recovery sequence. Oral Surg Oral Med Oral Pathol Oral Radiol Endod 2003;96:499–507.
12. Caldemeyer KS, Mathews VP, Righi PD, et al. Imaging features and clinical significance of perineural spread or extension of head and neck tumors. Radiographics 1998;18:97–110.
13. Escott EJ, Rao VM, Ko WD, et al. Comparison of dynamic contrast-enhanced gradient-echo and spin-echo sequences in MR of head and neck neoplasms. AJNR Am J Neuroradiol 1997;18:1411–9.
14. Branstetter BF 4th, Blodgett TW, Zimmer LA, et al. Head and neck malignancy: Is PET/CT more accurate than PET or CT alone? Radiology 2005;235:580–6.
15. Schoder H, Yeung HW, Gonen M, et al. Head and neck cancer: clinical usefulness and accuracy of PET/CT image fusion. Radiology 2004;231:65–72.
16. Schoder H, Yeung HW. Positron emission imaging of head and neck cancer, including thyroid carcinoma. Semin Nucl Med 2004;34:180–97.
17. Agarwal V, Branstetter BF 4th, Johnson JT. Indications for PET/CT in the head and neck. Otolaryngol Clin North Am 2008;4:23–49.

Computer-Assisted Craniomaxillofacial Surgery

Sean P. Edwards, DDS, MD, FRCD(C)

KEYWORDS
- Computer-assisted surgery • Computer-aided surgery
- Cone beam computed tomography
- Reconstructive surgery planning • Distraction osteogenesis
- Template

How often should results go according to plan? No surgeon is perfect all the time yet surgery is a discipline driven by results. Surgeons have therefore turned to technology to improve not only their outcomes but also how often they achieve high-quality results.

Computer-assisted surgery (CAS) is an umbrella term used to describe all forms of surgery planning or execution that incorporate various forms of advanced imaging, software, analysis, and planning and, in some cases, rapid prototyping (RP) technology, robotics, and image-guidance systems. Although these may represent the current state of affairs, innovation is progressing rapidly, and new forms of technology continue to be incorporated and evaluated for their value in improving operations.

As is often the case with the introduction of new technology, critics of CAS abound. The techniques are in their infancy and still have much to prove. Critics often point to the increased direct costs that may result from these technologies. Although the direct costs of an operation may be increased, the overall cost of care may be reduced. Decreased operative time, blood loss, complications, and the need for reoperative surgery are all potential cost-saving benefits. Minimally invasive, or at least less invasive, approaches may also result from improved planning and visualization. These are value-added components of care and may ultimately decrease hospitalization and

recovery time, thereby reducing morbidity and the indirect costs of care.

These techniques may also increase the time spent preparing for surgery. The value of planning is not lost on orthodontists and oral and maxillofacial surgeons. Each surgeon performs model surgery and diagnostic set-ups, makes splints, reviews clinical photographs, and performs ceph-analyses to prepare for surgery. The value of this time investment has been recognized for several decades as critical to achieving consistent high-quality results. Because these methods are new and not standardized, little effort has been directed at evaluating the benefits of CAS in cost and treatment time, although this evaluation needs to be accomplished before the techniques can become standard.

Interest in this field is broad. In addition to cranio-maxillofacial surgery, this technology has been incorporated into orthodontics, radiation oncology, neurosurgery, sinus surgery, joint replacement surgery, spine surgery, and dental implantology. The acceleration in interest in CAS is a result of the increased availability of lower-cost, low-radiation imaging technology and powerful, commercially available software packages that allow a surgeon, without sophisticated computer expertise, to visualize and simulate operations. RP and stereolithography (SLA) became commonplace in the late 1990s and have been coupled with enhanced software planning to push the technology forward.

Department of Pediatric Maxillofacial Surgery, C.S. Mott Children's Hospital, University of Michigan Health System, TC B1 208, 1500 East Medical Center, Dr Ann Arbor, MI 48109-0018, USA
E-mail address: seanedwa@med.umich.edu

Oral Maxillofacial Surg Clin N Am 22 (2010) 117–134
doi:10.1016/j.coms.2009.11.005

IMAGING

Although virtually any imaging system can be incorporated into CAS treatment schemes, cone beam computed tomography (CBCT) and conventional multislice computed tomography (CT) are the standard imaging modalities in craniomaxillofacial CAS. Skeletal surgery is particularly well suited to CAS. The skeleton is easy to image well with CT and, given its inflexible nature, represents an invariant data set that can be manipulated in the virtual environment.

CBCT is a medical imaging system that uses a cone-shaped X-ray beam centered on a two-dimensional detector (**Fig. 1**). The source-detector complex makes 1 rotation around the patient analogous to an orthopantomogram. These systems have found broad use in medicine and dentistry in radiation oncology, interventional radiology, otolaryngology, implantology, orthodontics, and craniomaxillofacial surgery. Dedicated scanners for the oral and maxillofacial region were introduced in the late 1990s and since then there has been increased interest in the imaging technique and applications to which it might be applied. Image quality in most cases lags behind conventional multislice scanners but is more than adequate for its intended need (**Fig. 2**A, B).

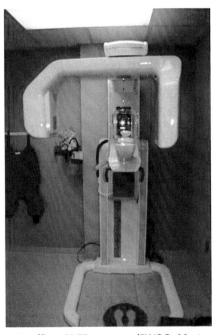

Fig. 1. In-office CBCT scanner (EWOO Master 3DS; EWOO Technology USA Inc, Houston, TX, USA). Note nonintimidating profile comparable with a conventional panoramic machine. This machine has a minimal footprint and is easily incorporated into the office environment.

Since the introduction of CAS, 2 general classes of scanners have emerged based on the size of their field of view. Field of view refers to the area imaged with a scan and is referenced in linear dimensions. Scanners with a smaller field of view (13 cm or smaller) lend themselves to implant dentistry and other dentoalveolar applications such as impacted teeth. Those scanners with broader fields of view (greater than 13 cm and up to 21 cm) allow the clinician to image the entire face. These larger data sets permit evaluation of a facial deformity, generation of cephalograms, airway analysis, and complex craniomaxillofacial surgery planning.

The CBCT scanners are cheap compared with conventional multislice scanners and many are purchased and situated in the surgeon's clinic under the surgeon's control. This proximity offers a better degree of control of how the images are acquired. Because most surgeons have a dental laboratory situated in or close to their clinic, the surgeon can fabricate guides for template-based surgery or even dental splints for surgical navigation. Having a dental radiology technician acquire the imaging data is useful in that the technician is already familiar with preparing the patient for orthopantomograms and cephalograms. As a result, concepts such as natural head position, Frankfort horizontal, centric relation, and resting lip posture are not unfamiliar to the technologist taking the images, which simplifies the process and improves the quality of the data set. Quality control in such an arrangement is also easier to maintain.

As computer processors improve in their power so does the time taken to acquire these scans. A full head scan can generally be performed in less than a minute, sometimes less than 20 seconds, with approximately the same amount of time taken to process the data for image display. From a workflow perspective, this is efficient, permitting these systems to be rapidly integrated into busy practices without any significant loss in productivity. Moreover, by avoiding a revisit after the image is obtained before presenting an operative plan to a patient, clinic time may in the end be reduced. As a result, these scanners are being quickly incorporated in oral and maxillofacial surgery and orthodontic offices.

Dosimetry is 1 of the biggest advantages of the cone beam technology. The dose reduction is partly because the image is acquired in a single sweep instead of multiple slices and partly because only images of the skeleton are acquired. Doses vary based on machine and scan specifications. Larger fields of view and higher-resolution scans (smaller voxel size) result in higher doses. The radiation source can deliver a continuous

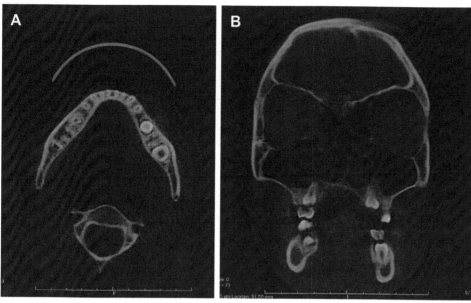

Fig. 2. (*A, B*) Typical image quality of CBCT with a large field of view. Quality of skeletal detail is more than adequate for diagnostic and treatment planning purposes.

beam or it may be pulsed, lowering the dose. Doses for full head scans range from 69 to 560 μSv. This range compares favorably with the 860 to 2000 μSv for a conventional head CT scan.[1–3] This is still a significant increase over conventional dental radiography at 4 to 43 times the dose of a conventional panoramic radiograph and should not be seen as a substitute for these films when they are adequate.[1,4]

ENHANCED THREE-DIMENSIONAL DIAGNOSTICS

To correct a deformity accurately, a surgeon must first be able to identify and quantify all the different components of the deformity. Using orthognathic surgery as an example, midline discrepancies are easily measured, whereas cants are more difficult to measure, and yaw deformities that result in asymmetric buccal corridors are even more difficult to quantify. Differences in the height of the mandibular body and ramus are also not easily measured with clinical means or with conventional two-dimensional radiographic techniques (**Fig. 3**). A three-dimensional data set obtained from a CT scan overcomes many of these difficulties.

Several software packages have been developed to display CT data sets for this type of analysis. Typically, images are reconstructed in axial, sagittal, and coronal planes along with three-dimensional views of the patient (**Fig. 4**A–C). All aspects of a patient's skeletal detail can be examined, permitting a qualitative assessment of

a deformity. This data set includes the soft-tissue mask, which may be viewed in the context of the skeletal deformity. Furthermore, two-dimensional and three-dimensional stereophotogrammetry

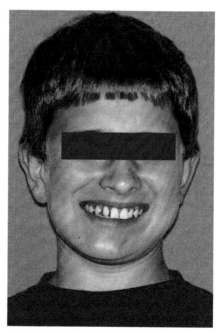

Fig. 3. Young adolescent with hemimandibular hyperplasia and facial asymmetry. The midline discrepancy is obvious and easy to measure. The difference in the height of the inferior border of the mandible is more difficult to quantify, as is the yaw/rotational deformity of the jaws.

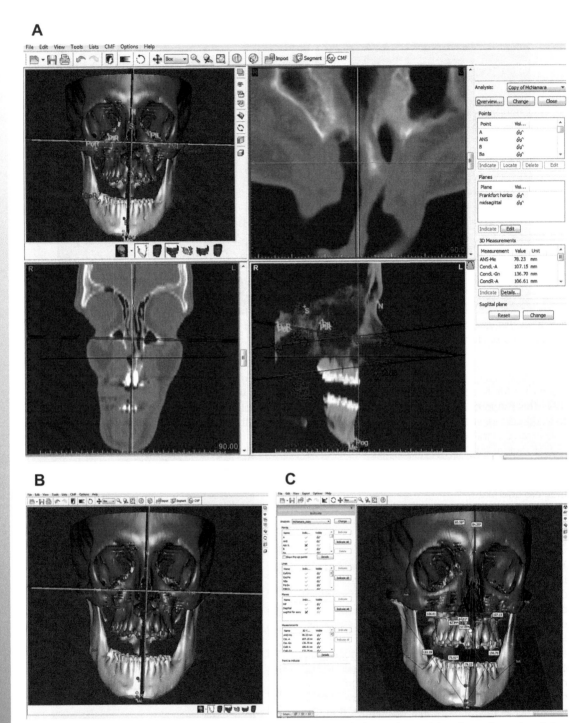

Fig. 4. (*A*) CT data reconstructed to show axial, coronal, and sagittal planes along with a three-dimensional view of the head. (*B*) Virtual skull is aligned according to sagittal, coronal, and axial planes to align the head for analysis. A natural head posture registration could also be used. (*C*) Three-dimensional reconstruction of CT data permits three-dimensional analysis to help the surgeon understand and quantify a complex deformity.

may be easily fused with the CT data set and create a lifelike, virtual-patient model. With most of these commercially available software packages, lateral cephalograms and orthopantomograms are easily generated, which remain useful because clinicians are comfortable viewing anatomy presented in this way, although cephalograms and orthopantomograms ignore some of the potential of a three-dimensional data set. Readers are referred to a thorough overview of three-dimensional cephalometry by Swennen and colleagues.[5] Despite there being standard landmarks and planes, a deformity can be quantified from virtually any orthogonal plane that the surgeon deems helpful in formulating an operative plan. These measurements can extend to almost any portion of the face, including the supraglottic airway. Maxillomandibular surgery may affect a patient's airway, creating or correcting sleep-disordered breathing. As the understanding of the relationship between maxillomandibular surgery and the airway improves, airway analyses and diagnostics may eventually be incorporated as a routine part of surgery planning.

The next step in the evolution of the treatment planning software and its usefulness with respect to CAS was the development of segmentation tools. Segmenting is analogous to creating an osteotomy and is a way to sequester portions of a patient's anatomy. The cutting planes for this function are arbitrary and defined by the user in most cases and can be chosen to define anatomic units, such as the airway or a tumor, or to simulate typical operations such a LeFort I osteotomy. With an osteotomy, the bones on either side of the cut, each with its own separate data set, can be repositioned according to the developed treatment plan, soft-tissue changes can be simulated, and adequacy of the treatment plan can be assessed (**Fig. 5**).

TACTILE MODELS

Tactile model technology, or RP, became commonplace in craniomaxillofacial surgery in the late 1990s. These models were immediately familiar and recognized as valuable diagnostic adjuncts to orthodontists and oral and maxillofacial surgeons, who had been working with stone dental models for decades; the new models gave the surgeon a full view of a patient's skeletal deformity and could be used to quantify the deformity and plan a patient's operation (**Figs. 6** and **7**). Osteotomies could be created and templates made to help transfer the desired treatment plan to the operating room.

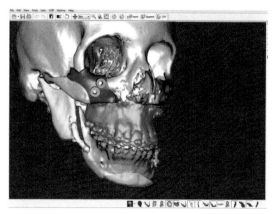

Fig. 5. Cutting planes are established and the data segmentation accomplished to simulate a LeFort I osteotomy, sagittal split of the mandible, and asymmetric sliding genioplasty.

These models were initially limited by cost and the availability of means to fabricate them. RP printers are now much more commonplace, which makes their routine use easier. Many hospitals have purchased the systems, engineering departments at most universities have the technology, and several companies now offer the service.

This technology involves several steps, beginning with data file conversion. Because RP was used primarily in the automotive and aerospace industries for design and prototyping, it was not originally conceived to work with medical imaging

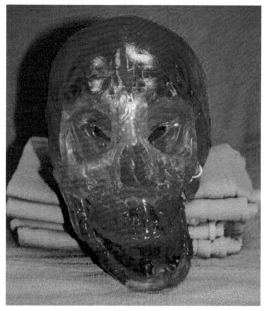

Fig. 6. Stereolithographic model of a complex asymmetry associated with type III hemifacial microsomia.

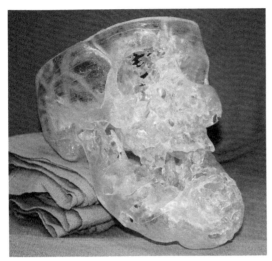

Fig. 7. Stereolithographic model of an adolescent severely affected with cherubism. Measurements can be taken from this model to plan and establish goals for the remodeling procedures.

data. CT scans and magnetic resonance imaging (MRI) scans are stored in digital imaging and communications in medicine (DICOM) format, which must be converted to a binary stereolithography (STL) file format for use in RP. In essence, the universal file format for imaging (DICOM) is converted to the universal file format for RP (STL).[6]

The quality of these data, which determines the quality of the model produced, primarily depends on the quality of the imaging data. Because CT scans give the best images of skeletal structures, this is the primary modality used to fabricate patient-specific tactile models. High-resolution, thin-slice CT scans acquired without motion artifact and distortion produce the best images and thereby the best models. Metal (eg, from dental restorations, orthodontic appliances, or fixation devices) produces streak artifacts that negatively affect the quality of every step of this process. Thin bones, such as the anterior wall of the maxillary sinus and the walls of the orbit, are often missed and poorly represented in three-dimensional data sets and so are not well represented in three-dimensional models without significant image processing. This finding is important because it directly affects a surgeon's ability to use these models for planning surgery in these regions. Procedures and software packages are available to process imaging data to improve the quality of the scan and reduce the effect of these issues on scan data, but the effort can be laborious.

Several methods exist to produce these models, each with its advantages and disadvantages. Each method converts a series of axial image slices into two-dimensional layers of some material that is layered on itself to make a model.[6]

SLA is the method best known to most surgeons and dentists. These models are translucent, and key anatomic structures can be inspected and even colorized and studied for their relevance to the desired treatment plan. The models are produced from a vat of liquid polymer that is photopolymerized a layer at a time. Selective application of additional ultraviolet energy colorizes the polymer red in desired areas. Typically, teeth and the inferior alveolar nerve are treated in this fashion. Time and high cost are the biggest drawbacks to this technique. It takes between 10 and 30 hours to produce such a model, depending on the size needed. These models, when made from high-quality CT scans, are accurate and are produced at a 1:1 size ratio so that planning can be similarly accurate.[6]

Other methods produce opaque models. Three-dimensional printing is analogous to ink-jet printing, with layers of a powder fused together with a liquid binder. This method yields opaque models, but it is fast and cheap. One drawback is that the models are fragile. Fused deposition modeling involves the extrusion of a melted plastic in layered fashion to create a model. These models are opaque and take a great deal of time to produce, but they are strong. Selective laser sintering (SLS) uses a CO_2 laser to sinter or fuse a given material 1 layer at a time into a model. This method is flexible in the materials that can be used, although nylon is the most common.[6] In the future, custom titanium devices could be produced by this method. Resorbable, patient-specific anatomic constructs made of polycaprolactone for tissue-engineering applications have also been produced with SLS.[7]

CAS CONCEPTS

In the broadest possible sense, CAS of the craniomaxillofacial skeleton exists in 2 forms: image-guided surgery and template-based surgery.

Image-guided surgery (**Fig. 8**), also known as navigational surgery, uses imaging data as a road map for the operating surgeon. It is analogous to the global positioning systems (GPSs) becoming ubiquitous in modern automobiles. The techniques pair well with minimally invasive approaches and operations in which broad exposure cannot be achieved, such as in the deep orbits. The surgeon uses various forms of probe to locate or guide instruments and correlates this position with the patient's anatomy in real time on a computer screen displaying the patient's

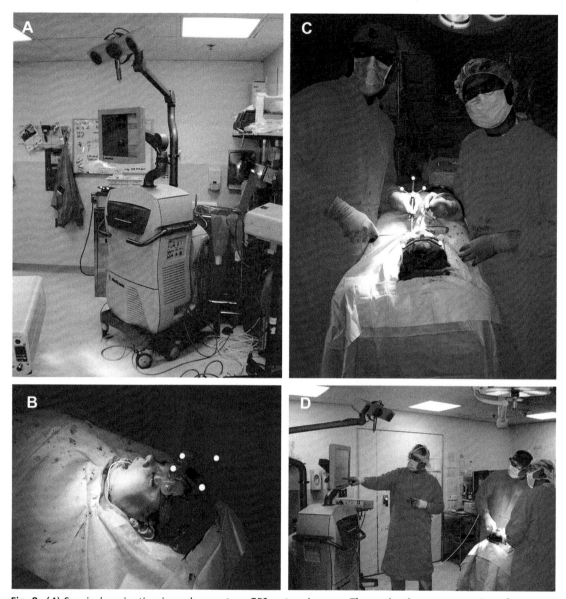

Fig. 8. (*A*) Surgical navigation is analogous to a GPS system in a car. The navigation tower consists of a camera and a monitor. The camera registers the position of the patient and the navigation probe and displays the position of the probe on the monitor. (*B*) At the beginning of a case, landmarks on a patient are registered to corresponding landmarks on their CT data set. To maintain this linkage, a system to track movement of the patient is required. In this case, the Medtronic Stealth System (Medtronic Navigation Inc, Minneapolis, MN, USA) uses a headband with 4 fiducial markers. Changes in the position of the patient's head are reflected in position changes in the markers that are tracked by the camera. (*C, D*) Instruments and probes with a similar fiducial system are tracked by the camera to display progress on the patient's CT scan.

imaging data in all 3 planes. Image guidance has been widely adopted by sinus surgeons and neurosurgeons to help them navigate the deeper structures of the head without broad surgical exposure. In craniomaxillofacial surgery, it has found use in orbital trauma and reconstruction and tumor extirpation, especially that of the skull base. Xia and colleagues[8] described various

applications combining navigation for reconstructive surgery planning. For routine use in reconstructive surgery, however, the techniques are unwieldy and this has limited their broader application. Improvements in intraoperative imaging systems will increase the value of image-guided surgery to the craniomaxillofacial surgeon because current systems do not reflect any anatomic changes as a result of surgery. The road map in these cases is invariant and only as current as the preoperative CT scan. Intraoperative CT scans are now available at some hospitals, including portable cone beam technology, and this offers the potential for real-time quality control, which can correct errors before the operation is completed. Accuracy has been a concern with these approaches but will likely be overcome as the technology progresses. Craniomaxillofacial surgery is a small market for navigation systems. As a result, most surgeons use those systems already available in their institution. Only 1 of the currently available navigation systems, BrainLab (Feldkirchen, Germany), has a software package (iPlan) that permits advanced treatment, surgical simulation, and export of treatment plans to the navigation system. If the field is to enjoy broader clinical application, such software applications need to be more commonplace.

Template-based surgery is a more familiar paradigm for craniomaxillofacial surgeons. Templates are routinely used for orthognathic surgery, dental implant placement, and even for alveoloplasty. Incorporation of improved imaging, diagnostics, and segmentation that leads to template generation is a straightforward and logical extension of current practice.

The general workflow is shown in **Fig. 9**. Although these enhanced diagnostics are valuable, templates are the key to translating this enhanced treatment planning to the operating room. The potential forms for the template are limited only by the imagination of the surgeon and engineer: they can be rapid prototyped guides for cutting osteotomies and repositioning bones; they can be customized models on which fixation plates are adapted; they may be traditional orthognathic occlusal wafers; and they can even be custom-made, implantable prostheses.

RECONSTRUCTIVE SURGERY

Unilateral defects (traumatic and oncologic) and asymmetries lend themselves well to CAS techniques. A mirror image of the unaffected side can be created and superimposed on the affected area. Segmenting the deformed portion of a patient's anatomy and replacing it with a mirror image of the opposite side creates the surgical objective. This technique has been well described for orbital trauma.[9–11] The difference between the 2 images can be used to quantify the deformity and help plan the reconstructive operation. It can also be used to fashion various templates. For example, a tactile model made of the reconstructed mandible can be used to adapt a reconstruction plate to which a bone graft will be fixed. Because the plate is adapted to the surgical objective, the bone graft or bone flap form will be exactly as desired. This planning has the potential to take into account not just facial form but also the eventual dental rehabilitation if the jaws are a part of the intended reconstruction. The step by step creation

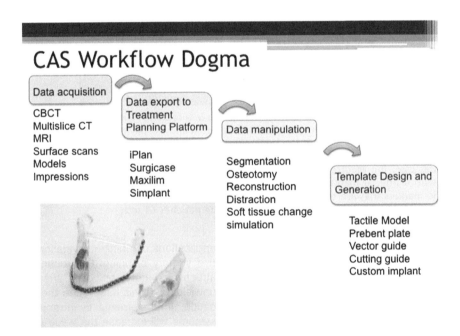

Fig. 9. CAS workflow dogma.

of a customized tactile model that was used to design the reconstruction in a patient in whom the normal reference points and planes were abrogated by a tumor is presented in **Fig. 10**A–L.

Bilateral and midline defects are more of a challenge in this regard because the opposite side cannot be used to determine the treatment objective. A treatment objective can be created virtually

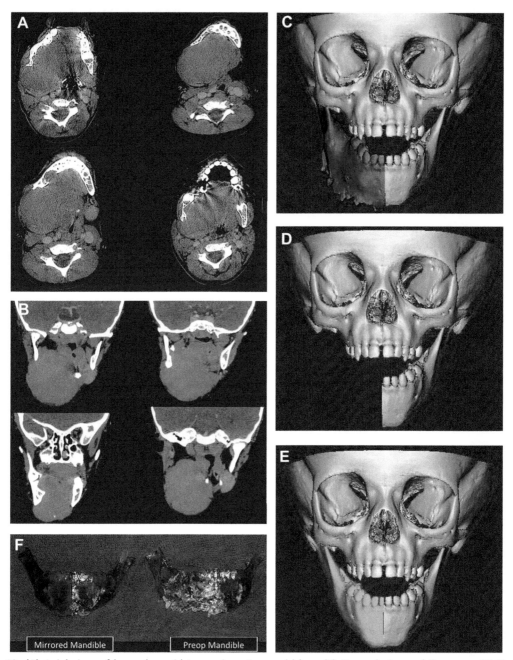

Fig. 10. (*A*) Axial view of large desmoid tumor in a 4-year-old boy. (*B*) Coronal views of the same. (*C*) Three-dimensional view with deformed mandibular half segmented. (*D*) Deformed half removed. (*E*) Mirrored left mandible aligned to replace the deformed right hemimandible. (*F*) Comparison of stereolithographic models of new mandible and deformed mandible. The new mandible model becomes the surgical objective and the template to guide the reconstructive process. (*G*) Reconstruction plate is adapted to the new mandible. It is then sterilized and taken to the operating room to guide the reconstruction. (*H*) Tumor is resected. (*I*) Specimen. (*J*) Plate fixed to residual mandible and rib grafts are then fixed to the plate. (*K*) Closure with resulting good symmetry and form of the new mandible after a three-quarter mandibulectomy, (*L*) Frontal view at closure.

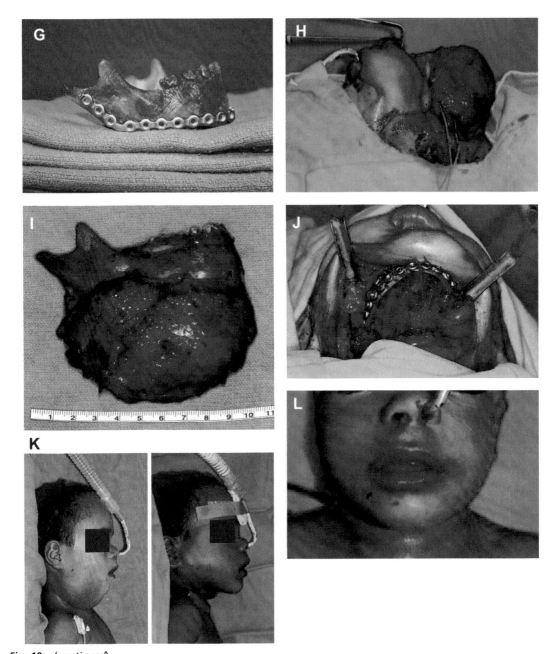

Fig. 10. (*continued*)

by using anatomic standards to create the desired structures that can then be used to generate a template. A case of a self-inflected gunshot wound resulted in a large composite tissue defect of the anterior mandible. In this case, the data sets from other patients' mandibles were virtually tried in until one with the appropriate intergonial width and chin projection was found. This mandible was aligned such that the alveolar ridges were appropriately positioned for future implant rehabilitation. A tactile model was then made of the reconstructed mandible such that a plate could be adapted to shape the reconstruction. Similar strategies have been devised for orbital reconstruction in which both orbits are deformed (**Fig. 11**A–F).[9]

BONE FLAP SHAPING

Templates can also be fashioned to help shape a flap or a graft precisely according to a preoperative virtual treatment plan. One of the most

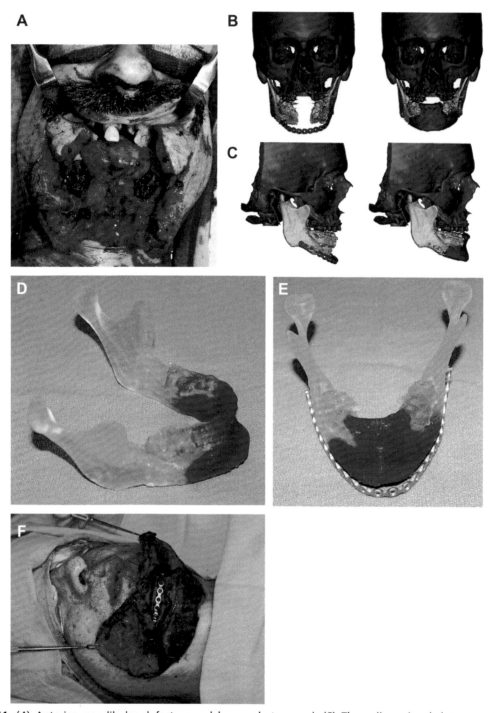

Fig. 11. (*A*) Anterior mandibular defect caused by gunshot wound. (*B*) Three-dimensional data sets of the mandibular defect. On the right is a frontal view of the treatment objective, which was developed by taking stock mandibular CT scan images and finding one that matched the desired gonial width and chin projection. (*C*) Lateral view of preoperative condition and treatment objective. (*D*) This treatment objective data set is used to fabricate a stereolithographic model that can then be used to adapt a reconstruction plate and bone flap and approximate the virtual treatment objective. (*E*) Plate adapted to the customized model. (*F*) Free fibula osteocutaneous flap osteotomized to adapt intimately to the plate, achieving the treatment objective.

common indications for such a guide is a fibula free flap for mandibular or maxillary reconstruction. The process generally begins with CT data set of the mandible. The planned resection is completed and either a CT or MRI of the patient's own fibula is then shaped virtually to create the desired mandible. A stock fibula may be used for the same process. Shaping of the graft requires creating 1 or more closing osteotomies in which a wedge of bone is removed to allow intimate adaptation of the bone edges. Attention is directed at replicating the gonial angle, intergonial width, chin projection, and chin width, and maintaining an adequate interarch space for dental

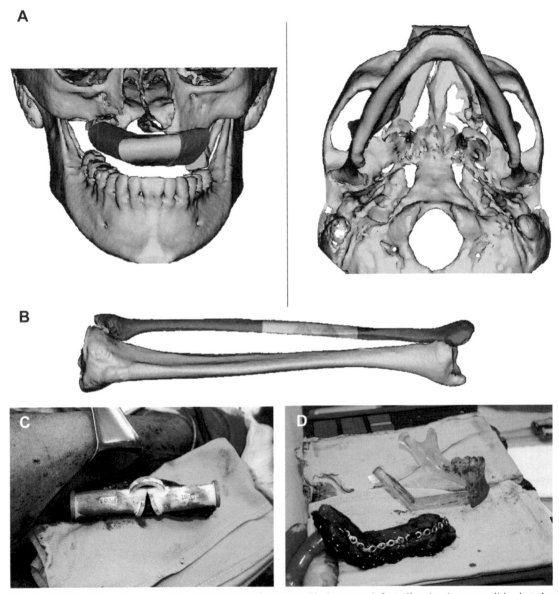

Fig. 12. (*A*) Fibula free flap harvest to reconstruct a hemimandibulectomy defect. Shaping is accomplished at the leg while the flap continues to be perfused. The fibula bone is cut according to the length of the template. The template can be held in place with a Kocher clamp. A wedge of bone is removed from the center of the fibula according to the plan to replicate the patient's gonial angle. (*B*) SLA model is fabricated to permit off field adaptation of the reconstruction plate. Shaped fibula matches the reconstructive plan. (*C*) Cutting template is positioned on the fibula, which sets the length of bone for the planned reconstruction. The middle cut-out sets the angle and amount of bone that needs to be removed for an accurate closing osteotomy. (*D*) Shaped and plated fibula flap. Stereolithographic model of the planned operation adjacent to the shaped flap, demonstrating concordance between the planning and the operation.

rehabilitation. Time savings with such a template are also gained because the flap can be precisely shaped and fixation applied while it continues to be perfused. Such techniques can also reduce the warm ischemia time of a flap (**Fig. 12**A, B).

DISTRACTION OSTEOGENESIS

Distraction osteogenesis is a powerful technique for the elongation of bones without the need for bone grafting. The process involves gradual elongation of the bony callus that forms at the site of an osteotomy. The force to create this movement can then be applied either internally or externally. An external system that sits external to the patient's face and its interface with the bones with rigid pins or wires offers the surgeon maximum control over the direction of bone movement and provides the potential for changes in the vector of movement as warranted by the clinical situation. Although favored for this element of control, these external devices are not well accepted by patients and their parents because they are unwieldy and must be worn 24 hours per day for several months during the phases of active treatment and consolidation of the newly generated bone. This is analogous to having a patient wear a protraction facemask all day for several months. As a result, many surgeons have turned to buried devices, in which the only hardware visible is an activation arm that emerges intraorally or in the upper cervical region. These devices are generally univector, which means that the vector of movement is set and immutable once it is installed at the time of surgery. Thus, the quality of the result achieved depends on the ability of the surgeon to place the device with the proper orientation in all 3 planes to achieve the desired result, particularly when bilateral devices are being placed. Convergence of the distraction vectors of devices on either side of the mandible leads to excessive lateral condylar torque. In the maxilla and upper facial skeleton, where the posterior elements are fixed, there may be device binding and ultimately failure. If the devices are not parallel in the vertical planes, this can also lead to cants, open bites, and other iatrogenic deformities (**Fig. 13**).

Accurate device placement and thereby distraction vector determination is not an easy task when the anatomy is abnormal because of the underlying deformity or previous surgery. Furthermore, because mandibular devices in toddlers are often placed through a transcervical approach, the surgeon seeks to limit the incision length to avoid an unsightly scar.

Computer-based planning systems now exist that permit a surgeon to perform the operation

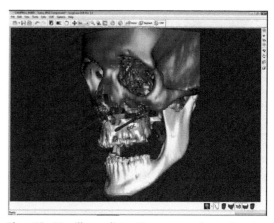

Fig. 13. Maxillary distraction case planned using buried distractors. Devices are virtually selected. Parallelism is assured, as is the angle of declination to achieve vertical lengthening of the maxilla while sagittal lengthening is ongoing.

virtually. There are many benefits to this process. Firstly, a multitude of devices may be virtually "tried in" until one of appropriate size and form is selected. The device may be positioned so as to avoid injury to developing tooth buds and other vital structures, such as the inferior alveolar nerve, with the osteotomy and screw placement. The distraction process can then be simulated and the reciprocal soft-tissue changes predicted, permitting the surgeon to pick a distractor with an appropriate length activation arm.

The application of the technique in a child with Treacher Collins syndrome is presented in **Fig. 14**A–J.

ORTHOGNATHIC SURGERY

Orthognathic surgery is 1 area of maxillofacial surgery already subject to extensive preoperative planning. A single-jaw surgical plan requires that the opposing arch be adequate in position, width, and symmetry; these cases generally yield predictable, satisfactory results without extensive planning. Two-jaw surgery, which involves surgically repositioning the maxilla and mandible in 3 planes, is more difficult. The decision to embark on 2-jaw surgery is predicated on neither jaw being in a satisfactory position, form, or symmetry. This is a difficult undertaking considering the submillimetric precision required to achieve a satisfactory result. Preoperative planning for a double-jaw case is more involved. The preoperative planning of a single-jaw case consists of a review of photographic records and cephanalysis with surgical prediction tracings, followed by the fabrication of a single interocclusal splint to guide the

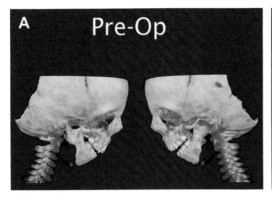

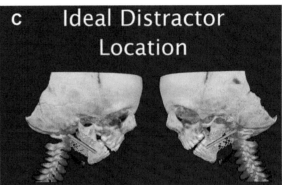

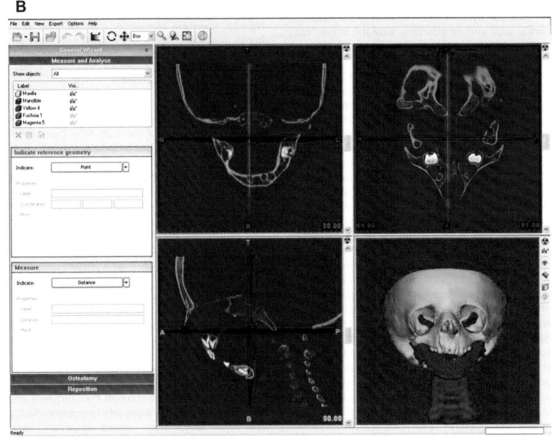

Fig. 14. (*A*) A 4-year-old boy with Treacher Collins syndrome and severe obstructive sleep apnea. He had previously undergone distraction at 11 months of age. His mandibular anatomy is markedly abnormal. (*B*) CT data are acquired and analytical stage is begun. (*C*) A buried, single-vector distraction device is chosen and positioned to achieve the desired result. (*D*) A vector transfer guide (*in red*) is then virtually designed. The design of this guide is such that it can easily be positioned on the native mandible and adapts well to the contours of the distractor. It is purposefully designed to be larger than will be used in the operating room to permit customizing the guide further as the operative situation dictates. (*E*) A model and transfer guide are fabricated using RP techniques. The mandibular model allows the distractor to be adapted for a precise fit, whereas the vector transfer guide ensures the desired orientation. (*F*) The mandible is exposed and the template seated. (*G*) The distractor is seated in the template, replicating the treatment objective. (*H*) Distraction is accomplished having avoided injury to developing tooth buds. (*I*) Predistraction lateral view. (*J*) Postdistraction lateral view.

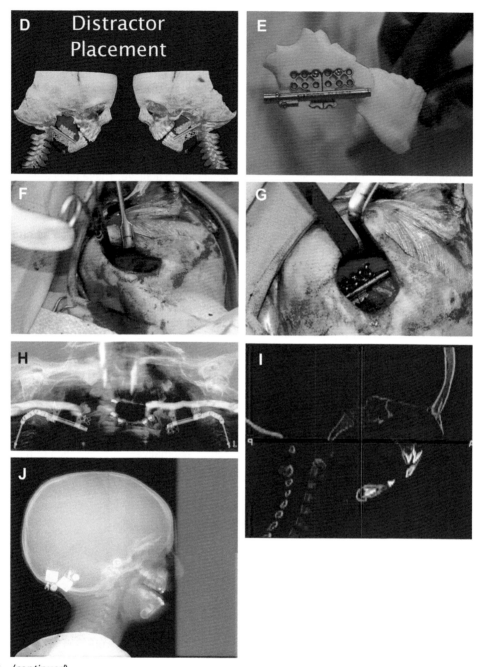

Fig. 14. (*continued*)

establishment of the final, desired occlusion. The time spent varies but is generally less than 1 hour for an experienced surgeon.

Preoperative planning for 2-jaw cases usually involves impressions, centric records, a facebow relation, a series of clinical measurements, and a mounting on a semiadjustable articulator. Surgery is then simulated on the articulated casts using a model block to register the desired changes. This procedure requires multiple steps, and small errors at each step can accumulate. There are components of a deformity, such as a yaw deformity, that are difficult to quantify with traditional diagnostic records and are therefore difficult to correct accurately. Several hours could be spent gathering the records and completing the treatment planning for such a case. Given the labor involved and the potential for error, surgeons try to incorporate technology that could reduce the time spent in preoperative planning and simultaneously improve surgical outcomes (**Fig. 15**A, B).

Several schemas have been devised for computer-assisted orthognathic surgery,[12–18] yet none has found its way into the mainstream. Establishing a final occlusion is a precise maneuver, with corrections of a fraction of a millimeter having a significant effect on the final outcome. Most surgeons are used to the tactile feedback that comes from hand articulating stone casts to get a sense of the presurgical orthodontic set-up. Enamoplasty is occasionally performed to improve a presurgical set-up; this could not be reliably performed in the virtual environment and then replicated in the operating room. Collision detection is a software property in which contact between 2 virtual objects (in this case, teeth) prevents them from passing through each other. Collision detection is an essential property in developing a final occlusion and is poorly developed in current software packages. As a result, the fabrication of surgical splints for a final occlusion is not yet routine.

The final splint notwithstanding, the intermediate splint is the site where the true benefit of this technology could be realized. CT scans allow for a true three-dimensional evaluation of a given deformity and permit three-dimensional cephanalysis such that asymmetries can be better quantified. Yaw deformities, which are notoriously difficult to measure clinically, can now be accurately measured in all 3 planes. A maxilla can be centered in the face as desired. An intermediate splint can be made to reposition the maxilla at this point. Collision detection is not relevant nor is the tactile appreciation of a set-up. This procedure could eliminate the error and labor required for the intermediate splint, the most time-consuming part of these cases. Difficulties arise when a maxilla must be segmented. This segmentation is based on the final occlusion; as stated earlier, because of the nontactile nature of the planning and the lack of collision detection, this is difficult to achieve. These techniques are slowly coming into clinical practice but much work remains to be done to show consistent accuracy before they become routine.

The general workflow for such an orthognathic case using commercially available systems is as follows.[16] A three-dimensional data set is acquired with a CT scanner (either a CBCT or conventional multislice scanner). This scan and data set must encompass all relevant anatomy for analysis and surgical simulation and will preclude the use of some limited field of view CBCT scanners. A set of models are scanned either with the CT scanner or a surface scanner. These image sets, the CT scan, and the stone models, are fused to yield a scatter-free image set for cephanalysis and surgical simulation. A Cartesian coordinate system then establishes a natural head posture and serves as a reference for aberrations in symmetry and form.[5] Alternatively, a registration of natural head posture can be incorporated into the treatment plan, as described by Xia and colleagues.[8] The

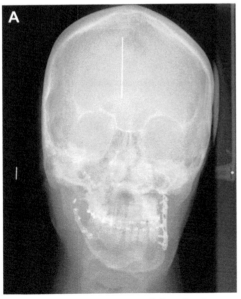
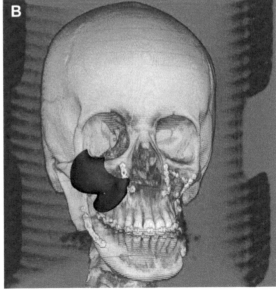

Fig. 15. (*A*) Complex asymmetric deformity that would be difficult to quantify from traditional two-dimensional imaging modalities. (*B*) Three-dimensional view of the same patient.

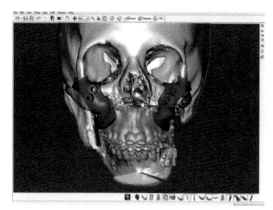

Fig. 16. Surgical treatment objective developed by segmenting and repositioning the mandible, chin, and maxilla.

anatomy can be surveyed, the deformity quantified, and a surgical plan devised to correct it. This plan is effected by segmenting the skeleton, as would be done intraoperatively **(Fig. 16)**. Once complete, and once 1 jaw is repositioned, an intermediate splint is virtually created and becomes its own data set, which is then rapidly prototyped and can be taken to the operating room to carry out the surgical plan. Several algorithms have been proposed for developing a final occlusion in the virtual environment but as mentioned earlier all have some limitations. Conventional stone models could be used to develop a final occlusion, and a final surgical splint could then be made by conventional means, potentially eliminating multiple laborious steps in surgical splint fabrication and reducing the potential for error that can accumulate over the many steps of model surgery.

Most studies have shown model surgery to be generally accurate at a submillimetric level. It is likely that asymmetric patients, especially those with cants and yaw deformities, may suffer poorer levels of accuracy with conventional means and may fare better in this new paradigm. Even if the results in accuracy are equivocal, this is a technology of interest to surgeons because of the resultant time savings in a climate of diminishing reimbursement for this type of surgery.

SUMMARY

Continuous quality improvement has been a mantra in health care for many years. Surgeons are always looking to improve not only the quality of their results but also the consistency with which these results are achieved. To this end, new technology is being incorporated into or replacing traditional diagnostics and treatment planning. The knowledge gleaned from this technology is being taken to the operating room, augmenting

conventional surgical techniques and improving the surgeon's eye. There has been much interest in the application of these technologies in many types of surgery and dentistry, and interest is particularly strong in craniomaxillofacial surgery.

REFERENCES

1. Ludlow JB, Ivanovic M. Comparative dosimetry of dental CBCT devices and 64-slice CT for oral and maxillofacial radiology. Oral Surg Oral Med Oral Pathol Oral Radiol Endod 2008;106:106.
2. Roberts JA, Drage NA, Davies J, et al. Effective dose from cone beam CT examinations in dentistry. Br J Radiol 2009;82:35.
3. Suomalainen A, Kiljunen T, Kaser Y, et al. Dosimetry and image quality of our dental cone beam computed tomography scanners compared with multislice computed tomography scanners. Dentomaxillofac Radiol 2009;38:367.
4. Ludlow JB, Davies-Ludlow LE, Brooks SL, et al. Dosimetry of 3 CBCT devices for oral and maxillofacial radiology: CB Mercuray, NewTom 3G, and i-CAT. Dentomaxillofac Radiol 2006;35:219.
5. Swennen GR, Swennen F, Hausamen JE. Three-dimensional cephalometry. Berlin: Springer; 2006.
6. Christensen A. Tactile surgical planning using patient-specific anatomic models. In: BWaG C, editor. Distraction osteogenesis of the facial skeleton. Hamilton (Canada): BC Decker; 2007. p. 99.
7. Smith MH, Flanagan CL, Kemppainen JM, et al. Computed tomography-based tissue engineering scaffolds in craniomaxillofacial surgery. Int J Med Robot 2007;3:207.
8. Xia JJ, Gateno J, Teichgraeber JF. Three-dimensional computer-aided surgical simulation for maxillofacial surgery. Atlas Oral Maxillofac Surg Clin North Am 2005;13:25.
9. Metzger MC, Schön R, Weyer N, et al. Anatomical 3-dimensional pre-bent titanium implant for orbital floor fractures. Ophthalmology 2006;113:1863.
10. Metzger MC, Schön R, Zizelmann C, et al. Semiautomatic procedure for individual preforming of titanium meshes for orbital fractures. Plast Reconstr Surg 2007;119:969.
11. Schramm A, Suarez-Cunqueiro MM, Rucker M, et al. Computer-assisted therapy in orbital and mid-facial reconstructions. Int J Med Robot 2009;5:111.
12. Fushiima K, Kobayashi M, Konishi H, et al. Real-time orthognathic surgical simulation using a mandibular motion tracking system. Comput Aided Surg 2007; 12:91.
13. Metzger MC, Hohlweg-Majert B, Schwarz U, et al. Manufacturing splints for orthognathic surgery using a three-dimensional printer. Oral Surg Oral Med Oral Pathol Oral Radiol Endod 2008;105:1.

14. Mischkowski RA, Zinser MJ, Kubler AC, et al. Application of an augmented reality tool for maxillary positioning in orthognathic surgery – a feasibility study. J Craniomaxillofac Surg 2006;34:478.

15. Olszewski R, Villamil MB, Trevisan DG, et al. Towards an integrated system for planning and assisting maxillofacial orthognathic surgery. Comput Methods Programs Biomed 2008;91:13.

16. Swennen GR, Mollemans W, De VClerq C, et al. A cone-beam computed tomography triple scan procedure to obtain a three-dimensional augmented virtual skull model appropriate for orthognathic surgery planning. J Craniofac Surg 2009;20:297.

17. Uechi J, Okayama M, Shibata T, et al. A novel method for the 3-dimensional simulation of orthognathic surgery by using a multimodal image-fusion technique. Am J Orthod Dentofacial Orthop 2006; 130:786.

18. Xia J, Ip HH, Samman N, et al. Three-dimensional virtual-reality surgical planning and soft tissue prediction for orthognathic surgery. IEEE Trans Inf Technol Biomed 2001;5:97.

Computer Planning and Intraoperative Navigation in Cranio-Maxillofacial Surgery

R. Bryan Bell, DDS, MD, FACS

KEYWORDS

- Cranio-maxillofacial surgery • Computer planning
- Intraoperative navigation • Computer-assisted surgery

Complex congenital, developmental, and acquired deformities of the cranio-maxillofacial skeleton are currently managed by reestablishing facial symmetry and projection through restoration of known horizontal, vertical, and sagittal buttresses using craniofacial techniques that have been developed and refined during the past 30 years.[1,2] Advances in diagnostic imaging, rigid internal fixation, and microvascular free tissue transfer have profoundly affected the predictability in which today's surgeons are able to restore patients to form and function. Despite notable successes, however, problems remain with regard to reestablishing facial symmetry, consistently restoring orbital volume, and accurately repositioning skeletal or composite tissue constructs into optimal anteroposterior, vertical, and sagittal relationships. These relationships should ideally result in favorable facial proportions and allow for successful implant-supported prosthetic rehabilitation.

Some patients with complex problems undergo surgical treatment with suboptimal results that are apparent to both patient and clinician, despite well-planned operations by experienced surgeons. There are several factors that contribute to poor outcomes, including the surgeon's reliance on 2-dimensional (2-D) imaging for treatment planning on a 3-dimensional (3-D) problem; difficulty in assessing the intraoperative position, projection, and symmetry of repositioned or deformed skeletal anatomy; poor visualization of deep skeletal contours involving the orbit, mandibular condyle,

and skull base; variability in the anteroposterior, vertical, and sagittal jaw and tooth position relative to each other and the skull base; and variations in head position and craniofacial development, as well as disproportionate growth.

Recently, surgeons have begun to adopt computer-aided design and computer aided modeling (CAD/CAM) software—initially engineered for applications in neurosurgery and radiation therapy—to assist in the planning and implementation of complex cranio-maxillofacial (CMF) procedures.[3] CAD/CAM software enables the clinician to import 2-D computed tomography (CT) data in DICOM format (Digital Imaging and Communications in Medicine) to a computer work station and generate an accurate 3-D representation of the skeletal and soft tissue anatomy. The data set can then be used to additively manufacture a stereolithographic model or it can be manipulated by segmentation, reflection, or insertion of specific anatomic regions for purposes of treatment planning.

Computer-aided CMF surgery can be divided into three main categories: (1) computer-aided presurgical planning; (2) intraoperative navigation; and (3) intraoperative CT/MRI imaging (**Fig. 1**). Presurgical planning software allows the surgeon to import CT data to provide a 3-D rendering of the skull for purposes of visualization, orientation, and diagnosis; analysis with 2-D and 3-D linear and volumetric measurements; manipulations or surgical simulation by mirroring, segmentation, or

Oral and Maxillofacial Surgery Service, Legacy Emanuel Hospital and Health Center, Head and Neck Surgical Associates, Oregon Health & Science University, 1849 NW Kearney, Suite 300, Portland, OR 97209, USA
E-mail address: bellb@hnsa1.com

Oral Maxillofacial Surg Clin N Am 22 (2010) 135–156
doi:10.1016/j.coms.2009.10.010
1042-3699/10/$ – see front matter © 2010 Elsevier Inc. All rights reserved.

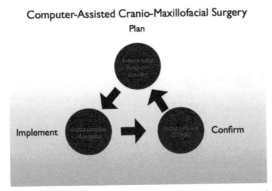

Computer-Assisted Cranio-Maxillofacial Surgery

Plan

Implement   Confirm

Fig. 1. Schematic describing computer evaluation and manipulation for treatment planning, intraoperative navigation for treatment implementation, and intraoperative or postoperative imaging for confirmation of accurate treatment.

insertion of anatomic structures; and creation of a planning model or custom implant. The virtual data can then be imported into a navigation system (frameless stereotaxy) that is used to provide guidance for the accurate and safe placement of hardware or bone grafts, movement of bone segments, resection of tumor, and/or osteotomy design. Finally, newly designed, mobile intraoperative CT scanners can be used to confirm the accuracy of the reconstruction before the patient leaves the operating room.

STEREOLITHOGRAPHIC MODELS

Using CT data sets to construct a stereolithographic model is a useful technique for evaluating and treatment planning complex facial deformities that was developed and popularized in the later part of the twentieth century.[4–9] As CT imaging has become more resolute, the quality of the additively manufactured model has likewise improved, resulting in a high-quality, precise representation of the patient's underlying skeletal anatomy. Two decades of experience has refined the indications for obtaining these models. In the author's opinion, they are most useful as an adjunct to maxillomandibular reconstruction, orbital reconstruction, and complex craniofacial/orthognathic surgery, primarily facial asymmetry.

Stereolithographic models are useful in maxillomandibular reconstruction as a guide to plate adaptation, jaw contouring, anteroposterior jaw positioning, and as an aid to constructing patient-specific custom implants.[10,11] They are equally as efficacious in orbital reconstruction by facilitating the planning of ideal osteotomy designs, allowing preoperative plate adaptation,

and enabling intraoperative bone graft contouring for precise inset into the patient at the time of surgery.[12] Craniofacial/orthognathic surgical planning is enhanced through stereolithographic modeling by giving the surgeon a tactile, 3-D representation of pitch, roll, and yaw; through vector planning in distraction osteogenesis; and as an aid to osteotomy design.[13,14] Unfortunately, modeling alone is limited by the fact that there is inadequate precision of the occlusal surfaces so as to eliminate the need for plaster casts or to provide a method for implementing the surgical plan in the patient; performing osteotomies is laborious; and there is no predictable method, when used alone, that the surgical plan as performed on the model can be transferred to the patient.

COMPUTER-ASSISTED SURGICAL SIMULATION

Computer planning systems have been developed for use in the craniofacial skeleton that provide individualized, 3-D manipulation of CT datasets,[15–18] which can then be combined with intraoperative navigation to facilitate accurate implementation of the virtual plan.[19,20] Virtual bone-based reconstruction can be performed through mirror imaging the opposite (presumably unaffected) side; by segmentation and virtual manipulation of deformed anatomic regions; or by inserting new anatomic structures into acquired, developmental, or congenital defects. Specifically, in maxillo-mandibular reconstruction, for example, mandibular contours can be *virtually* manipulated to accommodate for vertical, sagittal, and horizontal discrepancies, and the stereolithographic model can then be additively manufactured based on the virtual reconstruction.

Numerous CAD/CAM programs are currently commercially available for applications in craniofacial surgery, orthognathic surgery, head and neck reconstructive surgery, and dental implantology (**Box 1**). In the author's opinion, the ability to "back convert" data from their proprietary language to the standard DICOM format, so that digital reconstruction may then be imported into a surgical navigation system, is a distinct advantage of some systems over others. This also allows clinicians to transfer data back and forth for purposes of treatment planning or teaching. For example, iPlan and Voxim are both excellent software programs, but they do not offer the ability to be "back converted" into DICOM format, which can be understood by navigation systems other than their proprietary counterparts (BrianLab and Voxim, respectively). Analyze is an excellent research tool, but not very useful for routine clinical use. For this reason, the author prefers to use Surgi Case CMF (Materialise, Leuven, Belgium) for maxillo-mandibular reconstruction; and Simplant OMS (Materialise Dental, Ann Arbor, MI) for orthognathic surgery, both of which can then be "back converted" into the Intellect Cranial Navigation System (Stryker, Freiburg, Germany) for intraoperative guidance. The virtual reconstructions can be milled into a stereolithographic model, and a custom implant or surgical splint can be constructed and the final result is confirmed with intraoperative imaging.

INTRAOPERATIVE NAVIGATION

Intraoperative navigation is comparable to GPS systems commonly used in automobiles and is composed of three primary components: a localizer, which is analogous to a satellite in space; an instrument or surgical probe, which represents the track waves emitted by the GPS unit in the vehicle; and a CT scan data set that is analogous to a road map (**Fig. 2**). Intraoperative navigation systems were initially developed for use in neurosurgery[21,22] and are now commonly used in endoscopic sinus surgery.[23,24] Recently, several computer-aided surgical navigation systems became commercially available for use in cranio-maxillofacial surgery as well (**Box 2**).[25–28] All of these "frameless stereotaxy" systems allow precise location of an anatomic landmark or implant with a margin of error that is typically less than 1 to 2 mm.[29,30]

Early navigation systems, such as Instatrak, relied on electromagnetic fields, superimposed over the operative site, to achieve "satellite tracking" of the surgical instrument. The position of the tracking probe was determined by analyzing the effect of its ferromagnetic parts on the magnetic field. The problem with these systems lies in the variable stability of the magnetic field, such as that which can occur from metallic instruments. More contemporary navigation systems use optical instrument-based designs that rely on detection of light-emitting diodes (LEDs) by infrared cameras.

There are two types of commercially available optical instrument–based systems: active and passive. Active systems have battery-powered LEDs attached to the instrument probes that can be used anyplace in the body with a high degree of accuracy. Passive systems, on the other hand, replace the active light sources with reflectors, which are then illuminated by infrared flashes. The principal advantage of passive systems is that there is no need for electrical wires or batteries; thus, the handheld instrument is potentially lighter and more user friendly. The

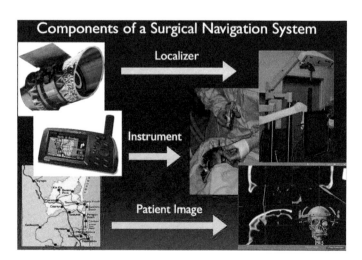

Fig. 2. Components of a surgical navigation system. Intraoperative navigation is comparable to GPS systems commonly used in automobiles and is composed of three primary components: A localizer, which is analogous to a satellite in space; an instrument or surgical probe, which represents the track waves emitted by the GPS unit in the vehicle; and a CT scan data set that is analogous to a road map.

disadvantage of passive systems is that artificial light sources may interfere with tracking, and they cannot be used within an enclosed cavity.

The position of the instrument relative to the patient is determined by the computer using the "local rigid body" concept, which states that "an object must have at least three fixed reference elements that span the coordinate system of the object in question."[3] The process of correlating the anatomic references to the digitalized data set constitutes the registration process. There are two types of registration: invasive and noninvasive. Invasive registration involves the placement of fixed markers that are secured to the patient's head with screws via small incisions in the scalp (or alternatively to the occlusion using a custom splint). The primary disadvantage of these fixed markers is the need for operative insertion and the need to immobilize the patient's head by attaching it to a Mayfield headset. Noninvasive registration methods, however, do not require head immobilization and can be performed by applying adhesive skin markers, either individually at various points on the face, or by using a commercially available LED mask. This technique is quick, simple, and accurate. Alternatively, a markerless technique called "surface matching" can be used in which a series of points on the face are scanned and correlated with the CT data set. The primary disadvantage of this approach is that it is time consuming. The author prefers noninvasive, mask registration whenever possible to avoid the use of a Mayfield head frame. Unfortunately, if a coronal flap is required, the LED mask cannot be used and either surface matching is required or the patient must be placed into a Mayfield and the registration completed using fixed skull markers.

Numerous clinical applications for these computer-based technologies are possible and will continue to be explored.[31–35] More than a decade of experience has led most surgeons to conclude that computer-aided CMF surgery is indicated in the circumstances listed in **Box 3**.

Orbital Reconstruction

High-velocity injuries often result in a "shattered orbit" with large volumetric increases internally, massive herniation of periorbital contents into the surrounding anatomic spaces, and cranial neuropathies. Although advances in craniomaxillofacial surgical approaches and biologic materials have improved our ability to more predictably restore these patients to form and function, a significant number of patients will still require revisional surgery despite the best efforts of an experienced surgeon.[36] When the entire orbit is disrupted and there are no posterior bony landmarks to guide in the reconstruction, accurate positioning of bone grafts or mesh plates becomes problematic. There is difficulty in establishing proper orbital contour, volume, and ethmoidal or antral bulge projection, as well as risk of encroachment upon the orbital apex and optic nerve (**Fig. 3**). Recently, preformed orbital mesh plates based on a composite of normal orbital CT data sets were developed and made commercially available for use in complex orbital trauma (Synthes, Paoli, PA) (**Fig. 4**). Presurgical planning using stereolithographic models to establish proper plate contour, as well as intraoperative navigation to ensure accurate and safe positioning of the plate in a poorly visualized anatomic region affords even the experienced surgeon greater confidence and predictability in the deep orbit (**Figs. 5** and **6**).[37–40]

In addition to navigating the orbital apex, computerized planning and pre-bent orbital mesh has the potential to predictably restore the difficult-to-access posterior medial bulge (ethmoidal bulge) region, also known as the key area, as well as the posterior orbital slope (antral bulge). Recently, Metzger and colleagues[39] described

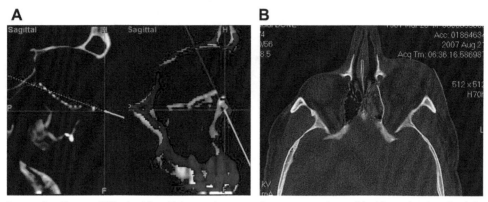

Fig. 3. Factors leading to difficulty identifying and accurately reconstructing orbital bony landmarks. (*A*) Sagittal CT scan demonstrating the normal ascending slope of the posterior orbit (*left*) and the common surgical error (*right*) of inadequate restoration of the height of the posterior orbit. (*B*) Axial CT scan demonstrating the normal postero-medial orbital bulge (*left, red*), and the common surgical error (*right, red*) or inadequate restoration of the postero-medial bulge. The green line represents optimal orbital contour.

a semiautomatic procedure for individual preforming of titanium meshes for orbital fractures. By using CT scan data, the topography of the orbital floor and wall structures can be recalculated. After

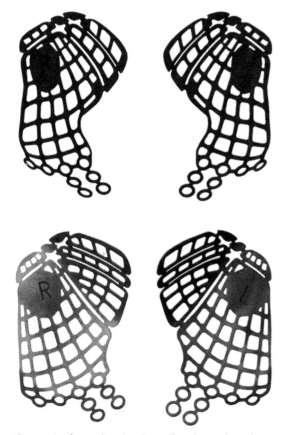

Fig. 4. Preformed orbital mesh plates based on a composite of normal orbital CT data sets are now commercially available for use in complex orbital trauma.

mirroring the unaffected side onto the affected side, the defect can be reconstructed virtually. Data of the individual virtual model of the orbital cavity are then sent to a template machine that reproduces the surface of the orbital floor and medial walls. A titanium mesh can then be adjusted preoperatively, or custom implant constructed, for exact 3-D reconstruction. It is then placed using intraoperative navigation to ensure accurate position within the orbit.

At the time of surgery, patients are typically approached via a transconjunctival incision alone or combined with an upper blepharoplasty or coronal approach depending on the clinical scenario. The internal orbit is reconstructed with the previously contoured titanium orbital plate or bone grafts. The external orbital frame is reduced or repositioned and stabilized using 1.3-mm and/or 1.5-mm titanium plates and screws (Stryker, Kalamazoo, MI; Synthes). Intraoperative navigation is then used to assess the accuracy of the restored internal and external orbital anatomy (Surgical Tool Navigation System, Stryker Navigation, Kalamazoo, MI).

Intraoperative navigation is performed by means of frameless stereotaxy with three infrared cameras controlling the pointer via integrated LEDs. The patient's position is identified with a digital reference frame that is fixed to an adhesive mask. The mask has a total of 31 LEDs that it uses for registration. A minimum of 21 of the LEDs are required to achieve optimal registration accuracy. Various points on the virtual image at the workstation and the patient are matched and compared with anatomic landmarks. An acceptable margin of error is defined as less than 1 mm. If a 1-mm margin of error is not obtained, then the registration is made using a fixed skeletal reference tool. Proper position of the bony

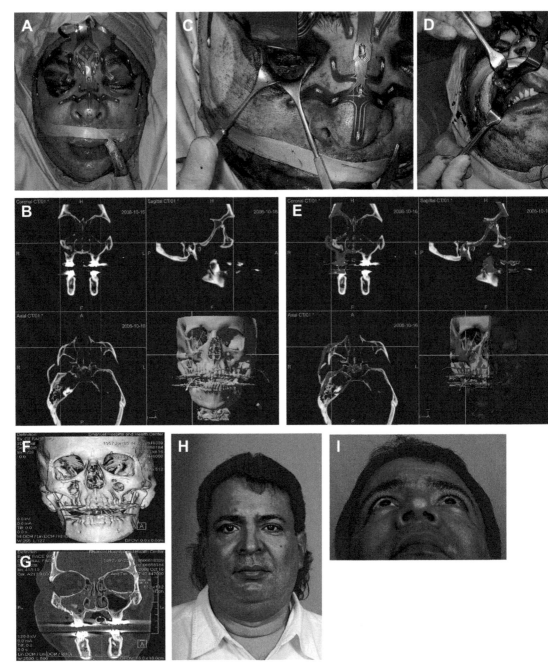

Fig. 5. A 35-year-old male involved in motor vehicle collision sustaining displaced right orbito-zygomaticomaxillary complex fracture and left orbital blowout fracture. (*A*) Preoperative appearance with LED mask applied. (*B*) Preoperative axial, coronal, sagittal, CT scans with 3-D reconstructions demonstrating medially displaced orbito-zygomaticomaxillary complex fracture with orbital displacement and increased orbital volume. (*C*) Intraoperative view following open reduction and internal fixation of the ZMC component with reconstruction of the orbital floor. (*D*) Intraoperative view of fixation at the maxillary buttress. (*E*) Virtual reconstruction by mirror imaging of the unaffected side with intraoperative navigation used to confirm accurate reduction of the malar buttress and restoration of orbital volume. (*F*) Postoperative 3D reconstruction. (*G*) Postoperative coronal CT scan demonstrating restoration of orbital volume with titanium mesh. (*H*) Postoperative appearance. (*I*) Postoperative appearance.

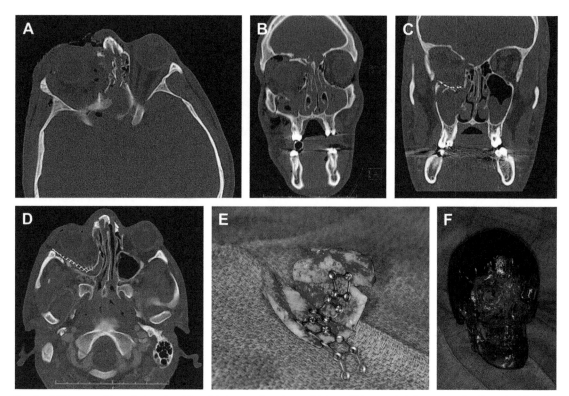

Fig. 6. A 21-year-old male involved in a high-speed motor vehicle collision sustaining severely disrupted fronto-basilar skull fractures involving the orbit and naso-orbital-ethmoidal complex resulting in significant increase in orbital volume and orbital apex syndrome. (*A*) Initial preoperative axial CT scan demonstrating increased orbital volume with complete disruption of posterio-medial skeletal landmarks. (*B*) Initial preoperative coronal CT scan demonstrating increased orbital volume with disruption of the entire orbit, herniation of periorbital contents and skull base involvement. (*C*) Postoperative coronal CT scan following initial orbital repair demonstrating inaccurate plate placement posterior to the equator of the globe, note increased orbital volume. (*D*) Postoperative axial CT scan following initial orbital repair demonstrating inadequate restoration of the postero-medial orbital bulge and significantly increased orbital volume. (*E*) Calvarial bone graft construct. (*F*) Bone graft "try-in" using stereolithographic model. (*G*) Bone graft inset into patient. (*H*) Intraoperative navigation images demonstrating increased, overcorrected globe position. (*I*) Intraoperative navigation demonstrating accurate placement of bone graft construct along the medial orbital wall based upon a mirror image (*red*) of the opposite (unaffected) side. (*J*) Intraoperative navigation demonstrating accurate placement of bone graft construct posterior to the equator of the globe along the antral bulge. (*K*) Postoperative coronal CT scan demonstrating favorable restoration of orbital volume. (*L*) Postoperative axial CT scan demonstrating favorable restoration of orbital volume posterior to the equator of the globe.

segments and internal orbit is confirmed in sequential fashion according to the following systematic protocol: malar eminence, infraorbital rim, lateral orbital rim, orbital floor, medial internal orbit/postero-medial orbital bulge, lateral internal orbit, posterior orbit/orbital apex, globe projection.

Maxillo-Mandibular Reconstruction

The loss of mandibular continuity or palatal integrity as a result of ablative tumor therapy or severe trauma is physiologically and psychologically debilitating. The utility of the free fibular osteocutaneous flap (FFOF) for mandibular reconstruction was recognized and subsequently popularized by Hidalgo in 1989.[41,42] Since that time, a series of surgeons throughout the world have shown the FFOF to be a highly reliable flap for reconstruction of mandibular and maxillary continuity defects.

Despite wide acceptance, there has been some controversy over the method of fixation used to stabilize the fibular constructs, with some authors advocating miniplates[43,44] and others advocating reconstruction plates.[10,45,46] One of the advantages of reconstruction plates is that an accurate shape of the neomandible may be created by bending the plate to the native mandible. In situ plate bending is time consuming, however, and a gap is formed between the straight fibula and

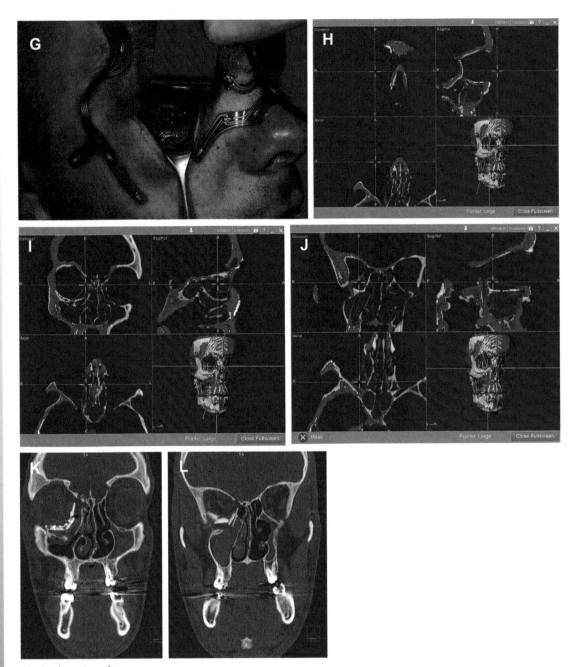

Fig. 6. (*continued*)

the curved mandible unless multiple osteotomies are performed. Increasing the number of fibular osteotomies further increases the complexity of the procedure and invites vascular complications. Additionally, in situ plate bending is not practical if tumor grossly invades soft tissue on the lateral mandible.

The use of stereolithographic models for plate adaptation before surgery has been used by the author for the past 5 years to aid in maxillo-mandibular reconstruction.[10] The model may be used to remove tumor deformation and eliminate mandibular convexities, and thus minimize fibular osteotomies. In addition to correcting transverse problems related to mandibular reconstruction, favorable anteroposterior relationships can be achieved by placing the reconstruction plate/fibular construct in an optimal relationship relative to the opposite jaw, at the correct occlusal plane angle. This will allow for more predictable implant-supported prosthetic rehabilitation and prevent overprojection of the mandible.

More recently, CAD/CAM software has been used to accomplish much of this "bench work" in a virtual environment (**Fig. 7**). All of the previously mentioned factors can be virtually altered and a stent is then constructed to provide a method for transferring the virtual reconstruction into reality.[47] Hirsch and colleagues described the use of CAD/CAM technology to produce orthognathically ideal surgical outcomes for patients with segmental mandibular defects undergoing reconstruction with fibular free flaps.[48] Using the Surgi Case CMF software (Leuven, Belgium), surgery is simulated on a computer workstation. The fibular and maxillary or mandibular osteotomies are transferred to a rapid prototyping instrument and a guide stent is constructed to allow for accurate placement of osteotomies (Medical Modeling, Inc, Golden, CO). The guide stent is sterilized and used during surgery (both fibular osteotomies and maxillary or mandibular osteotomies). In this fashion, the vascularized composite tissue is transferred into the appropriate anteroposterior, vertical, and transverse position, presumably with increased accuracy and efficiency (**Fig. 8**). Additionally, dental implants can be placed into the proper position based on optimal digital renderings. Proper positioning of the entire composite tissue construct is then confirmed intraoperatively using navigation. This "real time" intraoperative imaging also allows for immediate dental implant placement, and theoretically optimizes the chance for successful prosthetic restoration and decreases treatment time (**Fig. 9**).

Cranial Reconstruction

Reconstruction of cranial defects (cranioplasty) may be performed using autogenous bone or a number of alloplastic materials. Bone cranioplasty should generally be performed whenever possible, although success rates are proportional to the size of the defect.[49] However, if adequate bone is not available to cover the critical-sized defect, alloplastic cranioplasty is a viable option. Alloplastic cranioplasties may be performed with titanium (mesh or custom molded) and acrylics (polymethylmethacrylate),[50] ceramics (hydroxyapatite cement),[51,52] or high-performance thermoplastics (porous high-density polyethylene or polyetheretherketone [PEEK]).[53] The ultimate choice of material depends on the size and location of the defect, the presence or absence of infection, the quality and quantity of soft tissue coverage available, and the proximity to the paranasal sinuses.

CAD/CAM software can be used to construct custom-milled titanium plates or patient-specific implants constructed from high-performance thermoplastics such as PEEK.[54,55] The primary advantage of this technique over intraoperative molding of titanium mesh combined with hydroxyapatite, for example, is that it is potentially time saving and it provides an accurate, anatomic reconstruction of the defect. The significant disadvantage, however, is that it is difficult to manage the extradural dead space, when present, and the custom implants are expensive.

Tumor Resection

Intraoperative navigation has been advocated as a means to delineate resection margins during extirpative tumor surgery in the craniomaxillofacial skeleton.[56–58] Several reports have highlighted the value of this technology in improving the precision in which tumors are resected, while minimizing the amount of uninvolved tissues. In addition, surgery involving the skull base, pterygomaxillary fossa, or infratemporal fossa, including temporomandibular joint (TMJ) ankylosis release,[59] may be performed with an added degree of safety with respect to surrounding vital structures (**Fig. 10**). Finally, osteotomies may be accurately positioned based on a presurgical image so that preformed implants, bone grafts, or free flaps may be inset into the defect in an effort to increase operative efficiency and accuracy.

Surgery in the mandible deserves special mention because of the complexities of navigating a mobile structure. Accurate synchronization of the acquired CT data is made difficult because of the problems associated with determining a stable and reproducible mandibular position. There are three possible solutions to the problem.[60] The first approach is to place the patient in intermaxillary fixation before the CT scan. This method, however, is not feasible for transoral surgery. The second method is to position the mandible in centric relation or centric occlusion, either manually or using a dental splint. The strategy is sensitive to relative movements of the mandible, which in turn undermines the accuracy of the intraoperative navigation. A third approach has been described that uses a special sensor frame that is mounted onto the mandible, thereby allowing surgeons to optically track the jaw's position and to compensate for its continuous movement during surgery. Although time consuming, this method has the theoretical advantage of improved accuracy by monitoring the position of the

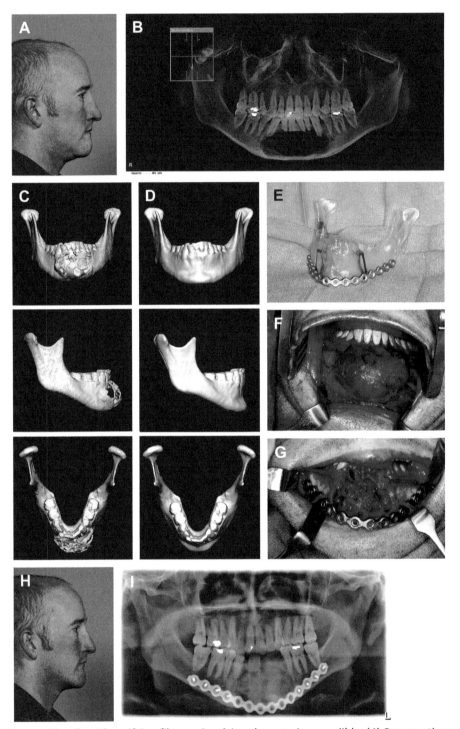

Fig. 7. A 29-year-old male with ossifying fibroma involving the anterior mandible. (*A*) Preoperative profile. (*B*) Preoperative panoramic radiograph. (*C*) 3-D CT image of the mandible, highlighting tumor deformation. (*D*) "Virtually corrected" 3-D CT image of the mandible, with tumor deformation removed and restoration of normal mandibular contours. (*E*) "Perfected" stereolithographic model with pre-bent reconstruction plate. (*F*) Intraoperative appearance of tumor before resection. (*G*) Intraoperative view following transoral tumor excision and application of pre-bent reconstruction plate. (*H*) Postoperative profile. (*I*) Postoperative panoramic radiograph.

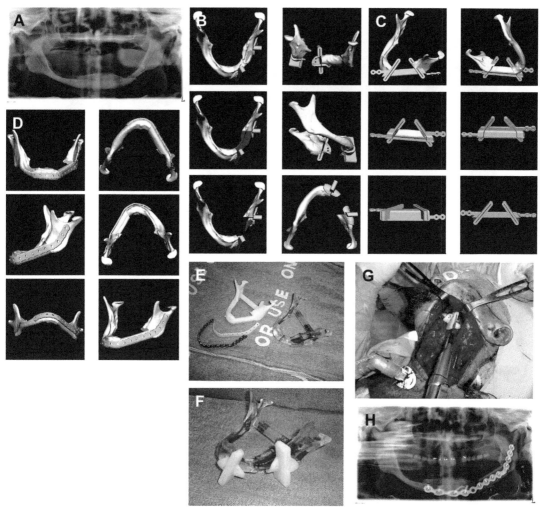

Fig. 8. Virtual planning for resection and fibular free flap reconstruction in a patient with osteoradionecrosis and pathologic fracture of the mandible. (*A*) Preoperative panoramic radiograph. (*B*) 3-D CT images a virtually planned resection with insertion of virtual cutting guides to assist in accurate placement of osteotomies. (*C*) Virtual fibula is inserted and cutting guides are designed to accurately transfer the virtual surgery into reality. (*D*) Virtual template of the reconstructed mandible with insertion of virtual reconstruction bar, which is then additively manufactured into an acrylic template or custom titanium reconstruction bar. (*E*) Stereolithographic model of unaltered mandible (*clear model*), the virtually reconstructed mandible (*white model*), and the reconstruction plate and acrylic template. (*F*) Unaltered stereolithographic model and mandibular cutting guide. (*G*) Intraoperative view with mandibular cutting guide. (*H*) Postoperative panoramic radiograph.

mandible directly, rather than by its relative position to other fixed cranial structures.

Craniofacial/Orthognathic Surgery

Preoperative computer imaging and intraoperative navigation are useful for planning complex surgical movements of the craniofacial skeleton. Using recently designed CAD/CAM software, osteotomies may be planned and the jaws or other anatomic structures can be virtually repositioned in any plane of space.[61–70] Maxillo-mandibular deformities of yaw, pitch, or roll can be accurately

repositioned into a more esthetic and functional position based on the individual clinical situation. Although clearly not necessary for routine orthognathic procedures, its potential in achieving improved accuracy in treatment planning complex facial asymmetry cases is self-evident.

Xia and colleagues[71,72] and Gateno and colleagues[73] have described computer-aided surgical simulation (CASS) for use in treatment planning of complex cranio-maxillofacial deformities. The first step of the CASS process is to create a composite skull model.[68] This is accomplished with a bite jig that is used to relate the

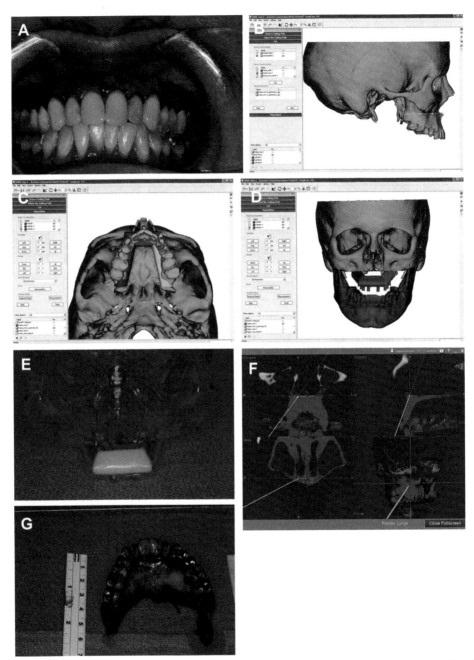

Fig. 9. A 67-year-old female with invasive mucosal melanoma involving the maxillary gingiva extending from the second molar to the contralateral second molar. (*A*) Preoperative appearance of lesion. (*B*) Virtual image based on CT data set of patient illustrating planned resection osteotomies. (*C*) Virtual reconstruction using a fibula (average female dimensions) illustrating inset with care to position fibular construct into a favorable position relative to the dental arch and into the pterygoid plates. (*D*) Virtual implants are placed into the virtual neomaxilla in a prosthetically favorable position relative to the opposing dental arches. (*E*) Stereolithographic model with neomaxilla template and dental implant stent additively manufactured based on the virtual reconstruction. (*F*) Navigated resection osteotomies. The virtual reconstruction is "back-converted" into the navigation system generating intraoperative navigation images that are used to transfer the virtual reconstruction into reality. (*G*) Resection specimen. (*H*) Closing-wedge fibular osteotomies are performed using cutting guides and templates from the virtual reconstruction. (*I*) Neomaxilla is formed from the fibula and implants are then placed using a stent constructed from the virtual images. (*J*) Accurate inset of the fibular construct is confirmed using intraoperative navigation. Planned anteroposterior and vertical position of the anterior neomaxilla is confirmed. (*K*) Following stabilization of the neomaxillary construct, the dental implants are placed under navigation guidance. (*L*) Postoperative panoramic image.

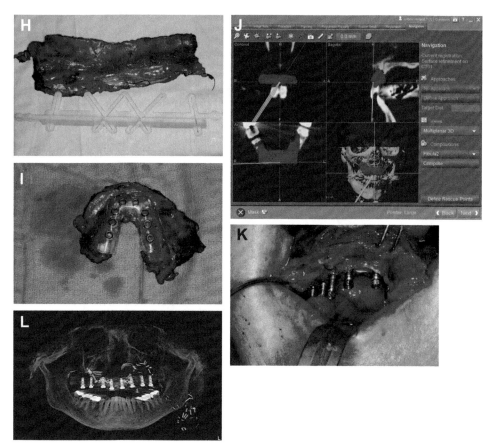

Fig. 9. (*continued*)

upper and lower dental casts to each other and to support a set of fiducial markers. The fiducial markers are then used to register the digital dental models to the 3-D CT skull model. After the bite jig is created, a CT of the patient's craniofacial skeleton is obtained with the patient biting on the bite jig. Digital dental models are then created by scanning the plaster dental models with a laser surface scanner. The result is a computerized composite skull model with an accurate rendition of the bone and teeth. The second step of the CASS is to quantify the deformity with cephalometric analyses and virtual anthropometric measurements. The third step in the process is to simulate the surgery in the computer by moving the bony segments to the desired position. Using this software, the maxilla and mandible can be repositioned in all three planes of space. Hence, deformities of yaw, pitch, and roll can be accurately corrected in a virtual environment. The final step is to transfer the virtual plan to the patient through surgical splints and templates that are created using a specialized CAD/CAM technique.

The author's preferred technique uses SimPlant OMS (Materialise Dental, Leuven, Belgium) in a fashion similar to the CASS described by Getano and colleagues[73] The patient is clinically examined in the usual fashion for orthognathic surgery and anthropometric measurements are obtained and analyzed. The bite jig is created (**Fig. 11**A), natural head position is virtually defined (**Fig. 11**B), plaster casts are obtained, and a CT scan with 1-mm cuts from the skull vertex to the clavicles is performed. Digital clinical photos, upper and lower stone casts, clinical anthropometric measurements, the acrylic bite jig, final occlusion registration, CT datasets, and the gyroscopic natural head position readings are then mailed to a software engineer for computer rendering (**Fig. 11**C) (Medical Modeling, Inc, Golden, Co). The software engineer then creates digital dental models by scanning the plaster casts with a laser surface scanner. The digital dental casts are "melded" to the digital CT skull using a best-fit model.[68] A tentative surgical plan is outlined and taken to a "live" Web conference with the software engineer. The maxillary and mandibular osteotomies are performed and movements are made with the patient's composite CT scan in the previously defined natural head position (**Fig. 11**E–G).

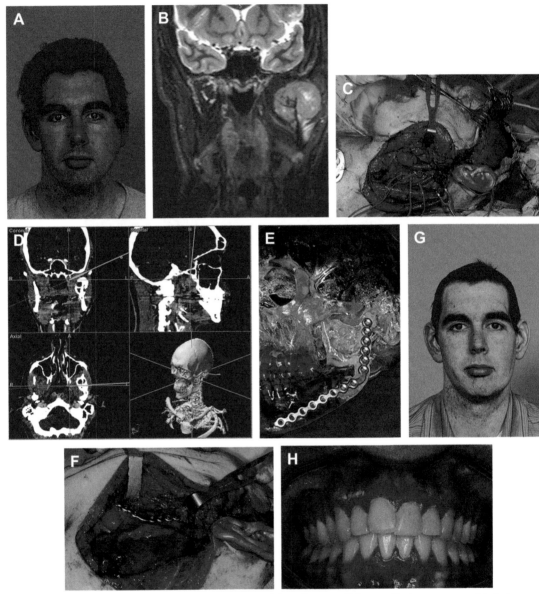

Fig. 10. A 25-year-old male with Ewing Sarcoma involving the mandible, masticator space, and infratemporal fossa. (*A*) Preoperative photograph. (*B*) Pretreatment sagittal MRI demonstrating large tumor emanating from the mandibular condyle with involvement of the masticator space and infratemporal fossa. (*C*) Intraoperative photograph demonstrating the approach for surgical resection to include composite resection of the mandible, masticator space, and infratemporal fossa via combined transcervical and infratemporal approach. (*D*) Intraoperative navigation used to assist in safe and accurate skull base resection. (*E*) Stereolithographic model used to plan resection and pre-bend reconstruction plate. (*F*) Inset of the fibular fascio-osseous free flap. (*G*) Postoperative photograph 12 months following surgery demonstrating resolving lymphedema, complete facial nerve function, and favorable esthetics. (*H*) Postoperative occlusion.

Deformities of yaw, pitch, and roll can be virtually corrected and accurately assessed using precise angular and linear digital measurements. Any inaccuracies in the virtual plan can then be corrected based on the virtual image analysis. Finally, the virtual reconstruction is transferred to the patient by construction of an intermediate and final splint using a CAD/CAM technique, which is mailed back to the surgeon before the planned procedure.

Temporomandibular Joint Surgery

Treatment of end-stage degenerative TMJ disease poses significant challenges to the surgeon

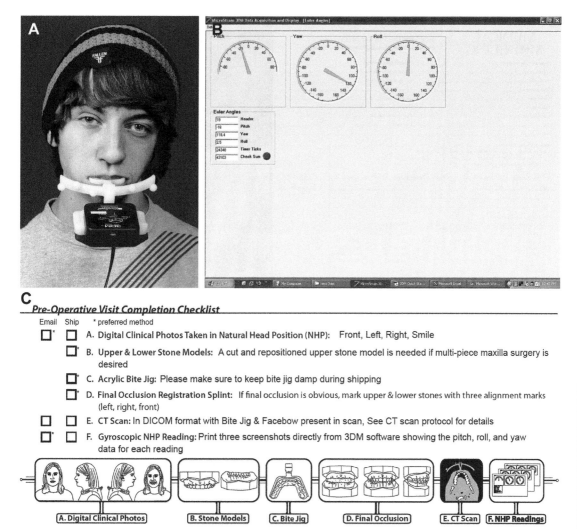

Fig. 11. Computer-aided surgical simulation with Simplant OMS and Medical Modeling Corporation. (*A*) Registration of natural head position with fiducial markers and gyroscope. (*B*) Gyroscope natural head position readings showing pitch, roll, and yaw data. (*C*) Preoperative checklist with required data necessary for virtual planning. (*D*) SimPlant OMS order form. (*E*) CT data set with 3D reconstructions and virtual plan for a patient with severe mandibular deficiency, retrogenia, and short ramus height. Patient is treatment planned for counter-clockwise maxillo-mandibular repositioning using bilateral inverted L osteotomies, Le Fort I, and genioplasty. (*F*) The mandible is virtually repositioned according to the preoperative plan, midlines are confirmed, and accurate and symmetrical correction of pitch, roll, and yaw is verified. A virtual intermediate splint is constructed from laser scanned plaster casts, which is then milled into an acrylic intermediate splint using a CAD/CAM technique. (*G*) The maxilla is virtually repositioned and a final splint is constructed intermediate splint following virtual repositioning of the mandible according to the preoperative plan (right mandibular sagittal osteotomy and left mandibular inverted L osteotomy). (*H*) Final splint following virtual reposition of the maxilla (Le Fort I ostoeotmy) and chin (genioplasty). (*I*) Post-prediction 3-D cephalometric analysis. Midlines are confirmed and accurate and symmetrical correction of pitch roll and yaw is verified (*J*) post-prediction 3-D CT images (*K*) post-prediction tereolithographic model for analysis and pre-bending of reconstruction plate (*L*) insert pre-bent reconstruction plate to stabilize inverted L osteotomy with interpositional bone graft (*M*) intermediate splint in place (*N*) final splint in place (*O*) preoperative appearance, frontal view (*P*) preoperative appearance, lateral view (*Q*) preoperative occlusion (*R*) postoperative appearance, frontal view (*S*) postoperative appearance, lateral view (*T*) postoperative occlusion. ([d] *From* Medical Modeling, Inc, Golden, Co; with Permission.)

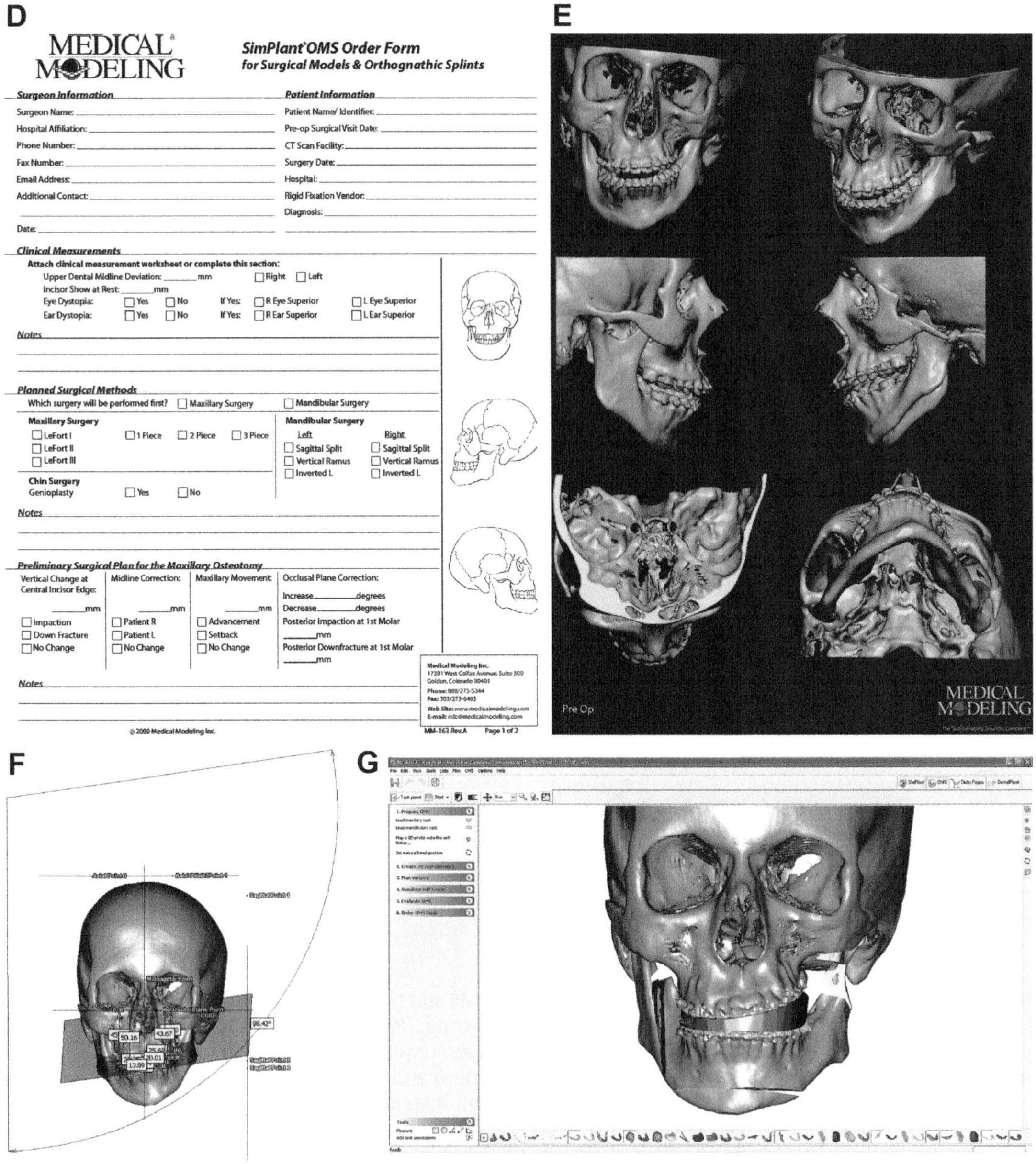

Fig. 11. (*continued*)

because of altered anatomy and carries the risk of injury to structures within the middle cranial fossa. Treatment is further complicated by the complex functional demands of the TMJ. Various methods have been described for total TMJ replacement, including gap arthroplasty with autogenous bone graft reconstruction, microvascular free tissue transfer, stock alloplastic condyle, and fossa prosthesis construction and custom, patient-specific TMJ condyle and fossa implants.

Traditionally, a two-stage approach has been used for total TMJ replacement in the presence of ankylosis or end-stage TMJ degeneration. Gap arthroplasties were performed, often with risk of neurovascular injury to structures in the middle cranial fossa, and a second-stage reconstruction was performed some time later. Navigation has been advocated for use in TMJ surgery for two primary reasons: (1) to promote safety during the ankylosis release, and (2) to

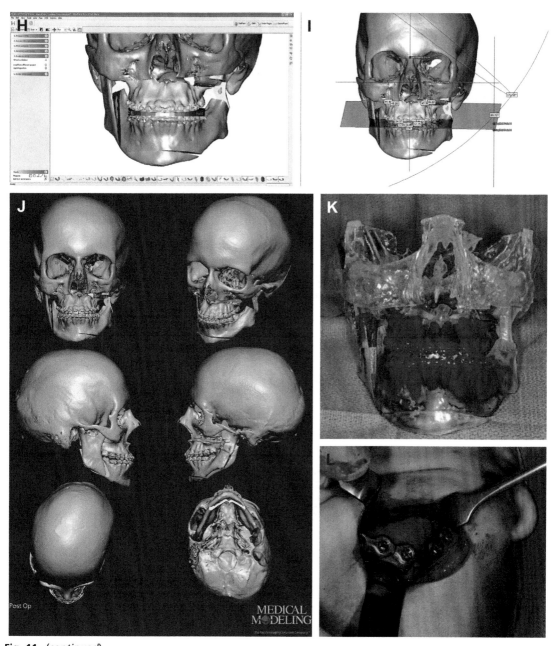

Fig. 11. (*continued*)

provide a predictable method by which one-stage ankylosis release and custom TMJ replacement can be facilitated.[59] Malis and colleagues[74] described a one-stage approach by which the navigation-assisted surgery is simulated on a stereolithographic model and a custom prosthesis is fabricated before surgery (**Fig. 12**).

Dental/Craniofacial Implants

Intraoperative navigation has for many years been advocated as a means to assist in the accurate placement of dental implants.[33,75–79] For a number of reasons, however, widespread acceptance of this technology for routine dental implant–supported prosthetic rehabilitation has not occurred. The reasons for this are primarily related to cost of the

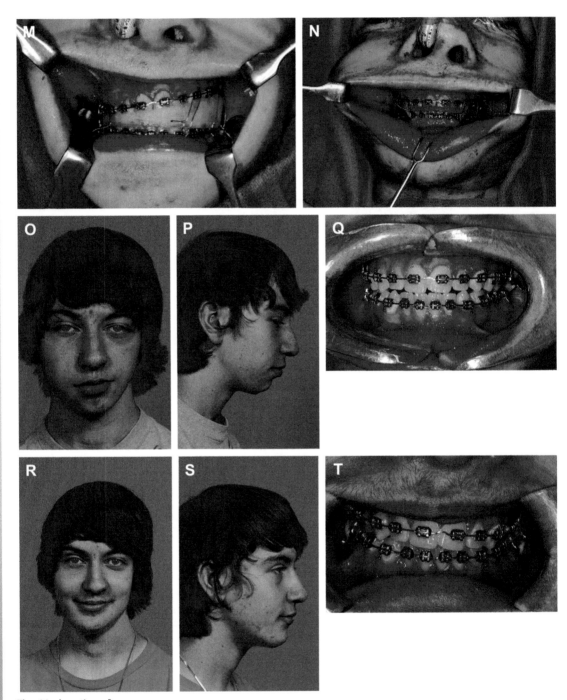

Fig. 11. (*continued*)

equipment in the context of the current US dental care delivery model—that being small, office-based private practices. The benefits probably do not outweigh the costs for routine cases of dental implantology. On the other hand, there are several important exceptions to this cost-benefit inequity, which are primarily related to completely edentulous and severely atrophic maxillo-mandibular rehabilitation[78]; composite tissue reconstruction of the maxilla and mandible following ablative surgery or posttraumatic deformity[57]; and for craniofacial implants used for prosthetic auricular reconstruction.[80]

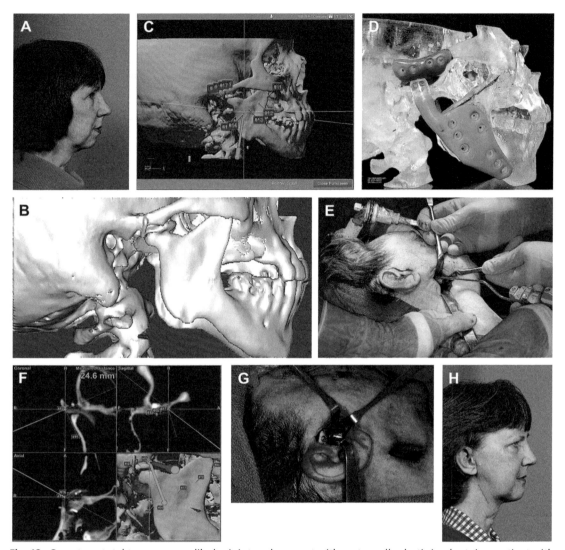

Fig. 12. One-stage total temporomandibular joint replacement with custom alloplastic implants in a patient with giant cell foreign body reaction secondary to failed Teflon-proplast implants. (*A*) Preoperative lateral view. (*B*) Preoperative 3D CT image demonstrating condylar degeneration with loss of ramus-condyle height and retained Teflon-proplast implant. (*C*) Virtual plan for resection before construction of custom TMJ condyle and fossa implants. (*D*) Stereolithographic model demonstrating "waxed up" custom condyle and fossa TMJ implant (TMJ Implants, Inc). (*E*) Intraoperative view of submandibular approach to the ramus facilitated navigation-assisted ramus osteotomy at the precise level as the virtual plan. Note navigation pointer. (*F*) CT images of intraoperative navigation with measurement of distance between glenoid fossa and planned ramus osteotomy, facilitating accurate osteotomy placement. (*G*) Inset of custom fossa and condyle implants. (*H*) Postoperative lateral view.

SUMMARY

Preoperative computer design and stereolithographic modeling combined with intraoperative navigation provide a useful guide for and possibly more accurate reconstruction of a variety of complex cranio-maxillofacial deformities. Although probably not necessary for routine use, the author's early experience confirms that of other surgeons with more than a decade of experience: computer-assisted surgery is indicated for complex posttraumatic or postablative reconstruction of the orbits, cranium, maxilla, and mandible; total TMJ replacement; orthognathic surgery; and complex dental/craniofacial implantology. Further study is needed to provide outcomes data and cost-benefit analyses for each of these indications.

ACKNOWLEDGMENTS

The author gratefully acknowledges the expertise of Katherine A. Weimer, MS (Chief Engineer, Medical Modeling Inc, Golden CO) for her tireless and dedicated technical assistance in computer planning.

REFERENCES

1. Manson PN, Hoopes JE, Su CT. Structural pillars of the facial skeleton: an approach to the management of Le Fort fractures. Plast Reconstr Surg 1980;66:54–61.
2. Gruss JS, Bubak PJ, Egbert MA. Craniofacial fractures. An algorithm to optimize results. Clin Plast Surg 1992;19:195–206.
3. Schramm A, Gellrich NC, Schmelzeisen R. Navigational surgery of the facial skeleton. Berlin, Heidelberg, New York: Springer; 2007.
4. Hemmy DC, David DJ, Herman GT. Three-dimensional reconstruction of craniofacial deformity using computed tomography. Neurosurgery 1983;13:534–41.
5. Vannier MW, Marsh JL, Warren JO. Three dimensional CT reconstruction images for craniofacial surgical planning and evaluation. Radiology. 1984;150:179–84.
6. Gillespie JE, Isherwood I. Three-dimensional anatomical images from computed tomographic scans. Br J Radiol 1986;59:289–92.
7. Komori T, Takato T, Akagawa T. Use of a laser-hardened 3D-replica for simulated surgery. Int J Oral Maxillofac Surg 1994;52:516–21.
8. Bill JS, Reuther JF, Dittmann W, et al. Stereolithography in oral and maxillofacial operation planning. Int J Oral Maxillofac Surg 1995;24:98–103.
9. Sader R, Zeilhofer HF, Kliegis U, et al. Uber die Genauigheit von 3D-gestutzten Operationsplanungen mit rapidprototping techniken. Mund Kiefer Gesichtchir 1997;1:61–4 [in German].
10. Bell RB, Dierks EJ, Potter JK, et al. A comparison of fixation techniques in oro-mandibular reconstruction utilizing fibular free flaps. J Oral Maxillofac Surg 2007;65(9):39.
11. Hannen EJM. Recreating the original contour in tumor deformed mandibles for plate adapting. Int J Oral Maxillofac Surg 2006;35:183–5.
12. Perry M, Banks P, Richards R, et al. The use of computer generated three-dimensional models in orbital reconstruction. Br J Oral Maxillofac Surg 1998;36:275–84.
13. Santler G. The Graz hemisphere splint: a new precise non invasive method of replacing the dental arch of 3D-models by plaster models. J Craniomaxillofac Surg 1998;26:169–73 [in German].
14. Linder A, Rasse M, Wolf HP, et al. Indikationen und Anwendung stereolithographischer Schadelrekonstruktionen in der Mund Kiefer Gesichtschirurgie. Radiologe 1995;25:578–82.
15. Altobelli DE, Kikinis R, Mulliken FB, et al. Computer-assisted three-dimensional planning in craniofacial surgery. Plast Reconstr Surg 1993;92:576–85.
16. Girod S, Keeve E, Girod B. Advances in interactive craniofacial surgery planning by 3D simulation and visualization. Int J Oral Maxillofac Surg 1995;37:120–5.
17. Vannier MW, Marsh JL, Tsiaras A. Craniofacial surgical planning and evaluation with computers. In: Taylor RH, Lavallee S, Burdea GC, et al, editors. Computer integrated surgery: technology and clinical applications. London (UK): MIT; 1995.
18. Bohner P, Holler C, Hassfeld S. Operation planning in craniomaxillofacial surgery. Comput Aided Surg 1997;5:153–61.
19. Hohlweg-Majert B, Schon R, Schmelzeisen R, et al. Navigational maxillofacial surgery using virtual models. World J Surg 2005;29:1530–8.
20. Schipper J, Klenzner T, Berlis A, et al. Objectivity of therapeutic results following skull base surgery using virtual model analysis. HNO 2006;54(9):677–83.
21. Drake JM, Joy M, Goldenberg A, et al. Computer and robot assisted resection of thalamic astrocytomas in children. Neurosurgery 1991;79:27–33.
22. Barnett GH. Surgical management of convexity and falcine meningeomas using interactive image guided surgery systems. Neurosurg Clin N Am 1996;7:279–84.
23. Mosges R, Klimek L. Computer assisted surgery of the paranasal sinuses. J Otolaryngol 1993;22:69–71.
24. Ossoff RH, Reinisch L. Computer assisted surgical techniques: a vision for the future of otolaryngology-head and neck surgery. J Otolaryngol 1994;23:354–9.
25. Hassfeld S, Muhling J. Computer assisted oral and maxillofacial surgery: a review and an assessment of technology. Int J Oral Maxillofac Surg 2001;30:2–13.
26. Wagner A, Ploder O, Enislidis G, et al. Virtual image guided navigation in tumor surgery: technical innovation. J Craniomaxillofac Surg 1995;23:271–3.
27. Ploder O, Wagner A, Enislidis G, et al. Computergestutzte intraoperative visualisierung von dentalen implantaten. Radiologe 1995;35:569–72.
28. Marmulla R, Niederdellmann H. Computer assisted bone segment navigation. J Craniomaxillofac Surg 1998;26:347–59.
29. Luebbers HT, Messmer P, Obwegeser JA, et al. Comparison of different registration methods for surgical navigation in cranio-maxillofacial surgery. J Craniomaxillofac Surg 2008;36:109–16.
30. Metzger MC, Rafii A, Holhweg-Majert B, et al. Comparison of 4 registration strategies for computer aided maxillofacial surgery. Otolaryngol Head Neck Surg 2007;137:93.
31. Heiland M, Habermann CR, Schmelzle R. Indications and limitations of intraoperative navigation in

maxillofacial surgery. J Oral Maxillofac Surg 2004; 62:1059–63, 99 2007.

32. Hejazi N. Frameless image guided neuronavigation in orbital surgery: practical applications. Neurosurg Rev 2006;29:118–22.

33. Ewers R, Schicho K, Undt G, et al. Basic research and 12 years of clinical experience in computer-assisted navigation technology: a review. Int J Oral Maxillofac Surg 2005;34:1–8.

34. Schramm A, Schon R, Rucker M, et al. Computer-assisted oral and maxillofacial reconstruction. J Computing and Information Technology CIT 2006; 14(1):71–6.

35. Pham AM, Rafii AA, Metzger MC, et al. Computer modeling and intraoperative navigation in maxillofacial surgery. Otolaryngol Head Neck Surg 2007;137: 624–31.

36. Hammer B, Kunz C, Schramm A, et al. Repair of complex orbital fractures: technical problems, state of the art solutions and future perspectives. Ann Acad Med Singap 1999;28:687–91.

37. Gellrich NC, Schramm A, Hammer B, et al. Computer-assisted secondary reconstruction of unilateral posttraumatic orbital deformity. Plast Reconstr Surg 2002;110:1417.

38. Schmelzeisen R, Gellrich NC, Schoen R, et al. Navigation-aided reconstruction of medial orbital wall and floor contour in cranio-maxillofacial reconstruction. Injury 2004;35:955–62 Int J Care Injured.

39. Metzger MC, Schon R, Schulze D, et al. Individual preformed titanium meshes for orbital fractures. Oral Surg Oral Med Oral Pathol Oral Radiol Endod 2006;102:442–7.

40. Klug C, Schicho K, Ploder O, et al. Point to point computer assisted navigation for precise transfer of planned zygoma osteotomies from the stereolithographic model into reality. J Oral Maxillofac Surg 2006;64:550–9.

41. Hidalgo DA. Fibula free flap: a new method of mandible reconstruction. Plast Reconstr Surg 1989;84(1):71–9.

42. Wei FC, Santamaria E, Chang YM, et al. Mandibular reconstruction with fibular osteoseptocutaneous free flap and simultaneous placement of osseointegrated dental implants. J Craniofac Surg. 1997;8:512.

43. Hidalgo DA, Pusic AL. Free flap mandibular reconstruction: a 10-year follow-up study. Plast Reconstr Surg 2002;110(2):438–49.

44. Cordeiro PG, Disa JJ, Hidalgo DA, et al. Reconstruction of the mandible with osseous free flaps: a 10-year experience. Plast Reconstr Surg 1999;104(5): 1314–20.

45. Kim Y, Smith J, Sercarz JA, et al. Fixation of mandibular osteotomies: comparison of locking and non-locking hardware. Head Neck 2007;29(5):453–7.

46. Futran ND, Urken ML, Buchbinder D, et al. Rigid fixation of vascularized bone grafts in mandibular reconstruction. Arch Otolaryngol Head Neck Surg 1995;121(1):70–6.

47. Leiggener C, Messo E, Thor A, et al. A selective laser sintering guide for transferring a virtual plan to real time surgery in composite mandibular reconstruction with free fibula osseous flaps. Int J Oral Maxillofac Surg 2009;38(2):187–92.

48. Hirsch DL, Garfein ES, Christensen AM, et al. Use of computer-aided design and computer-aided manufacturing to produce orthognathically ideal surgical outcomes: a paradigm shift in head and neck reconstruction. J Oral Maxillofac Surg 2009; 67(10):2115–22.

49. Grant GA, Jolley M, Ellenbogen RG, et al. Failure of autologous bone assisted cranioplasty following decompressive craniectomy in children and adolescents. J Neurosurg 2004;100:163–8.

50. Malis LI. Titanium mesh and acrylic cranioplasty. Neurosurgery. 1989;25(3):351–5.

51. Pompili A, Caroli F, Carpanese L, et al. Cranioplasty performed with a new osteoconductive osteoinducing hydroxyapatite derived material. J Neurosurg 1998;89(2):236–42.

52. Tadros M, Costantino PD. Advances in cranioplasty: a simplified algorithm to guide cranial reconstruction of acquired defects. Facial Plast Surg 2008;24(1): 135–45.

53. Frodel JL Jr. Computer designed implants for fronto orbital defect reconstruction. Facial Plast Surg 2008; 24(1):22–34.

54. Chim H, Schantz JT. New frontiers in calvarial reconstruction: integrating computer assisted design and tissue engineering. Plast Reconstr Surg 2005; 116(6):1726–41.

55. Dean D, Min KJ, Bond A. Computer aided design of large format prefabricated cranial plates. J Craniofac Surg 2003;14(6):819–32.

56. Schramm A, Suarez-Cunqueiro MM, Barth EL, et al. Computer assisted navigation in craniomaxillofacial tumors. J Craniofac Surg 2008;19(4):1067–74.

57. Schramm A, Gellrich NC, Gutwald R, et al. Indications for computer assisted treatment of cranio-maxillofacial tumors. Comput Aided Surg 2000;5(5):343–52.

58. To EW, Yuen EH, Tsang WM, et al. The use of stereotactic navigation guidance in minimally invasive transnasal nasopharyngectomy: a comparison to the conventional open transfacial approach. Br J Radiol 2002;75(892):345–50.

59. Schmelzeisen R, Gellrich NC, Schramm A, et al. Navigation guided resection of temporomandibular joint ankylosis promotes safety in skull base surgery. J Oral Maxillofac Surg 2002;60:1275–83.

60. Casap N, Wexler A, Eliashar R. Computerized navigation for surgery of the lower jaw: comparison of 2

navigation systems. J Oral Maxillofac Surg 2008; 66(7):1467–75.

61. Metzger MC, Hohlwe-Majert B, Schwarz U, et al. Manufacturing splints of orthognathic surgery using a three dimensional printer. Oral Surg Oral Med Oral Pathol Oral Radiol Endod 2008;105(2):e1–7.

62. Swennen GR, Mommaerts MY, Abeloos J, et al. The use of a wax bite wafer and a double computed tomography scan procedure to obtain a three dimensional model. J Craniofac Surg 2007;18(3):533–9.

63. Olszewski R, Villamil MB, Trevisan DG, et al. Towards an integrated system for planning and assisting maxillofacial orthognathic surgery. Comput Methods Programs Biomed. 2008;91(1):13–21.

64. Noguchi N, Tsuji M, Shigematsu M, et al. An orthognathic simulation system integrating teeth, jaw and face data using 3D cephalometry. Int J Oral Maxillofac Surg 2007;36(7):640–5.

65. Papadopoulos MA, Christou PK, Athanasiou AE, et al. Three dimensional craniofacial reconstruction imaging. Oral Surg Oral Med Oral Pathol Oral Radiol Endod 2002;93:382.

66. Xia J, Ip HH, Samman N, et al. Computer assisted three dimensional surgical planning and simulation: 3D virtual osteotomy. Int J Oral Maxillofac Surg 2000;29:11.

67. Gateno J, Teichgraeber JF, Xia JJ. Three dimensional surgical planning for maxillary and midface distraction osteogenesis. J Craniofac Surg 2003;14:833.

68. Gateno J, Xia J, Teichgraeber JF, et al. A new technique for the creation of a computerized composite skull model. J Oral Maxillofac Surg 2003;61:222.

69. Santler G. 3D COSMOS: a new 3D model based computerized operation simulation and navigation system. J Maxillofac Surg 2000;28:287.

70. Santler G. The Graz hemisphere splint: a new precise, non-invasive method of replacing the dental arch of 3D models by plaster models. J Craniomaxillofac Surg 1998;26:169.

71. Xia JJ, Gateno J, Teichgraeber JF. Three-dimensional computer-aided surgical simulation for maxillofacial surgery. Atlas Oral Maxillofac Surg Clin North Am 2005;13:25.

72. Xia JJ, Gateno J, Teichgraeber JF. New clinical protocol to evaluate craniomaxillofacial deformity and plan surgical correction. J Oral Maxillofac Surg 2009;67(10):2093–106.

73. Gateno J, Xia JJ, Teichgraeber JF, et al. Clinical feasibility of computer aided surgical simulation (CASS) in the treatment of complex craniomaxillofacial deformities. J Oral Maxillofac Surg 2007;65: 728–34.

74. Malis DD, Xia JJ, Gateno J, et al. New protocol for 1-stage treatment of temporomandibular joint ankylosis using surgical navigation. J Oral Maxillofac Surg 2007;65:1843–8.

75. Wagner A, Wanschitz F, Birkfellner W, et al. Computer aided placement of endosseous oral implants in patients after ablative tumour surgery: assessment of accuracy. Clin Oral Implants Res 2003;14:340–8.

76. Ruppin J, Popovic A, Strauss M, et al. Evaluation of the accuracy of three different computer aided surgery systems in dental implantology: optical tracking vs. stereolithographic split systems. Clin Oral Implants Res 2008;19(7):709–16.

77. Wittwer G, Adeyemo WL, Schicho K, et al. Navigated flapless transmucosal implant placement in the mandible: a pilot study in 20 patients. Int J Oral Maxillofac Implants 2007;22(5):801–7.

78. Ewers R, Schicho K, Truppe M, et al. Computer aided navigation in dental implantology: 7 years of clinical experience. J Oral Maxillofac Surg 2004; 62(3):329–34.

79. Casap N, Wexler A, Persky N, et al. Navigation surgery for dental implants: assessment of accuracy of the image guided implantology system. J Oral Maxillofac Surg 2004;62(9 Suppl 2):116–9.

80. Girod SC, Rohlfing T, Maurer CR Jr. Image guided surgical navigation in implant based auricular reconstruction. J Oral Maxillofac Surg 2008;66(6): 1302–6.

Endonasal Surgery of the Ventral Skull Base—Endoscopic Transcranial Surgery

Amol M. Bhatki, MD[a], Ricardo L. Carrau, MD[b,c,*],
Carl H. Snyderman, MD[a,c], Daniel M. Prevedello, MD[c],
Paul A. Gardner, MD[c], Amin B. Kassam, MD[a,c]

KEYWORDS

- Endoscopic • Skull • Base • Surgery
- Reconstruction • Tumors

Nearly every surgical specialty has witnessed an evolution toward minimal access techniques. In otolaryngology, neurologic surgery, skull base surgery, and in other fields, progress has been driven by the introduction of the endoscope. This, coupled with commensurate advancements in anatomic knowledge, instrumentation, and imaging technology (intraoperative computed tomography [CT], image-guidance surgery), facilitates approaches that "provide access and visualization through the narrowest practical corridor by providing the maximum effective action at the target with minimal disruption of normal tissues."[1,2]

Skull base surgery, as a subspecialty, has been slow to assimilate endoscopic techniques. However, endoscopic endonasal surgery has become commonplace for the treatment of expansile mucoceles and sinonasal tumors that involve the skull base and intracranial pathology, such as pituitary tumors, cerebrospinal fluid (CSF) fistulas, and encephaloceles.[3–6] Through experience and innovation, the expanded endonasal approach (EEA) currently provides a nasal corridor for the surgical treatment of various benign and malignant pathologies in any area of the ventral skull base.

A paradigm shift is happening with effective skull base surgery, including large resections, carotid artery mobilization, and complex intracranial dissection, being performed through a minimally intrusive transnasal corridor.

PRINCIPLES OF ENDONASAL SKULL BASE SURGERY

The origins of the EEAs to the skull base can be traced back to endoscopic approaches to the sella turcica. This seminal work arose from the combined efforts of otolaryngologists and neurosurgeons who used their experience and knowledge to take advantage of endoscopic technology for the treatment of pituitary tumors.[3] Even today, this collaboration is a central tenet of our paradigm.

The technique involves 2 cosurgeons, usually an otolaryngologist and a neurosurgeon, working simultaneously and side-by-side throughout the procedure. The operating surgeon uses a bimanual technique, an essential asset for hemostasis, vascular control, and intracranial dissection. The cosurgeon maximizes the visualization benefits of the

[a] Department of Otolaryngology – Head and Neck Surgery, University of Pittsburgh School of Medicine, 200 Lothrop Street, Suite 500, Pittsburgh, PA 15213, USA
[b] Department of Otolaryngology – Head and Neck Surgery, Eye and Ear Institute, University of Pittsburgh School of Medicine, 200 Lothrop Street, Suite 500, Pittsburgh, PA 15213, USA
[c] Department of Neurological Surgery, University of Pittsburgh School of Medicine, 200 Lothrop Street, Suite 500, Pittsburgh, PA 15213, USA
* Corresponding author. Department of Otolaryngology – Head and Neck Surgery, Eye and Ear Institute, University of Pittsburgh School of Medicine, 200 Lothrop Street, Suite 500, Pittsburgh, PA 15213.
E-mail address: carraurl@gmail.com (R.L. Carrau).

Oral Maxillofacial Surg Clin N Am 22 (2010) 157–168
doi:10.1016/j.coms.2009.10.005

endoscope by providing a dynamic, x"real-time" view with continual adjustments to provide the best view, appropriate magnification, and to guide instruments and assist with dissection. A skilled and experienced surgical duo working together is a major advantage for intraoperative decision-making, delineation of complex or distorted anatomy, and for the management of potentially catastrophic vascular injuries.

A rod-lens endoscope (Karl Storz, Tuttlingen, Germany), in itself, confers multiple advantages that allow a minimal-access approach. It has a narrow profile that is 4 mm in diameter, which allows its introduction through small apertures. This obviates extensive transfacial or transcranial approaches (typically required for microscopic visualization), with their resultant tissue disruption. Furthermore, the lens of a rod-lens endoscope is divergent and provides a panoramic view that greatly exceeds its 4-mm diameter. By changing the proximity of the scope to the operative field, magnification is simple and precise, and with the advent of high-definition camera systems, clarity of the image is unparalleled. Rod-lens endoscopes provide enhanced visualization, and the use of angled lenses avoids the "line-of-sight" limitations of the microscope. Although binocular 3-dimensional vision is lost, the surgeon's brain quickly adapts to working in 2-dimensional views by using proprioceptive cues and surgical landmarks.

The sinonasal cavity provides an ideal corridor for the surgical treatment of ventral cranial base lesions (**Fig. 1**). Conventional ("open") approaches consist of facial or scalp incisions combined with a craniotomy and/or maxillofacial osteotomies. Postoperative pain after conventional approaches is significant and convalescence may take weeks. Surgical scars and complications, such as wound infection, bone malunion, and loss of cranio-orbital bone grafts, can result in substantial facial disfigurement. In addition, transcranial approaches often mandate brain retraction and manipulation, which may result in cognitive or memory dysfunction.

Alternatively, the use of an EEA provides a direct caudal approach to the ventral skull base obviating brain manipulation. Furthermore, facial incisions, osteotomies, and bone grafts are unnecessary, greatly decreasing postoperative pain and eliminating facial scarring and disfigurement. Of greatest benefit, however, is that the EEA provides unhindered access to the midline corridor that is flanked by cranial nerves and internal carotid arteries.[7,8] Endonasal access thus obviates cranial nerve manipulation that beleaguers conventional lateral approaches.

Paramount to efficient and successful skull base surgery is choosing the best corridor or combination

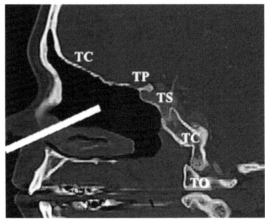

Fig. 1. Sagittal CT scan in a bone window showing the paramedian skull base. Septations of the ethmoid and sphenoid sinus and the floor of the frontal sinus have been digitally removed to simulate the breadth of the transnasal ventral skull base access (from the posterior table of the frontal sinus to body of C2). The endonasal skull base approach modules, including the transcribriform (TC), transplanum (TP), transsellar (TS), transclival (TC), and transodontoid (TO), are defined.

of corridors to address a specific pathology, which is not about whether to use direct visualization, a microscope, or an endoscope. However, the golden rule of endonasal surgery is to address the pathology without displacement of critical neural and vascular structures. If a tumor extends lateral or deep to the cranial nerves or a major blood vessel, a lateral conventional approach may be preferable. Extensive tumors often require the combination of an endonasal corridor and a traditional approach to access various components of the lesion (**Fig. 2**).

Principles of tumor dissection for endoscopic approaches are identical to those of traditional approaches. Critical neural and vascular structures are identified early, and when possible, the blood supply to the tumor is controlled. Tumors are first debulked so that precise dissection around the periphery can be performed. This allows for preservation of crucial submillimeter vessels and a precise dissection of the lesion from parenchymal pia mater (**Fig. 3**).

Critical to the success of surgery is the clearance of margins, especially when addressing malignancies. Intraoperative frozen-section analysis should confirm that microscopic negative margins have been achieved. A minimal access approach does not license the surgeon to be a minimalist. EEA may be less destructive to normal tissue and provide a more anatomically sound corridor, but the invasiveness of the procedure is commensurate with the pathology, the

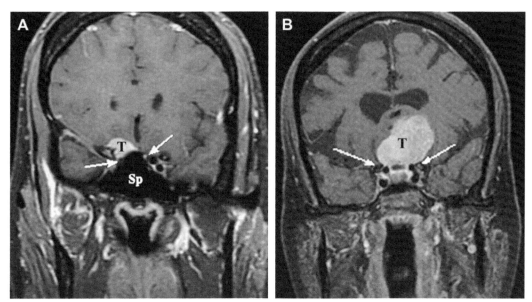

Fig. 2. (A) T1-weighted, contrast-enhanced, coronal magnetic resonance image (MRI) of a patient with a right anterior clinoid meningioma (T). The white arrows indicate the location of both optic nerves as they course lateral to the sphenoid (Sp) sinus. The right optic nerve, which lies medial and inferior to the tumor, would obstruct endonasal (transsphenoidal) access. Because the nerve cannot be mobilized, this case is best done through an "open," pterional craniotomy. (B) T1-weighted, contrast-enhanced, coronal MRI of a patient with an olfactory groove meningioma tumor (T). White arrows locate the optic nerves lateral to the tumor. Because the optic nerves are not interposed between the skull base and the lesion, this tumor is amenable to EEA.

needs of the patient, and the intended goals, whether it be cure or palliation. When treating malignancies, the resultant skull base defect after complete tumor extirpation is identical to that of

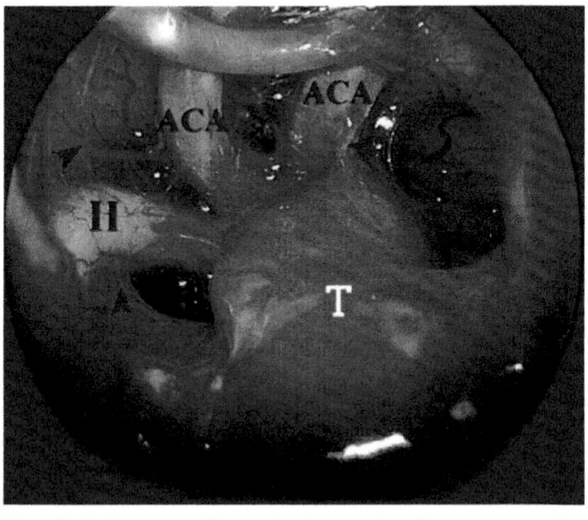

Fig. 3. Intraoperative photograph of a suprasellar tumor (T) being dissected off the optic apparatus. The right optic nerve (II), anterior cerebral arteries (ACA), and left posterior cerebral artery (PCA) are shown. The arrowheads demonstrate the crucial submillimeter vessels that can be preserved with microdissection, maintaining vascularity to important structures, such as the optic nerve and chiasm.

a traditional approach (**Fig. 4**). However, facial tissues disruption, craniotomy, and brain manipulation are obviated with EEAs.

PREOPERATIVE EVALUATION

Patients with skull base lesions may present with otolaryngological, neurologic, ocular, or endocrine symptoms. Despite the patient's specific symptoms, all 4 of these axes should be investigated. For example, a patient with epistaxis secondary to an extensive sinonasal tumor may have an undiagnosed optic neuropathy. Alternatively, a patient with headache and visual disturbance from a tuberculum sella meningioma may have a concomitant sinonasal inflammatory disease that must be addressed before the EEA. Therefore, a multidisciplinary skull base team is critical to optimizing the diagnosis and outcomes.

Besides a thorough history and physical examination, which includes a nasal endoscopy, skull base imaging is an essential aspect of the preoperative evaluation. This often includes a CT and a magnetic resonance imaging (MRI) scan. An imaging algorithm must be applied to obtain fine cuts (1–2 mm) through the entire skull base. CT angiography (CTA) provides excellent anatomic detail of proximity and distortion of vascular structures (**Fig. 5**). MRI sequences with different

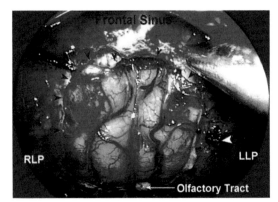

Fig. 4. Endonasal view after endoscopic anterior craniofacial resection of an esthesioneuroblastoma. The resection extends from the right lamina papyracea (RLP) to the left lamina papyracea (LLP) and from the frontal sinus to the planum sphenoidale. The olfactory tract has been transected to obtain negative tumor margins. The white arrowhead indicates the ligated left anterior ethmoidal artery.

relaxation times (T1-weighted versus T2-weighted) help in characterizing the lesions, formulating a differential diagnosis, determining the brain-tumor interface, and delineating adjacent neural and vascular structures. In addition, malignant tumors with potential for regional or distant metastasis may mandate a positron emission tomography (PET)/CT or CT of neck, lungs, and abdomen. Malignant sinonasal tumors with parameningeal involvement require a lumbar spinal tap for cytology and a spine MRI to rule out "drop metastasis" or carcinomatosis.

INTRAOPERATIVE STRATEGIES

Several intraoperative factors are instrumental in successful endoscopic endonasal skull base surgery. First, the administration of appropriate general neuroanesthesia with intra-arterial blood pressure monitoring and venous access is a basic requirement. Contrary to hypotensive anesthesia, which is a common practice during inflammatory sinonasal surgery,[9] the patient is maintained normotensive or mildly hypertensive to ensure perfusion of neural tissues (mean arterial pressure >85 mmHg). This is critical when compression or edema manifests as a preoperative neurologic defect. Compressed neural tissues are inherently ischemic; therefore, even transient perfusion fluctuations may cause prolonged or sustained deficits. To further assess neurologic function and perfusion, all patients undergo intraoperative monitoring of somatosensory evoked potentials and, when indicated, electromyography of muscles innervated by cranial nerves that are considered at risk.

The progressive expansion of endonasal skull base surgery beyond the sella would not be safely possible without the concomitant technological advancement of intraoperative image guidance. Real-time correlation of the operative field to

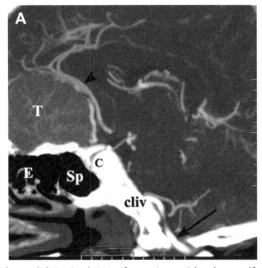
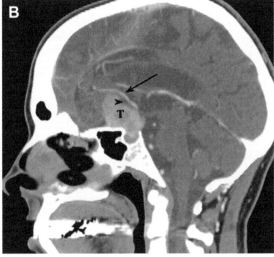

Fig. 5. (*A*) Sagittal CTA of a patient with a large olfactory groove meningioma tumor (T). The A2 segments of both anterior cerebral arteries (*arrowheads*) have been displaced superiorly and directly juxtapose the superior aspect of the tumor, making the tumor-brain interface dissection technically difficult. The parasellar internal carotid artery (C), sphenoid sinus (Sp) and vertebral artery (*arrow*) are also seen. (*B*) A sagittal CTA of another patient with a meningioma (T). A cuff of brain parenchyma (*arrowhead*) intercedes between the tumor and the A2 arteries (*arrow*). Dissection of the brain tumor interface is technically easier in such cases.

preoperative CT, CTA, MRI and magnetic resonance angiography precisely reflects and corroborates the surgeon's impression of the surrounding anatomy (**Fig. 6**). It is possible to identify and preserve critical structures and anticipate the position of others while focusing on the endonasal exposure and tumor dissection,[10] especially in the presence of anatomic variants or distortion of normal anatomy and surgical landmarks by the tumor.

The lack of specialized surgical instruments initially presented a technical challenge for endonasal skull base surgery. Many of the instruments were designed for endoscopic sinus surgery and did not have the length, angles, touch, and precision necessary for endoscopic skull base surgery. Now commercially available, these endoscopic instruments emulate conventional neurosurgical instruments and allow for efficient and precise manipulation of tissues. Similarly, instruments, such as bipolar electrocautery, high-speed drills, and ultrasonic aspirators, have been lengthened and made slimmer to accommodate the endonasal corridor.

Hemostasis, in particular, provides a special technical challenge for the endoscopic skull base surgeon. Prevention, the optimal solution, is best accomplished by visualization, cauterization, and sharp dissection, and by simultaneously limiting blunt dissection and traction. Realistically, bleeding from either the tumor or the surrounding vasculature is often unavoidable.

Low-flow bleeding from either the mucosa, bone, or from a venous source is best controlled using warm-water irrigation. It is a common misconception that cold-water irrigation provides effective hemostasis; the modest resultant vasoconstriction is often insufficient to significantly reduce bleeding. Warm-water irrigation, in contrast, is nearly as effective as surgery for epistaxis.[11] Proposed mechanisms of action include platelet activation, interstitial edema, and enhanced enzymatic activity of coagulation.[12] The ideal temperature for this is 48°C,[13] but 40°C is used to avoid hyperthermia of the neural structures. For example, brisk venous bleeding from a dural sinus requires application of a hemostatic agent, such as FloSeal (Baxter International, Inc, Deerfield, IL, USA), Avitene (Ethicon

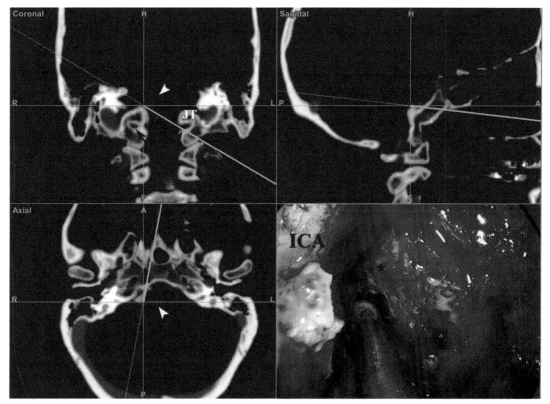

Fig. 6. Intraoperative snapshot of the image-guidance system for a patient with a right petroclival meningioma (*white arrowhead* and *asterisk*). The tumor emanates from the jugular tubercle (JT) just above the hypoglossal canals (*black arrows*). After the vidian canal (*black arrowhead*) was drilled away, the internal carotid artery (ICA) was mobilized to obtain access to the tumor.

[Johnson and Johnson], Somerville, NJ, USA), or Syvek (Marine Polymer, Boston, MA, USA).

In the case of high-flow arterial bleeding, direct application of bipolar cauterization or hemostatic or aneurysms clips is paramount. Although packing may provide temporary hemostasis, the potential for delayed intracranial bleeding mandates definitive control. Collaborative experience with the 2-surgeon approach is requisite for maintaining adequate visualization in a bloody field. Similarly, a bimanual approach facilitates suctioning with concomitant cautery (**Fig. 7**). On occasion, in the face of significant operative blood loss, tumor resections may be staged to allow hemodynamic recovery.

SURGICAL APPROACHES

The concept of surgical corridors typical of open skull base surgery can also be adopted for endoscopic skull base surgery; therefore, the endoscopic approaches to the ventral skull base have been defined by a series of surgical modules. These modules define the sinonasal exposure, the location and extent of skull base osteotomies, and the anticipated extracranial and intracranial anatomy. Furthermore, these modules can be combined to control multiple areas of the skull base and, segmentally, address a large, complex tumor as necessary. These modules have been categorized based on their relationship to the internal carotid artery (ICA); the sagittal plane modules define corridors medial to the ICA, whereas paramedian corridors lateral to the ICA are addressed by coronal plane modules.

Sagittal Plane Modules

The sagittal plane modules are divided into transsellar, transplanum, transcribriform, transclival, and transodontoid approaches (see **Fig. 1**).[7,14] The transsellar module provides exposure to the pituitary gland, the dorsum sella, and the medial aspects of the cavernous sinus. Sinonasal exposure with bilateral sphenoidotomies and posterior ethmoidectomies allows an adequate working corridor. This approach is most commonly used to address pituitary adenomas and Rathke cleft cysts.

The transplanum module exposes the dura overlying the planum sphenoidale, with the lateral limits defined by the optic nerves. Removal of the tuberculum and control of the superior intercavernous sinus augments this approach by providing access to the suprasellar cistern and the optic apparatus, distal ICA, and anterior cerebral and anterior communicating arteries. Meningiomas, craniopharyngiomas, and gliomas, involving the suprasellar cistern and planum sphenoidale, are approached via this module.[8,15]

The transcribriform module provides access to the anterior cranial fossa. A complete ethmoidectomy, sphenoidotomy, and wide endoscopic frontal sinusotomy (Draf III or endoscopic Lothrop) exposes the bone of the posterior table of the frontal sinus, ethmoid roof, and sphenoid roof. The cribriform plate can then be removed after the anterior and posterior ethmoidal arteries are ligated. Dura, frontal lobes, and olfactory bulbs and tracts may be exposed thereafter. This module is commonly used for meningiomas, schwannomas, and sinonasal malignancies (eg, esthesioneuroblastoma,

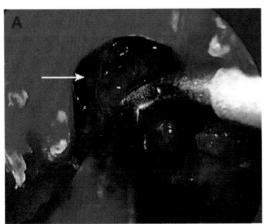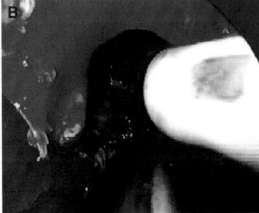

Fig. 7. (A) Intraoperative photograph of a suprasellar tumor (T) dissection. A small vessel feeding the tumor is present (*arrowhead*). The A2 segment of the anterior cerebral artery (*white arrow*) is adjacent to the tumor. (B) Bipolar microcautery is meticulously applied to the vessel before transection.

squamous cell carcinoma) (**Fig. 8**).[16] The bony and dural resection is identical to an open anterior craniofacial resection.

The clivus separates the sphenoid sinus and nasopharynx from the posterior fossa. Tumors, such as chordomas, chondrosarcomas, and meningiomas, can be successfully approached by the transclival module (**Fig. 9**).[17] Cranial nerves VI and XII and the vertebral and basilar arteries are encountered during the dural dissection of the posterior fossa. By further exposing the nasopharynx, removing the body of C1, and resecting the odontoid process, one can approach the ventral aspect of the craniocervical junction.[18] This transodontoid module allows for decompression of the spinal cord for rheumatoid diseases and also serves as a transnasal approach for limited intra-axial tumors.

Coronal Plane Modules

Approaches to tumors that are lateral to a virtual plane created by the paraclival ICA require an understanding of the coronal plane modules. These approaches are considered in 3 different depths from anterior (superficial) to posterior (deep). The anterior coronal plane has an intimate relationship with the orbits and anterior cranial fossae. The mid-coronal plane addresses the pterygopalatine, infratemporal, and middle cranial fossa (temporal lobe). The posterior coronal plane gives access to the lateral nasopharynx, jugular foramen, and posterior fossa.[19] Because the ICA demarcates the boundary, mastering its anatomic relationships, variations, and landmarks is essential for successfully and safely addressing these tumors.[19]

Several critical landmarks help the surgeon around the ICA. The plane of the anterior genu of the carotid artery is marked by the plane of the medial pterygoid plate. Clival bone removal lateral to this plane should be avoided until the ICA is definitively identified. A critical landmark for the more proximal petrous portion of the carotid artery is the vidian (pterygoid) canal (see **Fig. 9**).[20] Dissection along the lower half of this canal provides safe exploration until the ICA is identified; then, the superior portion and, if required, the bone of the carotid canal may be removed (**Fig. 10**). The cartilaginous eustachian tube provides a reliable landmark for the parapharyngeal ICA and the carotid canal.

The working corridor to the most anterior coronal module, the transorbital approach, is via a total ethmoidectomy and medial orbital decompression. Once the periorbita is incised, the medial compartment of the orbit is accessed. Vessel loops may be slung around the medial rectus and inferior oblique muscles via a transconjunctival incision, if necessary, allowing them to be stretched to further open the endonasal window to the intraconal compartment. Extension of the orbital decompression posteriorly provides for optic nerve decompression

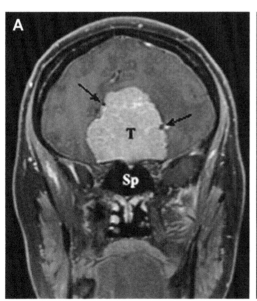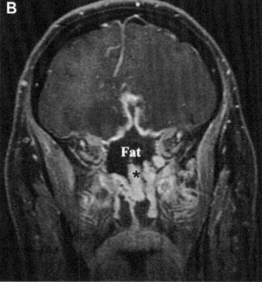

Fig. 8. (*A*) T1-weighted coronal MRI scan postcontrast demonstrates a large olfactory groove meningioma (T) with the A2 segments of the anterior cerebral arteries (*arrows*) flanking the tumor. (*B*) Postresection MRI, 3 months postoperative, shows complete tumor excision. The sphenoid is obliterated with fat and the skull base was reconstructed with a nasoseptal flap (*asterisk*).

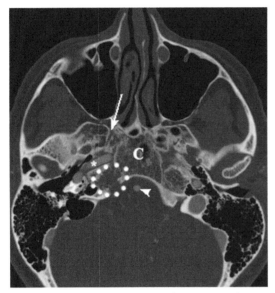

Fig. 9. Enclosed within the dotted lines is a right pet-roclival chondrosarcoma seen in the CTA. A transclival (C) module was used to approach and resect this tumor. The internal carotid artery (*asterisk*), vidian canal (*white arrow*), and basilar artery (*arrowhead*) are shown in relation to the tumor. Note the vidian canal's relationship to the anterior portion of the petrous ICA (*asterisk*).

and access to the dura of the superior orbital fissure. Although fibro-osseous tumors and meningiomas are common conditions requiring a transorbital approach, intraconal tumors, such as schwanno-mas, orbital pseudotumor, lymphoproliferative

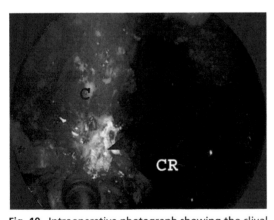

Fig. 10. Intraoperative photograph showing the clival recess (CR) and the right pterygoid fossa. Drilling along the inferior aspect (from 3 o'clock to 9 o'clock) along the vidian nerve (*asterisk*) is the safest tech-nique for identifying the petrous ICA and the anterior genu (*arrowhead*), which is often medial to the vidian nerve. The protrusion of the paraclival ICA (C) is seen within the right lateral wall of the sphenoid sinus.

lesions, and cavernomas, may also be addressed (**Fig. 11**).

The midcoronal plane modules specifically allow access to the pterygopalatine, infratemporal, and middle cranial fossa. The petrous portion of the ICA and its anterior genu must be successfully negotiated.[21] However, the width of the native nasal passage is insufficient to provide the required lateral access; an endoscopic medial maxillectomy (sometimes combined with an endo-scopic Denker extension) and transpterygoid dissection is often necessary. The sphenopalatine artery is ligated and the posterior antral wall and pterygoid plates are removed flush to the middle cranial fossa and foramen rotundum, to fully access the pterygopalatine and medial aspect of the infratemporal fossa.[22,23] Such exposure is essential to access large juvenile nasopharyngeal angiofibromas (JNA) that extend into the infratem-poral fossa (**Fig. 12**).[24] Tumors of Meckel cave and sinonasal malignancies with lateral extension are also addressed via this approach (**Fig. 13**).[23]

The posterior component of the coronal plane provides access from the occipital condyle medi-ally to the jugular foramen laterally. This working corridor is medial to the parapharyngeal ICA and the hypoglossal nerve, and nerves IX, X, and XI may be in the field of dissection. Commonly treated pathologies include nasopharyngeal carci-nomas, jugular foramen tumors, and chordomas.

RECONSTRUCTION

As endoscopic skull base resections have continued to increase in complexity, new chal-lenges have been presented for the reconstruction of these defects. Indeed, the continued evolution of the EEA to successfully and safely address larger and more intricate lesions has been commensurate with the development and growing experience with vascularized reconstructions.

All skull base reconstructions strive to recreate a separation of the cranial cavity from the sino-nasal cavity to prevent CSF fluid leakage, pneu-mocephalus, and intracranial infection. Small skull base defects and CSF fistulas can be recon-structed with various free-grafting techniques, re-sulting in a success rate greater than 95%.[25,26] However, for large dural defects, free grafts are associated with unacceptably high rates of post-operative CSF leakage typical after an EEA. The lack of supporting structures and high flow of CSF in cisterns and ventricles pose further chal-lenges to the reliability of reconstruction.

Initial reconstructions strategies consisted of suturing of allografts, buttressing the dural repair with free fat grafts, and supporting the reconstruction

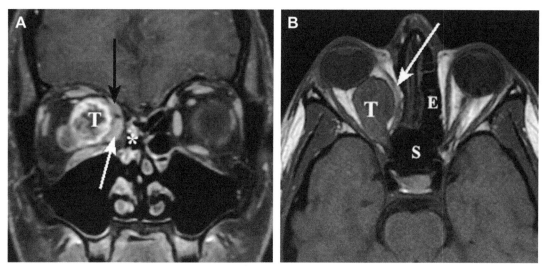

Fig. 11. 20 year-old patient with a right intraconal optic nerve glioma. (*A*) Coronal contrasted, T1-weighted MRI showing the heterogeneously-enhancing tumor (T). Note how the medial rectus (*white arrow*) and superior oblique (*black arrow*) obstruct the transorbital corridor from the ethmoids (*asterisk*). These muscles must be splayed by gentle traction to accommodate endoscopic endonasal instrumentation. The patient's left side provides comparative normal ethmoid and orbital anatomy. (*B*) Axial T1-weighted MRI showing the tumor (T) displacing the medial rectus (*white arrow*) medially. Septations within the sphenoid (S) and ethmoid (E) sinuses on the affected side must be removed to provide adequate exposure.

with balloon stents.[27] These techniques provided only modest improvements in outcomes. The greatest advance has been the development of vascularized, pedicled flaps that provide several advantages over traditional reconstructions. Compared with rotation or advancement flaps that recruit a random blood supply from a wide-based pedicle, an axial blood supply allows the flap to be mobilized over a larger arc of rotation and to conform better to irregular surfaces. A robust, reliable blood supply supports a large tissue surface area and expedites healing. In the authors' experience, the incidence

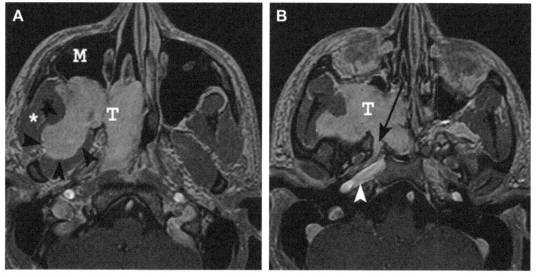

Fig. 12. Axial T1-weighted, contrast-enhanced, MR of a patient with a large JNA. (*A*) The tumor (T) fills the right nasal cavity, nasopharynx and extends into the infratemporal fossa (*arrowheads*) displacing the medial pterygoid and temporalis muscles (*asterisk*) laterally. (*B*) Adjacent section shows the tumor (T) expanding the vidian canal (*arrow*) proximally toward the petrous portion of the carotid artery (*white arrowhead*).

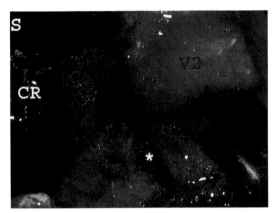

Fig. 13. Intraoperative photograph after a left ptery-gopalatine osteosarcoma resection. The sella (S) and clival recess (CR) are seen medially. Again, the vidian nerve (*arrowhead*) is seen just anterior to the paracliv-al carotid artery (C). The lingular process of the sphe-noid bone has been removed (*asterisk*) exposing the bony canal of the petrous carotid artery. Cranial nerve V2 is seen emanating from foramen rotundum and projecting anterolaterally and V3 is found just distal to foramen rotundum and travels inferolaterally.

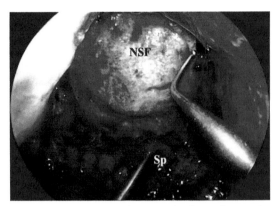

Fig. 14. Intraoperative photograph of anterior cranio-facial defect (from **Fig. 4**) with complete reconstruc-tion by the NSF in an onlay fashion. The sphenoid (Sp) is seen posteriorly.

of postoperative CSF leaks has reduced significantly to less than 5% from 20% to 30% with vascularized tissue reconstruction.[28]

The Hadad-Bassagasteguy nasoseptal flap (NSF)is the workhorse for endonasal skull base reconstruction.[29] Its large surface area and wide arc of rotation, coupled with a robust blood supply and technical ease, make for a reliable, versatile, and hardy reconstruction. The pedicle of this flap is the posterior septal artery (PSA), a terminal branch of the sphenopalatine artery (SPA), which traverses the sphenoid rostrum inferior to the sphenoid natural ostium. The reconstructive paddle incorporates the mucoperichondrium and mucoperiosteum of the nasal septum, which contains a highly vascular submucosal arcade of vessels derived from the PSA.

The large surface area of the nasal septum provides a flap that is capable of reconstructing virtually any skull base defect. In a radioanatomic study of the cranial base and flap dimensions, the authors' group demonstrated that the NSF could adequately reconstruct any single segment of the ventral skull base including the sella/planum, cli-vus, or cribriform.[30] In its largest dimensions, the NSF can reconstruct an entire anterior craniofacial defect from the frontal sinus to the planum sphenoi-dale and from orbit to orbit (**Fig. 14**). However, the flap length may not adequately cover defects re-sulting from combined approaches (eg, from frontal sinus to sella turcica or clivus). In such cases, adju-vant flaps, free fat grafts, or a shorter contralateral

NSF may be necessary to provide adequate recon-struction. The reach of the flap is maximized when it is on a planar surface instead of following the curves of the sinuses and skull base. Obliteration of a sphenoid or clival defect with a fat graft will allow the NSF to reliably reach the posterior table of the frontal sinus, if necessary.

If the NSF is not available because of tumor invasion, septal perforation, or prior sacrifice of the pedicle, adjuvant vascularized flaps may be used to provide a reliable reconstruction. Local en-donasal pedicled flaps include inferior turbinate and middle turbinate mucoperiosteal flaps.[31,32] Both flaps are pedicled posteriorly on respective branches of the SPA. Although both flaps provide a more limited surface area than the NSF, they may be sufficient for small defects of the planum sphenoidale and sella (middle turbinate flap) or the clivus (inferior turbinate flap).

For large skull base defects where the NSF is unavailable, regional axial flaps may be used for reconstruction: the endoscopic pericranial flap and the transpterygoid temporoparietal fascia flap.[33,34] Although both flaps require scalp inci-sions, they can be transposed endonasally and placed onto the skull base defect without the use of a craniotomy. For the endoscopic pericranial flap, the loose areolar tissue and pericranium of the scalp are harvested, much the same as for open cranial base surgery. The flap is pedicled on the supratrochlear and supraorbital vessels and transposed endonasally via a narrow glabellar osteotomy, obviating craniotomy.[33] A Draf III endoscopic frontal sinusotomy, requisite for this procedure, accommodates the pedicle as it is transposed. Tissue from this flap is ideal for large defects secondary to transcribriform, transpla-num, or transsellar modules.

The temporoparietal flap incorporates the pericranium, loose areolar tissue, and aponeurosis (which is continuous with the temporoparietal fascia). This flap is based on the superficial temporal artery and is harvested via a hemicoronal incision. Mobilization of the pterygopalatine fossa contents and removal of the pterygoid plates provides an endoscopic transpterygoid corridor that accommodates the pedicle of the flap.[34] Once the flap is transposed via the infratemporal/pterygopalatine fossae, it provides a large surface area of tissue capable of reconstructing clival and sellar defects.

Although vascularized flaps provide the cornerstone, skull base reconstruction is best performed using a multilayered technique. A collagen matrix synthetic graft is placed intradurally (inlay graft), which is then covered with the vascularized flap. Oxidized methylcellulose and DuraSeal (Confluent Surgical, Inc, Waltham, MA, USA) are applied as a tissue glue and sealant. The reconstruction is then bolstered with a balloon or expandable sponge nasal packing. Lumbar spinal drains are not routinely used; rather, they are reserved for cases where a cistern or ventricle has been exposed and a high-flow CSF leak is present.

CONTROVERSIES

One of the major controversies surrounding endoscopic skull base surgery is the oncological validity of endoscopic techniques. Critics of the EEA cite that en bloc resection is essential for surgical tumor control.[35] However, numerous examples in current medical practice refute this claim. Endoscopic removal of inverting papilloma of the sinonasal cavity has shown to have equivalent or even superior results to conventional en bloc partial maxillectomy.[36] Tumor debulking, in this case, provides for better exposure and delineation of normal and abnormal anatomy. The stalk or base of the tumor can be easily identified and resected totally, providing an equally complete extirpation. Mohs micrographic surgery for dermatologic neoplasms and transoral supraglottic laryngectomy for laryngeal neoplasms have similarly shown that en bloc resection is not needed to achieve adequate and appropriate tumor control. In reality, given the proximity to neural and vascular structures and friability of tumors, en bloc resection of skull base malignancies is often not possible even with a traditional open approach.

However, EEA techniques must conform to oncological principles. It is of utmost importance to achieve clear surgical margins, as confirmed by intraoperative analysis. To address a sinonasal tumor with skull base invasion, the portion of the tumor not attached to the skull base is first debulked to provide visualization of areas of tumor invasion. Bony margins of the skull base are identified and osteotomies are created to surround the tumor. Once the bone is removed, the underlying involved dura is resected en bloc (sometimes with the olfactory bulbs, such as in esthesioneuroblastoma). In this way, a sequential, layered resection of the tumor is performed to provide complete tumor excision.

SUMMARY

The continued progression of the EEA to cranial base lesions has been spurred by advances in instrument and imaging technology, growth in anatomic knowledge and surgical experience, and innovations in reconstructive techniques. Currently, a wide variety of malignant and benign lesions may be treated via the endonasal corridor without using facial incisions, craniotomy, or brain retraction. Understanding the complex, 3-dimensional anatomy is essential for success and safety. Although the endonasal route provides a less intrusive corridor, the surgical principles of resection, especially for malignancies, are not violated; tumor resections and resultant skull base defects mirror those of traditional "open" approaches.

REFERENCES

1. Jho HD. Endoscopic transsphenoidal surgery. J Neurooncol 2001;54(2):187–95.
2. Prevedello DM, Doglietto F, Jane JA Jr, et al. History of endoscopic skull base surgery: its evolution and current reality. J Neurosurg 2007;107(1):206–13.
3. Jho HD, Carrau RL. Endoscopic endonasal transsphenoidal surgery: experience with 50 patients. J Neurosurg 1998;87(1):44–51.
4. Zuckerman J, Stankiewicz JA, Chow JM. Long-term outcomes of endoscopic repair of cerebrospinal fluid leaks and meningoencephaloceles. Am J Rhinol 2005;19(6):582–7.
5. Mattox DE, Kennedy DW. Endoscopic management of cerebrospinal fluid leaks and cephaloceles. Laryngoscope 1990;100(8):857–62.
6. Lanza DC, O'Brien DA, Kennedy DW. Endoscopic repair of cerebrospinal fluid fistulae and encephaloceles. Laryngoscope 1996;106:1119–25.
7. Kassam AB, Snyderman CH, Mintz A, et al. Expanded endonasal approach: the rostrocaudal axis. Part I. Crista galli to the sella turcica. Neurosurg Focus 2005;19(1):E3.
8. Gardner PA, Kassam AB, Thomas A, et al. Endoscopic endonasal resection of anterior cranial base meningiomas. Neurosurgery 2008;63(10): 36–52.

9. Wormald PJ, van Renen G, Perks J, et al. The effect of the total intravenous anesthesia compared with inhalational anesthesia on the surgical field during endoscopic sinus surgery. Am J Rhinol 2005;19(5): 514–20.

10. Leong JL, Batra PS, Citardi MJ. CT-MR image fusion for the management of skull base lesions. Otolaryngol Head Neck Surg 2006;134(5):868–76.

11. Stangerup SE, Dommerby H, Lau T. Hot-water irrigation as a treatment of posterior epistaxis. Rhinology 1996;34(1):18–20.

12. Kassam A, Snyderman CH, Carrau RL, et al. Endoneurosurgical hemostasis techniques: lessons learned from 400 cases. Neurosurg Focus 2005; 19(1):E7.

13. Stangerup SE, Thomsen HK. Histological changes in the nasal mucosa after hot-water irrigation. An animal experimental study. Rhinology 1996;34(1):14–7.

14. Kassam A, Snyderman CH, Mintz A, et al. Expanded endonasal approach: the rostrocaudal axis. Part II. Posterior clinoids to the foramen magnum. Neurosurg Focus 2005;19(1):E4.

15. Gardner PA, Kassam AB, Snyderman CH, et al. Outcomes following endoscopic, expanded endonasal resection of suprasellar craniopharyngiomas: a case series. J Neurosurg 2008;109(1):6–16.

16. Carrau RL, Snyderman CH, Kassam AB, et al. Endoscopic transnasal anterior skull base resection for the treatment of sinonasal malignancies. Op Tech Otolaryngol 2006;17:102–10.

17. Stippler M, Gardner PA, Snyderman CH, et al. Endoscopic endonasal approach for clival chordomas. Neurosurgery 2009;64(20):268–77.

18. Nayak JV, Gardner PA, Vescan AD, et al. Experience with the expanded endonasal approach for resection of the odontoid process in rheumatic disease. Am J Rhinol 2007;21(5):601–6.

19. Kassam AB, Gardner P, Snyderman C, et al. Expanded endonasal approach: fully endoscopic, completely transnasal approach to the middle third of the clivus, petrous bone, middle cranial fossa, and infratemporal fossa. Neurosurg Focus 2005; 19(1):E6.

20. Vescan AD, Snyderman CH, Carrau RL, et al. Vidian canal: analysis and relationship to the internal carotid artery. Laryngoscope 2007;117(8):1338–42.

21. Herzallah IR, Casiano RR. Endoscopic endonasal study of the internal carotid artery course and variations. Am J Rhinol 2007;21(3):262–70.

22. Fortes FS, Sennes LU, Carrau RL, et al. Endoscopic anatomy of the pterygopalatine fossa and the transpterygoid approach: development of a surgical instruction model. Laryngoscope 2008;23(1):95–9.

23. Kassam AB, Prevedello DM, Carrau RL, et al. The front door to meckel's cave: an anteromedial corridor via expanded endoscopic endonasal approach- technical considerations and clinical series. Neurosurgery 2009;64(Suppl 3):71–82.

24. Hackman T, Snyderman CH, Carrau R, et al. Juvenile nasopharyngeal angiofibroma: the expanded endonasal approach. Am J Rhinol Allergy 2009; 23(1):95–9.

25. Hegazy HM, Carrau RL, Snyderman CH, et al. Transnasal endoscopic repair of cerebrospinal fluid rhinorrhea: a meta-analysis. Laryngoscope 2000; 110(7):1166–72.

26. Zweig JL, Carrau RL, Celin SE, et al. Endoscopic repair of cerebrospinal fluid leaks to the sinonasal tract: predictors of success. Otolaryngol Head Neck Surg 2000;123(3):195–201.

27. Kassam A, Carrau RL, Snyderman CH, et al. Evolution of reconstructive techniques following endoscopic expanded endonasal approaches. Neurosurg Focus 2005;19:E8.

28. Zanation AM, Carrau RL, Snyderman CH, et al. Nasoseptal flap reconstruction of high flow intraoperative CSF leaks during endoscopic skull base surgery. Am J Rhinol Allergy 2009;23(5):518–21.

29. Hadad G, Bassagasteguy L, Carrau RL, et al. A novel reconstructive technique after endoscopic expanded endonasal approaches: vascular pedicle nasoseptal flap. Laryngoscope 2006;116(10): 1882–6.

30. Pinheiro-Neto CD, Prevedello DM, Carrau RL, et al. Improving the design of the pedicled nasoseptal flap for skull base reconstruction: a radioanatomic study. Laryngoscope 2007;117(9):1560–9.

31. Prevedello DM, Barges-Coll J, Fernandez-Miranda JC, et al. Middle turbinate pedicled flap for anterior skull base reconstruction: Cadaveric feasibility study. Laryngoscope 2009;119(11):2094–8.

32. Fortes FS, Carrau RL, Snyderman CH, et al. The posterior pedicle inferior turbinate flap: a new vascularized flap for skull base reconstruction. Laryngoscope 2007;117(8):1329–32.

33. Zanation AM, Snyderman CH, Carrau RL, et al. Minimally invasive endoscopic pericranial flap: a new method for endonasal skull base reconstruction. Laryngoscope 2009;119(1):13–8.

34. Fortes FS, Carrau RL, Snyderman CH, et al. Transpterygoid transposition of a temporoparietal fascia flap: a new method for skull base reconstruction after endoscopic expanded endonasal approaches. Laryngoscope 2007;117(6):970–6.

35. Levine PA. Would Dr. Ogura approve of endoscopic resection of esthesioneuroblastoma? An analysis of the endoscopic resection data versus that of craniofacial resection. Laryngoscope 2009;119(1):3–7.

36. Nicolai P, Battaglia P, Bignami M, et al. Endoscopic surgery for malignant tumors of the sinonasal tract and adjacent skull base: a 10-year experience. Am J Rhinol 2008;22(3):308–16.

Endoscopic Techniques in Oral and Maxillofacial Surgery

Fred Pedroletti, DMD[a],*, Brad S. Johnson, DMD[a,b],
Joseph P. McCain, DMD[a,c]

KEYWORDS

- Endoscopy • Minimally Invasive • Teaching
- Sialoendoscopy • Orthognathic • Trauma

There have been many advancements in endoscopic surgery since Takagi first used the technique in 1918.[1] The endoscope has been described as an "extra set of eyes," and is the basis for innovation across multiple surgical disciplines and the fabrication of a new class of instruments and surgical techniques. As a teaching tool, endoscopically assisted surgery allows trainee surgeons to follow the surgery, and for the teaching surgeons to describe the procedure in real time and preserve the experience on video. Although there is a learning curve, teaching of the technique is improving, and various other techniques continue to be introduced with this surgical adjunct.[2–4] Some surgical procedures may also be completed with less morbidity and, perhaps, with a greater margin of safety (ie, avoiding technical error) with the use of an endoscope.[5,6] Increasingly, more endoscopic procedures are being described in the craniomaxillofacial region. This article reviews the present use of endoscopic techniques for the treatment of craniomaxillofacial trauma, orthognathic deformities, obstructive salivary gland disease, maxillary sinus disorders, trigeminal nerve injury, and temporomandibular joint (TMJ) disorders.

TRAUMA

Accurate repair of complex craniomaxillofacial trauma can be a challenge. Access can be difficult, and endoscopic techniques can expand the surgeon's view and capabilities in certain situations. The endoscope is a useful tool in these situations, and advances in this technology have provided some new opportunities in the management of patients. The use of this unique tool has been described in a wide range of surgical treatments, including fractures and orbital, frontal sinus, and other maxillofacial injuries.

Orbital Floor Fractures

Techniques for the use of the endoscope in orbital fractures have been refined since the 1970s.[7] With this tool, a minimally invasive procedure can be performed to evaluate the extent and severity of the fracture from a transantral approach. A surgeon can easily identify the location and size of the defect without invading the content of the orbit.[8] With superior visualization a well-informed decision can be made regarding the extent of reconstruction necessary and the approach to repairing the fracture.

[a] Oral and Maxillofacial Surgery, Broward General Medical Center/Nova Southeastern University, Fort Lauderdale, FL 33301, USA
[b] Currently in Private Practice in Eastern Tennessee, USA
[c] 8940 N. Kendall Dr #604E, Miami, FL 33176, USA
* Corresponding author.
E-mail address: fpedroletti@yahoo.com

Oral Maxillofacial Surg Clin N Am 22 (2010) 169–182
doi:10.1016/j.coms.2009.11.002

In traditional periorbital approaches, the posterior margin of the defect may be difficult to visualize.[9] These approaches require significant manipulation of the orbital tissues, and result in inflammation and the possibility of an ectropion or entropion. By using the transantral approach, these disadvantages are minimized. The transantral approach is technique sensitive and requires training and experience to be performed proficiently. Once experience is gained, the result can be comparable with that of the periorbital approaches.[9]

TRANSANTRAL ORBITAL FRACTURE REPAIR TECHNIQUE

The literature illustrates multiple approaches for repair of orbital floor fractures, including the use of a pure periorbital approach, a purely transantral approach, or a combination of the two.[10,11] The authors recommend that a purely transantral approach can be effective for the repair of the orbital blow-out fracture. With this technique, the posterior shelf of bone may be easily visualized (**Fig. 1**), and an implant placed transantrally to reconstruct the floor. This approach has the potential benefit of less manipulation of the orbital contents and periorbital tissues. Care is taken when manipulating the intraorbital contents from the antrum to avoid impingement of the musculature, periorbita, and optic nerve. It is important to reconstruct the posterior bulge of the orbital floor to restore orbital volume appropriately and avoid enophthalmos. Based on intraoperative findings, the surgeon should be prepared to access the

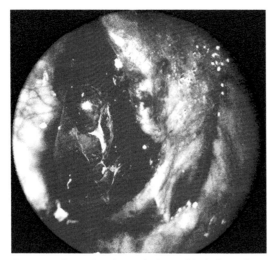

Fig. 1. Endoscopic view of the orbital floor from a transantral approach. Note the orbital content herniation into the sinus cavity.

orbital floor from a periorbital approach as needed.[10]

A simple maxillary vestibular incision is used. An osteotomy in the anterior antral wall is performed. The endoscope is placed into the sinus, which acts as a natural optical cavity. A 30°, 4-mm-diameter endoscope (Karl Storz, Tuttlingen, Germany) with a xenon light source is preferred; a 0°, 45°, or 70° endoscope may also be used. A sinusotomy of the sinus roof/orbit floor is completed, sharp bone fragments are removed, and the margins of the fracture are identified. Each shelf is carefully dissected and the orbital contents replaced back into the orbit. If fractured segments can be reduced, they can be stabilized with a titanium mesh or other material. If the fractured bone cannot be salvaged, the orbital contents are reduced, and an implant placed onto the orbital side of the fracture. The implant is tested for stability with a forced duction test and an ocular pulse test. Mesh or other implant material can be adapted onto the antral side of the fracture and stabilized. It is important to provide adequate support for the orbital contents by recreating the appropriate anatomy with suitable material.

Mandibular Angle Fractures

The mandibular angle fracture is one of the most common injuries of the maxillofacial region,[12] and may be treated in various ways.[13] Several factors contribute to the high reported rate of complications.[14] When using an intraoral approach, it may be difficult to position fixation with a high degree of precision because of limited access. With the adjunct of the endoscope, a surgeon may fixate the mandible with a superior and inferior border plate with a higher degree of certainty of its placement. With the aid of the endoscope, anatomic reduction by visualization of the entire fracture line to include the inferior border is simple.

Endoscopically assisted mandibular angle fractures all but eliminate the risk of injury to the facial nerve. The authors' experience shows that the procedure can have several advantages, including efficiency, when compared with the extraoral technique. In the authors' opinion, advantages include allowing the patient to function immediately rather than endure closed reduction, the patient suffers less pain than with extraoral incisions, and the scar is much less visible.

TECHNIQUE

There has been limited discussion of endoscopic-assisted open reduction and internal fixation (ORIF) of the mandibular angle fracture. When using the endoscope, the incision is similar to that of the standard intraoral incision for ORIF of the mandibular angle. A subperiosteal dissection is performed for creation of the optical cavity. The 30°, 4-mm-diameter endoscope, xenon light source, and a standard mandibular fracture instrumentation tray are used. A recommended specialized instrument is a retractor with an endoscopic sleeve to improve visualization and decrease instrumentation in the cavity. The endoscope allows for easy visualization of the fracture and inferior border of the mandible. Superior tension and inferior fixation plates are positioned and fixated using a single transbuccal trocar technique. The authors prefer a locking cannula as it aids in precise placement of the fixation hardware. Once optimal fixation is placed and the reduction is confirmed with the scope, appropriate documentation may be recorded, and closure is completed.

Subcondylar Fractures

When considering the management of all craniomaxillofacial fractures, the greatest controversy concerns the management options of the subcondylar fracture. The incidence of this fracture is significant, representing 9% to 45% of mandibular fractures.[15–17] The literature about subcondylar fracture repair supports open and closed reduction techniques.[15,18–25] Indications for ORIF of this type of fracture have been debated at length,[26–30] and are beyond the scope of this article. Level I evidence is lacking to provide a definitive answer regarding which modality is better in a particular clinical scenario.

The endoscope has changed the discussion and debate in that there is now a third choice for the management of this type of fracture with the advantages of the open technique, but without the major disadvantages (ie, external scar, facial nerve injury).

Endoscopically assisted reduction and internal fixation of subcondylar fractures have many purported advantages over conventional ORIF. Miloro[30] reported that the technique improved visibility in an illuminated and magnified field of view, with decreased bleeding, and better anatomic reduction, and decreased postoperative morbidity (ie, pain, edema, and limited opening). He further suggested that these reasons make endoscopy an attractive surgical adjunct. Because the technique is mostly performed with intraoral incisions, there is minimal risk for facial nerve injury, salivary fistula formation, or visible scarring. Although the advantages have been presented by many, endoscopic-assisted repair does have some disadvantages. As with many new technologies, and especially when dealing with this type of fracture, there is a steep learning curve. Operative times can be expected to double when first attempting this technique.[31] Despite the sensitivity of the technique, this surgical option has significant advantages once the surgeon becomes proficient (**Table 1**).

TECHNIQUE

Endoscopic-assisted treatment of the subcondylar fracture can be performed as an extraoral or a transoral procedure.[32] The authors recommend a transoral approach whenever possible to avoid the disadvantages of an open incision. The extraoral approach should be performed when the complexity of the fracture eliminates the transoral

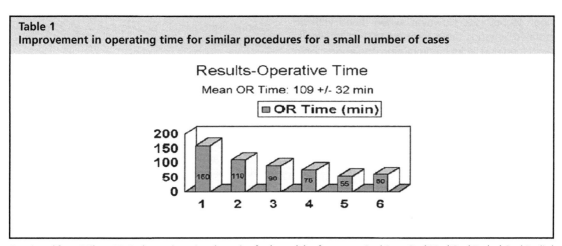

Table 1
Improvement in operating time for similar procedures for a small number of cases

Results-Operative Time

Mean OR Time: 109 +/- 32 min

⬜ OR Time (min)

Reprinted from Miloro M. Endoscopic-assisted repair of subcondylar fractures. Oral Surg Oral Med Oral Pathol Oral Radiol Endod 2003;96(4):387–91; with permission.

approach as a feasible technique (ie, severe fracture override, severely oblique fracture, or comminution).

The incision for the transoral approach consists of a lateral vestibular incision similar to that for a sagittal split osteotomy. A subperiosteal dissection to the proximal mandibular segment is performed for creation of the optical cavity. The authors prefer a 30°, 4-mm-diameter endoscope and a xenon light source. The Synthes subcondylar fracture tray (Synthes, ADI/AO Development Institute, Davos, Switzerland) has helpful retractors and instruments designed specifically for this procedure. It is important not to place the patient into maxillomandibular fixation to allow for manipulation of the proximal and distal segments of the mandible to facilitate reduction. Helpful points include the use of the specialized curved retractors, reduction-manipulation forceps, and placement of a clamp at the angle of the mandible percutaneously for control of the distal segment. A trocar is used to deliver the drill and screws for rigid fixation. The number of plates used for fixation can vary. Although use of this technique remains controversial, those individuals who become proficient may be able to avoid external incisions and provide stable fixation for various mandible fractures.

Frontal Sinus Fractures

Frontal sinus fractures represent about 5% of all facial fractures,[33] and one-third of those are isolated to the anterior table.[34] Frontal sinus fractures are typically associated with a significant force and usually involve other intracranial or facial injuries. Bicoronal, open-sky, or gull-wing approaches allow for proper reduction and reconstruction under direct visualization. Fractures that are complex or require detailed reduction and fixation techniques to gain stability should be repaired with open techniques. However, when faced with an isolated anterior table fracture that is minimally displaced and lacks comminution, the endoscopic approach may provide an alternative surgical option. The endoscopic approach avoids large incisions that may cause alopecia, paresthesia, scarring, or nerve injury.[35] This technique provides visualization of the sinus wall fracture, and can be used to evaluate the integrity of the nasofrontal duct (**Fig. 2**) and posterior wall of the sinus.[36]

TECHNIQUE

Limited incisions in the scalp or a transnasal approach may be used. As with the other techniques, a 30°, 4-mm-diameter endoscope and a xenon light source are used. An endoscopic brow-lift instrumentation tray or other endoscopic

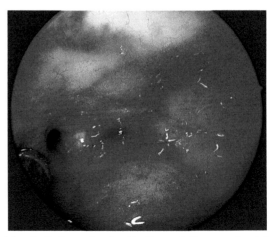

Fig. 2. Endoscopic visualization of the nasofrontal duct.

surgical instruments should be used to help manipulate the fracture segments.

One approach is via transnasal reduction after frontal sinusotomy[37] and insertion of a balloon catheter for reduction and support of the fractured segments. Another technique includes an incision through the eyebrow and a trephine bur hole into the sinus with endoscopic examination of the frontal sinus and subsequent reduction of the fracture.[36] The brow-lift approach, in which 2 incisions are placed in the hair-bearing area, can also be used. A subperiosteal dissection to the fracture followed by reduction with endoscopic instruments and plating may be performed for stability.[37–39] At times, particularly with younger individuals, reduction and fixation can be technically difficult because of the greensticking that typically occurs in this anatomic region.

ORTHOGNATHIC SURGERY

The endoscope has been used to assist with various orthognathic procedures in an attempt to gain better visualization and improve technical aspects of the procedure. The authors' experience suggests that this increased ability to visualize various aspects of the osteotomy can minimize complications. Visualizing the inferior border or medial cut during a sagittal split osteotomy may prevent an improper split. In addition, evaluating the posterior maxillary or mandibular anatomy before or after the osteotomy can aid the surgeon during positioning or fixation procedures. As the technology improves, the adjunctive uses of the endoscope become increasingly more common.

Sagittal Split Osteotomy

A deficient medial cut is often responsible for unfavorable fractures during a sagittal split osteotomy.

At times, an unfavorable fracture anterior to the lingula leaves the inferior alveolar nerve in the proximal segment.[40] A poorly oriented medial osteotomy puts the coronoid process at risk of fracture.[41] Another area of potential complication is at the inferior border osteotomy. An insufficient osteotomy in this area often leads to a buccal cortical plate fracture.[42,43]

Kim and McCain[5] reported the use of an endoscope during mandibular orthognathic surgery. After dissecting medially and visualizing the lingula with the endoscope, the surgeon can then apply soft-tissue protection and direct the angulation of the medial cut with appropriate anatomic cues. Aside from the small risk for inferior alveolar nerve stretch injury, the authors have seen few associated complications as a result of the isolation and direct visualization of the osteotomy site.

This report also described the ability to verify the inferior border osteotomy with the help of number 3 myringotomy suction. The surgeon can reduce complications at this site by visualizing a completed inferior border osteotomy, thereby reducing the possibility of a buccal plate fracture (**Fig. 3**).

Vertical Ramus Osteotomy

The traditional vertical ramus osteotomy is frequently used for mandibular setback. The location of the osteotomy is based on radiographic interpretation of the mandibular canal, and a landmark, the antilingula, which identifies the entry of the inferior alveolar nerve.[44] However, the antilingula is not reliable in this regard. It was reported in 2006 that the antilingula has no anatomic relationship to the mandibular canal, but rather serves as a muscular attachment tubercle.[45,46] Complications of the traditional technique include bleeding, nerve damage, or an unfavorable osteotomy, often based on poor anatomic judgments at the time of osteotomy. Excessive bleeding is typically associated with transection of the inferior alveolar, masseteric, or maxillary arteries. Similarly, nerve damage usually involves transection of the inferior alveolar nerve as it enters the mandible, secondary to an osteotomy completed too far anteriorly. In an effort to protect these structures by overcompensating, sometimes the osteotomy is placed too far posteriorly, and a subcondylar osteotomy may occur. Using the endoscope can limit these misjudgments and improve visualization before making the osteotomy.

Endoscopically assisted vertical ramus osteotomies have been described via a modified Risdon approach,[47] and via intraoral incisions.[48] The authors prefer the intraoral approach. If intraoral incisions are used, not only is visualization improved with the endoscope, but the medial aspect of the ramus can be explored, and appropriate protection of neurovascular structures improves accuracy of the osteotomy (**Fig. 4**).

LeFort I Osteotomy

Lefort I osteotomy is a predictable operation for repositioning the mid-face and upper arch of dentition. However, there are occasional complications, such as significant bleeding or unfavorable fractures. The endoscope can be used as a teaching tool during this procedure to allow trainees to visualize various aspects of the posterior anatomy and various views not typically available to assistants or

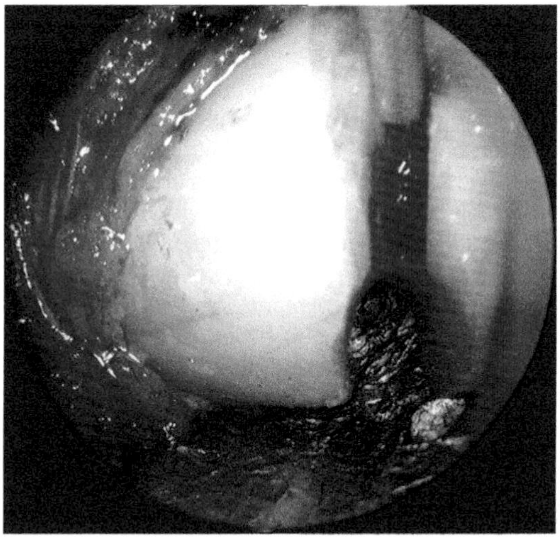

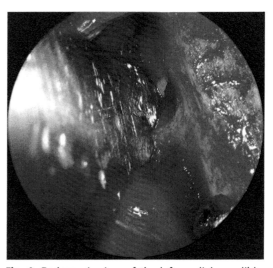

Fig. 3. Endoscopically assisted cut of the inferior border of the mandible in a sagittal split osteotomy.

Fig. 4. Endoscopic view of the left medial mandible. Isolation for a vertical ramus osteotomy or medial cut of a sagittal split is completed from this view.

observers. With 30° and 70° endoscopes, the pterygomaxillary junction, ptyergoid plates, nasal septum, and other relevant anatomic points can be visualized. A 0° scope can be used to visualize the posterior maxillary wall and the neurovascular bundles. Although not necessary to complete the procedure, the endoscope can be a useful aid for teaching the procedure and avoiding complications as trainees learn the relevant anatomy associated with this and other osteotomies.

SIALOENDOSCOPY

Surgical treatment of obstructive pathologic conditions of the salivary gland were, until recently, limited to open surgery. Although complications of salivary gland excision occur at a low rate (from 2% to 9%),[49] some of these sequelae are problematic for patients. Potential complications such as excessive scarring, nerve damage, hemorrhage, xerostomia, and gustatory sweating are reported with open techniques.[50]

Like other minimally invasive techniques for oral and maxillofacial surgery, endoscopic assistance in the treatment of pathologic conditions of the salivary gland is new, as endoscopes only recently achieved the degree of miniaturization necessary to navigate these fine structures. First described in 1991 by Katz,[51] the technique is still developing as optics and instrumentation improve. Nahlieli, Marchal, and other endoscopists have contributed significantly to this development.[52]

Sialoendoscopy provides the ability to diagnose and treat obstructive salivary gland disease without subjecting the patient to redundant testing and more invasive procedures.

Various modalities are available to diagnose an obstructive salivary gland condition. Various imaging techniques have been used with success, such as plain film, ultrasound, magnetic resonance imaging, computed tomography, and sialography. Each of these has its drawbacks. Some are cost prohibitive, whereas others do not have positive predictive value to warrant regular use. Approximately 20% of submandibular stones, 60% of parotid stones, and 80% of sublingual obstructions are not visualized with typical diagnostic tools.[53]

Sialoendoscopy allows the surgeon to visualize the duct system and contents to diagnose the problem. Nahlieli and Marchal have independently reported success rates greater than 80%[52] in treating obstructive pathologic conditions of the salivary gland using minimally invasive techniques. The growth of sialoendoscopy began with Katz[54] and the use of a flexible endoscope combined with a blind technique to grab the obstruction from the ductal system. The technique was considered blind because of the poor quality of the picture. These issues resolved as optics improved. Some argued that a flexible scope would be more beneficial when approaching the duct at the severe turn around the submandibular gland, a torturous duct, or a tight piercing of a duct through the buccinator. However, Arzoz[55] reported success using a rigid urethroscope to navigate the duct. He favored the working channel to fit other instruments for treatment purposes. By using a rigid scope, lighting was no longer a problem. Nahlieli followed with his rigid endoscope, although it occasionally caused trauma to the duct and other soft tissues.

Subsequently, the rigid scope was modified to be semirigid or semiflexible, and the addition of a working channel and improved diameter of the endoscope made this technique more practical. Since Marchal[56] introduced the semiflexible design in 1998, there have been few modifications. Diagnostic and interventional sialoendoscopy kits are available. The irrigation channel was introduced to the design in 1999 by Nahlieli.[55] The diameter of the scope varies (0.8–2.7 mm). The considerable variability in size is usually because of the presence of a working port.

The most used designs are semiflexible, with a 0.25-mm irrigating channel, a 0.8-mm working channel, and a diameter of 1.6 mm.[51] The authors prefer an endoscope that has a 0.90-mm optic and a 1.3-mm channel.[51] Wire baskets, grasping forceps, microburs, catheters, and stents are all available.

In many cases, imaging is still necessary in the diagnostic process to exclude contributory pathologic conditions. However, diagnostic sialoendoscopy can sometimes replace the need for expensive, often nondiagnostic studies. Situations remain in which sialoendoscopy is not warranted. These situations include nonobstructive sialadenitis that resolves with antibiotics, spontaneous expulsion of the obstruction, and large stone size, and proximal location of a stone. Stones that are seen within the gland, or extraglandular, are not amenable to endoscopic treatment. These stones are usually managed with excision of the gland, and sialodochoplasty.[57] However, for routine obstruction, if medical management is unsuccessful, sialoendoscopy can be considered. Marchal and colleagues[58] showed no correlation between frequency or duration of infection and glandular histology. They inferred that the gland had normal function even after chronic obstructive disease. This finding contradicts an accepted indication for gland removal after chronic obstruction, and consequently may allow some patients to undergo a sialoendoscopy procedure to salvage the gland.

Definitive management can be determined based on diagnostic sialoendoscopy. Mucous plugs, strictures, and radiolucent stones may be visualized during the diagnostic phase, allowing for intervention when appropriate. Smaller stones or obstructions can be washed out (**Fig. 5**), or retrieved using simple techniques. If larger stones are present or the location is more proximal (eg, within the hilum of the duct) open surgery may be indicated, but lithotripsy can also be considered.

Extracorporeal shock wave lithotripsy is a noninvasive technique that has been described in the urologic literature and applied to salivary gland stones. The lithotripsy uses shock wave therapy to ablate the obstruction. Problems include the need for repeat treatment and the need for retrieval of the stones that do not flow freely out of the system.[59–63] Intracorporeal lithotripsy (endoscopically assisted) is a minimally invasive technique used in the treatment of salivary gland stones.[64] An 0.8-mm pneumoblastic lithotriptor probe is used in the working channel to ablate the stone. Laser lithotripsy with endoscopic assistance was initially described by Konigsberger[65] in 1990, and successful results were reported by Arzoz[66] in 1994.

Techniques

Sialoendoscopy begins with preoperative evaluation of the patient to ensure that the procedure can be performed with an expectation of success. Trismus from pathologic conditions of the TMJ or active infection are contraindications for this technique. In the authors' experience this procedure can be performed with local anesthetic, intravenous sedation, or general anesthesia. More difficult cases warrant an operative field that is well controlled and gives the surgeon the opportunity for conversion to open surgery as needed. General anesthesia is suggested for obstruction that has significant complexity. Patients with submandibular gland obstruction are approached by locating and cannulating the duct. The use of methylene blue to help locate the duct has been described, and the authors find this technique particularly useful.[67] The dilating process using probes allows the surgeon to prepare the duct for the introduction of the endoscope. There are situations in which the duct does not dilate, and a papillotomy can be used. An 11-blade incision is made through 1 edge of the duct, allowing for a larger aperture to accept the scope. Once the scope is passed into the duct, forceps can be used to maintain countertension on the duct. Water-soluble lubrication may help during the dilation and scope placement. Isotonic saline is used as irrigation and navigation through the ductal system is achieved.

Multiple paths may be found during the procedure, and each must be evaluated for obstruction. In cases of chronic sialodenitis, copious irrigation through the ductal system is helpful.[68] If the obstruction is visualized, a Fogarty catheter may be passed through the working port beyond the obstruction, instrumented, and retrieved. Otherwise, a basket or clasp may be used. If a holmium laser is available, laser lithotripsy can be completed at this time as needed (**Fig. 6**).[68]

To prevent ductal stenosis, a 2-mm polyethelene stent is placed into the duct and stabilized with

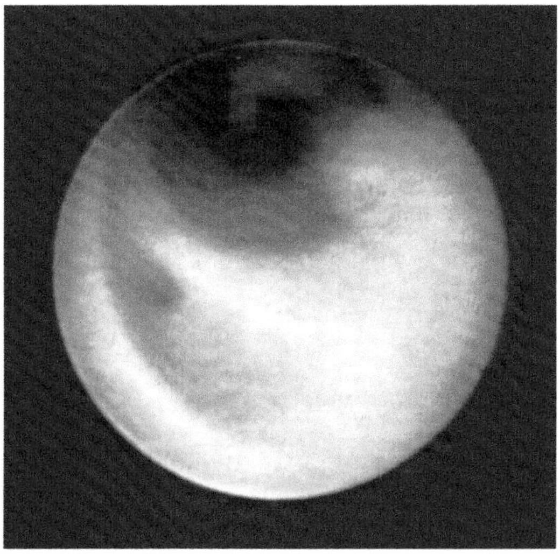

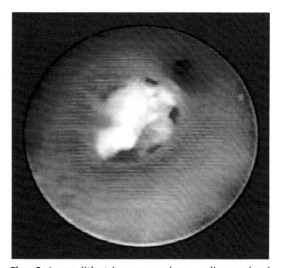

Fig. 5. Recurrent sialodenitis, without radiographic findings. View of a mucous plug. Note the field of view is smaller with sialoendoscopy equipment.

Fig. 6. Laser lithotripsy on a large salivary gland stone. The stone is obstructing 1 of the canals of the ductal system.

a temporary nonresorbable suture. The stent should remain in place for 4 weeks postoperatively. The patient is given appropriate antibiotics and postoperative instructions to optimize salivary flow.

Although the technique is safe and effective, complications may arise. The incidence of complications is reported to be less than 10%, and most complications are considered minor.[69] Most frequently, swelling of the gland is seen secondary to the copious irrigation process. Extravasation of irrigation fluid can occur into the floor of the mouth and the surrounding tissues. This extravasation can occur with an iatrogenic perforation of the duct. Transient paresthesia to the lingual nerve may occur, usually from instrument manipulation beyond the confines of the duct. If a perforation is suspected, the endoscopic technique should be aborted and another treatment modality considered. An iatrogenic ranula or infection may also result. The papilla may experience local trauma from manipulation and become ulcerated. Stricture of the duct may occur, and has been noted in 4% of cases.[70]

Sialoendoscopy is a technique-sensitive procedure that can be used for the treatment of obstructive salivary gland disease. Advances in the armamentarium are making this procedure more frequent. Thus far, the complication rates have bee low and good outcomes have been achieved. Sialoendoscopy will likely play a larger role in the treatment of obstructive salivary gland disease.

TMJ SURGERY

TMJ pathology is 1 of the areas of oral and maxillofacial surgery that has gone through a considerable transformation in recent decades. The use of technology in this area has not always provided positive outcomes. Since the Teflon-Proplast joint prosthesis failures became evident, the profession has been slowly making advances, and a new viewpoint on incorporation of technology has developed.

Various individuals have contributed to understanding of the pathophysiology present in TMJ disease, and understanding continues to grow.[71–76] For the most part, surgery of the TMJ has been directed at the physical manipulation of tissues that have anatomic abnormalities, such as degenerative joint disease and internal derangements. Among these procedures is endoscopic TMJ surgery. Arthroscopic surgery has been a mainstay in the diagnosis and treatment of TMJ problems for the past 25 years, and its advancements have paralleled those in the orthopedic literature. The armamentarium has steadily improved in design, as have the optics, making operative intervention via the scope more possible.

As a diagnostic tool, arthroscopy provides the surgeon with information not currently available via imaging modalities. It is also a straightforward procedure. Surgical techniques have improved as the technological advancements of smaller instrumentation and better optics have been applied from other areas. Some experience has shown that minimally invasive techniques seem to have similar results compared with their open counterparts.[77]

TMJ arthroscopy equipment remains relatively unchanged in the United States secondary to its small commercial market. Various techniques have been described using this instrumentation.[77] However, the advances in technology have made these devices less expensive and portable, and office systems are now available. The OnPoint system (**Fig. 7**) (Biomet, Jacksonville, FL, USA) is among the most recent additions. OnPoint is a diagnostic arthroscopy system that uses a 1.2-mm scope at 0°. With a high-quality resolution and a portable unit amenable to surgical operation, this system makes diagnostic arthroscopy useful in the outpatient setting, with considerable cost savings for the patient.

The goal of treating all surgical arthroscopy patients in the office is impractical because of the complications that may occur requiring more extended surgical techniques. However, further advances may allow for double-puncture surgery in the office setting.

A thorough understanding of the pathologic conditions of TMJ is necessary before initiating surgical treatment. Chronic facial pain of various

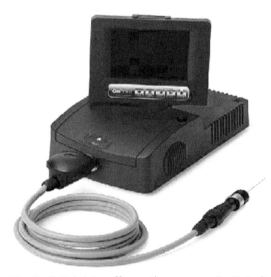

Fig. 7. OnPoint in office arthroscopy unit. Note its simple design and portability. (*Courtesy of* Biomet, Jacksonville, FL; with permission.)

types, such as temporal arteritis and trigeminal neuralgia, may have the same symptoms as TMJ conditions. Other types of pathologic conditions, such as tumoral, neurogenic, muscular, or psychological conditions, must also be evaluated appropriately and treated by other means. However, patients with intra-articular TMJ conditions may be candidates for endoscopic surgery.

For patients with internal derangement, nonsurgical treatment, including medical management, physical therapy, and orthotic treatments, can be initiated. Once evaluation is completed, definitive diagnosis can be attained via arthroscopic surgery. The Wilkes classification is used to evaluate and treat patients with internal derangements of the TMJ.[78] The literature supports arthoscopic lysis and lavage as an effective treatment in 70% of Wilkes III, IV, and V patients for decreasing pain, increasing mobility, improving diet, and reducing the use of medication.[79] For patients with mild synovitis or other inflammatory-type pathosis, synovectomy and reducing inflamed tissue can be completed with a laser.[80] For antiinflammatory therapy, endoscopically assisted injection of corticosteroids or hyaluronic acid into the retrodiscal tissue allows for placement of intra-articular medical therapies.

Geert Boering's thesis on the natural progression of disease[81] should be considered before making the decision of immediate debridement or observation after lysis and lavage. If after initial lysis and lavage, decreased function and pain are no longer complaints, proceeding to a debridement may be harmful. However, when indicated, debridement of the joint space can be achieved with the use of various instruments placed through the working port, including forceps, motorized shavers, electrocautery, or the holmium:yttrium-aluminum-garnet laser.[82,83] The use of the additional instrumentation allows for effective removal of adhesions and fibrocartilagenous scuff and sculpting of disk perforation margins. These surgical maneuvers are designed to optimize the motion of the joint and remove impediments to smooth function.

If diagnostic arthroscopy yields a Wilkes II to IV diagnosis, then the patient may benefit from a disk-repositioning procedure. McCain and Podransky[84] and Tarro[85] have described the technique endoscopically. The learning curve is considerable, but the technique may have advantages that warrant a discussion with patients considering open procedures. The authors have had excellent experience with this technique. Level III evidence is available in the literature to support its use, and additional outcome studies are under way in several centers.

At times the patient may have functional problems because of a hypermobile joint. These patients can frequently have open lock, which requires active reduction by a health care practitioner. Treatment modalities include bone augmentation of the eminence,[86] eminectomy,[87] injection of a sclerosing agent,[88] injection of autologous blood into the joint space,[89,90] or a posterior contraction procedure.[1] Of these options, all but the block graft and eminectomy procedures can be completed with arthroscopic assistance (**Fig. 8**). Posterior contraction of the retrodiscal tissue can be completed with the assistance of a laser, followed by a period of elastophysiotherapy.

Complications associated with athroscopy are rare. Complications occur in 1.3% of cases, and most are minor.[91] The most common complication is scuffing of the fibrocartilage during placement of the instruments into the joint, causing an iatrogenic injury.[92] Trauma to this tissue can lead to hypomobility of the joint. Extravasation of fluid can occur during prolonged surgeries. Severe complications such as pulmonary edema have also been reported after TMJ arthroscopy.[93] Careful attention to the pressure of irrigation and the functioning irrigating ports throughout the procedure can minimize these events. The periorbital tissues, masseter, and soft palate are common locations of collection. The surgeon should consider evaluating the oral cavity for soft-tissue edema post surgery. Deviation of the uvula can indicate extravasation. Temporary facial nerve paresis can be noted postoperatively, and in most cases is from local anesthetic injection around the major branches of the facial nerve.[94] It has also been hypothesized that prolonged paresis is the result of scar tissue that has formed near branches of the facial nerve near the surgical site.[1] Iatrogenic injury secondary to placement of

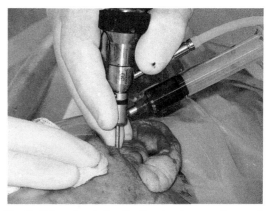

Fig. 8. Using direct visualization to place medicament. In this case, autologous blood was injected into the superior joint space. Endoscopic view confirms the precise placement.

the portals can also result in damage to facial nerves, but this is usually avoided with careful technique.[94] Appropriate patient positioning is helpful to appreciate appropriate landmarks and avoid technical complications.[1,80]

Damage to the cartilaginous or bony ear canal is also possible. This damage can occur because of patient positioning and a lack of perspective when the patient is fully draped. Occasionally, patients with complex degenerative joint diseases and other orthopedic issues present with limited neck mobility. If patients with limited neck mobility require TMJ arthroscopy, the surgeon may consider arthroscopy in a hospital setting to facilitate a more appropriate bed-tilt maneuver, which allows for a more appropriate operative field with good anatomic cues.

Bleeding can occur during an arthroscopy procedure, particularly during an anterior release procedure. This complication has been noted in 2% of cases.[95] Closing the patient's mouth to tamponade the bleed may be helpful. The authors suggest that the joint be re-entered and the clots removed as hemarthrosis can negatively affect mobility. Alternatively, persistent bleeds may be addressed with the placement of an occlusive balloon catheter via the second puncture portal into the anterior disk space for 5 to 7 minutes. However, the surgeon must always be prepared for open surgery or the use of interventional radiologic techniques if there is uncontrollable bleeding.

Perforation into the glenoid fossa has also been reported.[95,96] Although there have been no reports of death, appropriate imaging, neurosurgical consultation, and close observation are required. The failure of instrumentation is a rare complication but it does occur occasionally; it is important to have good visibility of the instrument and to retrieve it endoscopically if possible. Open

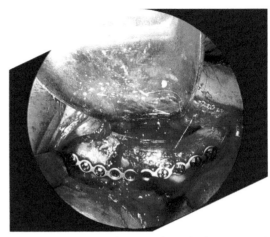

Fig. 10. By removing the scope from the lens, any unit can be used as a camera during surgery. This image served as our postreduction documentation of a lower rim and orbital floor repair.

procedures can be considered if the fragments are not easily retrieved through the working port.[1,97] Careful patient positioning, attention to detail, and understanding surgical anatomy help prevent many of these complications.

Arthroscopic management of pathologic conditions of the TMJ requires a thorough understanding of the mechanical principles and anatomy of the system, and the pathophysiology of TMJ disease. In the authors' opinion, effective management can be completed with the aid of an endoscope in most cases. Although some of the procedures described are technically challenging and require special skills of the surgeon, they often have clear benefits compared with their open counterparts.

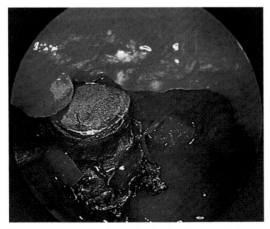

Fig. 9. Endoscopic view of a bullet fragment during initial debridement of a self-inflicted gunshot wound.

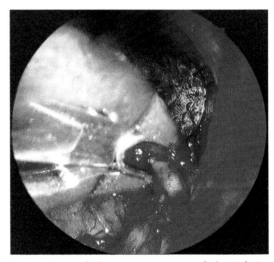

Fig. 11. View during a neurectomy of the inferior alveolar nerve to treat a patient suffering from peripheral trigeminal neuralgia.

REMOVAL OF FOREIGN BODIES

Occasionally, the endoscope can be used to help retrieve foreign bodies. A Smith & Nephew (Dyonics, Andover, MA, USA) scope (2.7 mm or 4.0 mm diameter) gives a larger field of vision and can be used as an adjunct in the removal of foreign bodies in the craniomaxillofacial region (**Fig. 9**). Its use as a sterile still image and video camera (**Fig. 10**) (Video 1, see online within this article at http://www.oralmaxsurgery.theclinics. com, February 2010 issue), allows visualization of important anatomy without extensive incisions (**Fig. 11**).

SUMMARY

The oral and maxillofacial surgeons are finding advantages and new applications for endoscopically assisted maxillofacial surgical procedures. Decreased complication rates, comparable success rates, diverse functionality, and efficiency make the endoscope a helpful instrument in a surgeon's armamentarium.

APPENDIX: SUPPLEMENTARY MATERIAL

Supplementary material can be found, in the online version, at doi:10.1016/j.coms.2009.11.002

REFERENCES

1. McCain JP, Williams L. Principles and practice of temporomandibular joint arthroscopy. St Louis: Mosby; 1996. p. 1–11.
2. Loukota RA. Endoscopically assisted reduction and internal fixation of condylar neck/base fractures–the learning curve. Br J Oral Maxillofac Surg 2006;44: 480–1.
3. Ally JR Jr, Stucky CC, Moncure M. Teaching surgical residents dome-down laparoscopic cholecystectomy in an academic medical center. JSLS 2008; 12(4):368–71.
4. Fritsch M. A new sialoendoscopy teaching model of the duct and gland. J Oral Maxillofac Surg 2008;66: 2409–11.
5. Kim K, McCain JP. Use of the endoscope in bisagittal split osteotomy. J Oral Maxillofac Surg 2008; 66(8):1773–5.
6. Westphal D, Kreidler JF. Sinuscopy for the diagnosis of blow-out fractures. J Maxillofac Surg 1977;5(3):180–3.
7. Saunders CJ, Whetzel TP, Stokes RB, et al. Transantral endoscopic orbital floor exploration: a cadaver and clinical study. Plast Reconstr Surg 1997; 100(3):575–81.
8. Strong EB. Endoscopic repair of orbital blow-out fractures. Facial Plast Surg 2004;20(3):223–30.
9. Wallace TD, Moore CC, Bromwich MA, et al. Endoscopic repair of orbital floor fractures: computed tomographic analysis using a cadaveric model. J Otolaryngol 2006;35(1):1–7.
10. Jin HR, Yeon JY, Shin SO, et al. Endoscopic versus external repair of orbital blowout fractures. Otolaryngol Head Neck Surg 2007;136(1):38–44.
11. Ellis E. Management of fractures through the angle of the mandible. Oral Maxillofac Surg Clin North Am 2009;21(2):163–74.
12. Gear AJL, Apasova E, Schmitz JP, et al. Treatment modalities for mandibular angle fractures. J Oral Maxillofac Surg 2005;63(5):655–63.
13. Ellis E. Treatment methods for fractures of the mandibular angle. J Craniomaxillofac Trauma 1996; 2(1):28–36.
14. Walker RV. Traumatic mandibular condyle fracture dislocation: effect of growth in the Macaca monkey. Am J Surg 1960;100:850.
15. Brandt MT, Haug RH. Open versus closed reduction of adult mandibular condyle fractures: a review of the literature regarding the evolution of current thoughts on management. J Oral Maxillofac Surg 2003;61:1324.
16. Schon R, Roveda SI, Carter B. Mandibular fractures in Townsville, Australia: incidence, aetiology and treatment using the 2.0 AO/ASIF miniplate system. Br J Oral Maxillofac Surg 2001;39:145.
17. Lindahl L. Condylar fractures of the mandible: classification and relation to age, occlusion, and concomitant injuries of the teeth and teeth-supporting structures, and fractures of the mandibular body. Int J Oral Surg 1977;6:12.
18. Walker RV. Condylar fractures: nonsurgical treatment. J Oral Maxillofac Surg 1994;52:1185.
19. Baker AW, McMahon J, Moos KF. Current consensus on the management of fractures of the mandibular condyle. Int J Oral Maxillofac Surg 1998;27:258.
20. Ellis E III, Simon P, Throckmorton GS. Occlusal results after open or closed treatment of fractures of the mandibular condylar process. J Oral Maxillofac Surg 2000;58:260.
21. Haug RH, Assael LA. Outcomes of open versus closed treatment of mandibular subcondylar fractures. J Oral Maxillofac Surg 2001;59:370.
22. Sorel B. Management of condylar fractures. Oral Maxillofac Surg Knowledge Update 2001;3:47.
23. Assael LA. Open versus closed reduction of adult mandibular condyle fractures: an alternative interpretation of the evidence. J Oral Maxillofac Surg 2003;61:1333.
24. Walker RV. Management of subcondylar fractures. Presented at the 86th annual meeting of the Association of Oral and Maxillofacial Surgery 2003. Orlando (FL), September.
25. Ellis E III, Moos KF, el Attar A. Ten years of mandibular fractures: an analysis of 2,137 cases. Oral Surg Oral Med Oral Pathol 1985;59:120.

26. Zide MF, Kent JN. Indications for open reduction of mandibular condyle fractures. J Oral Maxillofac Surg 1983;41:89.

27. Zide MF. Open reduction of mandibular condyle fractures. Clin Plast Surg 1989;16:69.

28. Kent JN, Neary JP, Silvia C, et al. Open reduction of mandibular condyle fractures. Oral Maxillofac Surg Clin North Am 1990;2:69.

29. Zide MF. Outcomes of open versus closed treatment of mandibular subcondylar fractures. J Oral Maxillofac Surg 2001;59:375 [discussion].

30. Miloro M. Endoscopic-assisted repair of subcondylar fractures. Oral Surg Oral Med Oral Pathol Oral Radiol Endod 2003;96(4):387–91.

31. Schon R, Gutwald R, Schramm A, et al. Endoscopy-assisted open treatment of condylar fractures of the mandible: extraoral vs intraoral approach. Int J Oral Maxillofac Surg 2002;31:237.

32. Cole P, Kaufman Y, Momoh A, et al. Techniques in frontal sinus fracture repair. Plast Reconstr Surg 2009;123(5):1578–9.

33. Hewitt DK, Scheidt TD, Calhoun KH. Depressed anterior table fracture: a minimally invasive method of reduction. Ear Nose Throat J 2009; 88(1):734–5.

34. Chen DJ, Chen CT, Chen YR, et al. Endoscopically assisted repair of frontal sinus fracture. J Trauma 2003;55(2):378–82.

35. Steiger JD, Chiu AG, Francis DO, et al. Endoscopic-assisted reduction of anterior table frontal sinus fractures. Laryngoscope 2006;116(10):1936–9.

36. Yoo MH, Kim JS, Song HM, et al. Endoscopic trans-nasal reduction of an anterior table frontal sinus fracture: technical note. Int J Oral Maxillofac Surg 2008; 37(6):573–5.

37. Schubert W, Jenabzadeh K. Endoscopic approach to maxillofacial trauma. J Craniofac Surg 2009; 20(1):154–6.

38. Mueller R. Endoscopic treatment of facial fractures. Facial Plast Surg 2008;24(1):78–91.

39. Strong EB, Kellman RM. Endoscopic repair of anterior table–frontal sinus fractures. Facial Plast Surg Clin North Am 2006;14(1):25–9.

40. Reyneke JP. Essentials of orthognathic surgery. Chicago: Quintessence Publishing; 2003. p. 251.

41. Iwai T, Matsui Y, Tohnai I, et al. Endoscopic-assisted medial osteotomy during sagittal split ramus osteotomy. J Plas Reconstr Aesthet Surg 2008; 61(12):1547–8.

42. Turvey TA. Intraoperative complications of sagittal osteotomy of the mandibular ramus. J Oral Maxillofac Surg 1985;43:504–9.

43. MacIntosh RB. Experience with the sagittal osteotomy of the mandibular ramus: a 13 year review. J Oral Maxillofac Surg 1981;8:151–65.

44. Martone CH, Ben-Josf AM, Wolf SM, et al. Dimorphic study of surgical anatomic landmarks of the lateral ramus of the mandible. Oral Surg Oral Med Oral Pathol 1993;75:436–8.

45. Pogrel MA, Schmidt BL, Ammar A. The presence of the antilingula and its relationship to the true lingula. Br J Oral Maxillofac Surg 1995;33:235–8.

46. Hogan G, Ellis E. The "antilingula": fact or fiction. J Oral Maxillofac Surg 2006;64:1248–54.

47. Troulis MJ, Kaban LB. Endoscopic vertical ramus osteotomy: early clinical results. J Oral Maxillofac Surg 2004;62:824–8.

48. Robiony M, Polini F, Costa F, et al. Endoscopically assisted intraoral vertical ramus osteotomy and piezoelectric surgery in mandibular prognathism. J Oral Maxillofac Surg 2007;65:2119–24.

49. Eisele D, Smith R. Complications of surgery of the salivary glands. Complications in head and neck surgery. 2nd edition. St Louis: Mosby; 2009. p. 221–39.

50. Bailey BM, Pearce DE. Gustatory sweating following submandibular salivary gland removal. Br Dent J 1985;158:17–8.

51. Iro H, Zenk J, Koch M, et al. The Erlangen salivary gland project; 2007. p. 12–3.

52. Nahlieli O, Shacham R, Bar T, et al. Endoscopic mechanical retrieval of sialoliths. Oral Surg Oral Med Oral Pathol Oral Radiol Endod 2003;95:396–402.

53. Miloro M. The surgical management of submandibular gland disease. Atlas Oral Maxillofac Surg Clin North Am 1998;6:29–50.

54. Katz P. Nouvelle thérapeutique des lithiases salivaire [New therapy for sialolithiasis]. Inf Dent 1991;73: 3975–9 [in French].

55. Nahlieli O. Endoscopic techniques for the diagnosis and treatment of salivary gland disease. Carl Stortz: Silver Books; 2009. p. 23.

56. Marchal F. The endoscopic approach to salivary gland ductal pathologies. Carl Stortz: Silver Books; 2005.

57. Marchal F. Sialolith management: the state of the art. Arch Otolaryngol Head Neck Surg 2003;129:951–6.

58. Marchal F, Kurt AM, Dulguerov P, et al. Histopathology of submandibular glands removed for sialolithiasis. Ann otol Rhinol Laryngol 2001; 110:464–9.

59. Iro H, Schneider HT, Fodra C, et al. Shockwave lithotripsy of salivary gland duct stones. Lancet 1992; 339:1333.

60. Marmary Y. A novel and non-invasive method for the removal of salivary gland stones. Int J Oral Maxillofac Surg 1992;15:585.

61. Iro H, Waitz G, Nitsche N, et al. Extracorporeal piezoelectric shock-wave lithotripsy of salivary gland stones. Laryngoscope 1992;102:492.

62. Hauser R, Vahlensieck W, Maier W, et al. Extracorporeal piezoelectric lithotripsy in the treatment of a parotic calculus with recurrent parotiditis. Laryngorhinootologie 1990;69:464.

63. Kater W, Hurst A, Schilck R, et al. Salivary gland stones: chances, risks and limits of ESWL. 10th World Congress on Endourology and ESWL 1992. Singapore 03-06.

64. Arzoz E, Santiago A, Esnal F, et al. Endoscopic intracorporeal lithotripsy for sialolithiasis. J Oral Maxillofac Surg 1996;54:847–50.

65. Konigsberger R, Feyh j, Goetz A, et al. Die endoscopisch Kontrollierte Laser lithotripsy zur behandlung der sialolithiasis [Endoscopic controlled laser lithotripsy in the treatment of sialolithiasis]. Laryngorhinootologie 1990;69:322 [in German].

66. Arzoz E, Santiago A, Garatea J, et al. Removal of a stone with endoscopic laser lithotripsy: report of a case. J Oral Maxillofac Surg 1994;52:1329.

67. Luers J, Vent J, Beutner D. Methylene blue for easy and safe detection of salivary duct papilla in sialoendoscopy. Otolaryngol Head Neck Surg 2008;139:466–7.

68. Nahlieli O, Baruchin A. Endoscopic technique for the diagnosis and treatment of obstructive salivary gland disease. J Oral Maxillofac Surg 1999;57:1394–401.

69. Nahlieli O, Baruchin AM. Long term experience with endoscopic diagnosis and treatment of salivary gland inflammatory diseases. Laryngoscope 2000;110:988–93.

70. McGurk M, Makdissi J, Brown JE. Intra-oral removal of stones from the hilum of the submandibular gland: report of technique and morbidity. Int J Oral Maxillofac Surg 2004;33:683–6.

71. Milam S, Schmitz J. Molecular biology of temporomandibular joint pathology: proposed mechanisms of disease. J Oral Maxillofac Surg 1995;53:1448–54.

72. Nitzan D. The process of lubrication impairment and its involvement in the temporomandibular joint disc displacement: a theoretical concept. J Oral Maxillofac Surg 2001;59:36–45.

73. Nitzan DW, Goldfarb A, Dan P, et al. Hyaluronic acid protects surface active phospholipids from lysis by exogenous phospholipase A2. Rheumatology 2001;40:336–40.

74. Sheets DW Jr, Okamoto T, Dijkgraaf LC, et al. Free radical damage in facsimile synovium: correlation with adhesion formation in osteoarthritic TMJs. J Prosthodont 2006;15:9–19.

75. Quinn J, Kent J, Moise A. Cyclooxygenase-2 in synovial tissue and fluid of dysfunctional temporomandibular joints with internal derangement. J Oral Maxillofac Surg 2000;58:1229–32.

76. Quinn JH, Bazan NG. Identification of prostaglandin E2 and leukotriene B4 in the synovial fluid of painful, dysfunctional temporomandibular joints. J Oral Maxillofac Surg 1990;48:968.

77. McCain JP, Sanders B, Koslin MG, et al. Temporomandibular joint arthroscopy: a six year multicenter retrospective study of 4831 joints. J Oral Maxillofac Surg 1992;50:926–30.

78. Wilkes C. Internal derangements of the temporomandibular joints. Arch Otolaryngol Head Neck Surg 1989;115(4):469–77.

79. Gonzales-Garcia R, Rodriguez-Campo FJ. Operative versus simple arthroscopic surgery for chronic closed lock of the temporomandibular joint; a clinical study of 344 arthroscopic procedures. Int J Oral Maxillofac Surg 2008;37:790–6.

80. Koslin M. Advanced arthroscopic surgery. Oral Maxillofac Surg Clin North Am 2006;18:329–43.

81. DeLeeuw R, Boering G, Stegenga B, et al. Symptoms of temporomandibular joint osteoarthrosis and internal derangement 30 years after non-surgical treatment. J Craniomandibular Pract 1995;13:81–8.

82. Indresano AT, Bradrick J. Arthroscopic laser procedures. In: Clark G, Sanders B, Bertolami C, editors. Advances in diagnostic and surgical arthroscopy of the temporomandibular joint. Philadelphia: WB Saunders; 1993. p. 129–37.

83. Koslin M. Laser applications in temporomandibular joint surgery. Oral Maxillofac Surg Clin North Am 2004;16:269–75.

84. McCain JP, Podransky AE. Arthroscopic disc repositioning and suturing: a preliminary report. J Oral Maxillofac Surg 1992;50:568.

85. Tarro AW. A fully visualized arthroscopic suturing technique. J Oral Maxillofac Surg 1994;52:362.

86. Fernandez-Sanroman J. Surgical treatment of recurrent mandibular dislocation by augmentation of the articular eminence with cranial bone. J Oral Maxillofac Surg 1997;55:333.

87. Norman JE. Glenotemporal osteotomy as definitive treatment for recurrent dislocation of the jaw. J Craniomaxillofac Surg 1997;25:103.

88. Ohnishi M. Arthroscopic surgery for hypermobile and recurrent temporomandibular dislocations. Oral Maxillofac Surg Clin North Am 1989;1:153.

89. Hooiveld M, Roosendaal G, Vianen N, et al. Blood-induced joint damage: longterm effects in vitro and in vivo. J Rheumatol 2003;30:339.

90. Machon V, Abramowicz S, Pasca J, et al. Autologous blood treatment for chronic recurrent temporomandibular joint dislocation. J Oral Maxillofac Surg 2009;67:114–9.

91. Gonzales-Garcia R, Rodriguez-Campo FJ. Complications of temporomandibular joint arthroscopy: a retrospective analytic study of 670 arthroscopic procedures. J Oral Maxillofac Surg 2006;64:1587.

92. Wilk BR, McCain JP. Rehabilitation of the TMJ after arthroscopic surgery. Oral Surg Oral Med Oral Pathol 1992;73(5):531–6.

93. Hendler BH, Levin LM. Postobstructive pulmonary edema as a sequela of temporomandibular joint arthroscopy: a case report. J Oral Maxillofac Surg 1993;51(3):315–7.

94. Westesson P, Eriksson L, Liedberg J. The risk of damage to the facial nerve, superficial temporal vessels, disk, and articular surfaces during arthroscopic examination of the temporomandibular joint. Oral Surg Oral Med Oral Pathol 1986;62: 124–7.

95. Carter JB, Testa L. Complications of TMJ arthroscopy: a review of 2225 cases: review of the 1988 annual scientific session abstracts. J Oral Maxillofac Surg 1988;46:M14.

96. McCain JP, DeLaRua H, LeBlanc N. Puncture technique and portals of entry for diagnostic and operative arthroscopy of the TMJ. Arthroscopy 1991;7(2): 221–32.

97. Sanders B, Buonchristiani RD. A 5-year experience with arthroscopic lysis and lavage for the treatment of painful temporomandibular joint hypomobility. In: Clark G, Sanders B, Bertolami C, editors. Advances in diagnostic and surgical arthroscopy of the temporomandibular joint. Philadelphia: WB Saunders; 1993. p. 51.

Molecular Diagnostics for Head and Neck Pathology

Elizabeth Bilodeau, DMD, MD[a], Faizan Alawi, DDS[b],
Bernard J. Costello, DMD, MD, FACS[a],
Joanne L. Prasad, DDS[c],*

KEYWORDS

- Head and neck squamous cell carcinoma
- Oral cancer • Polymerase chain reaction
- Microsatellite instability • Loss of heterozygosity
- Comparative genomic hybridization • Proteomics

Currently, clinical and radiologic findings and standard histopathologic techniques are relied on to detect, diagnose, and treat most pathologic lesions of the head and neck. Although useful, such techniques have significant drawbacks. For example, clinical examination may fail to detect early cancerous lesions or precancerous changes. Standard histologic evaluation may also fail to reveal mutated cells at normal-appearing margins of resection and biopsy techniques are prone to sampling error. Such techniques do not allow for recognition of genotypically different tumors with identical phenotypes, which could affect prognosis, because certain genetic mutations may be predictive of behavior or prognosis.

Molecular diagnostic techniques are quickly finding a role in the detection and diagnosis of tumors, and in predicting their behavior. They may also prove useful in developing new therapeutic approaches to head and neck cancer. Many of these advances have already translated into changes in the practice of pathology, oncology, and surgery, although, for the most part, molecular diagnostic techniques are still experimental and have limited current clinical application in head and neck pathology. Nonetheless, some possible practical applications of these newer molecular

techniques include (1) screening for risk of cancer; (2) earlier detection of premalignant and malignant changes, resulting in earlier treatment; (3) development of new treatment approaches; (4) monitoring treatment response; and (5) evaluation of margins of resection for residual disease. Surgeons treating patients with craniomaxillofacial pathology may use this new information to customize current treatment regimens in the future. Much like other diagnostic innovations, such as advances in imaging, redefining the pathology alters the surgical and medical approaches to therapy.

The surgeon working in the craniomaxillofacial region should have an understanding of these technologies, their availability in various settings, and how they affect various aspects of treatment, particularly in the detection and treatment of malignancies. This article offers an overview of recent advances in molecular diagnostic techniques, with their implications for diagnosis and management of head and neck tumors.

DNA-BASED TECHNOLOGIES
Polymerase Chain Reaction

Before 1985, when polymerase chain reaction (PCR) was first described,[1] analysis of DNA and

[a] Department of Oral and Maxillofacial Surgery, University of Pittsburgh School of Dental Medicine, 3501 Terrace Street, Pittsburgh, PA 15261, USA
[b] Department of Pathology, University of Pennsylvania School of Dental Medicine, 240 South 40th Street, Philadelphia, PA 19104, USA
[c] Department of Diagnostic Sciences, University of Pittsburgh School of Dental Medicine, 3501 Terrace Street, Pittsburgh, PA 15261, USA
* Corresponding author.
E-mail address: jlp92@pitt.edu (J.L. Prasad).

Oral Maxillofacial Surg Clin N Am 22 (2010) 183–194
doi:10.1016/j.coms.2009.10.006
1042-3699/10/$ – see front matter © 2010 Elsevier Inc. All rights reserved.

RNA was limited to conventional karyotyping, Southern blot, and Northern blot. PCR-based technologies have since proved to be excellent tools to study both RNA and DNA. Because it is more stable than RNA, DNA is commonly used as the starting material. PCR offers the following advantages over other techniques: (1) smaller specimen requirements because DNA can be readily amplified, (2) automation, (3) the ability to study tissue extracted from paraffin-embedded specimens, (4) the ability to process larger specimen numbers, and (5) increased quantitative ability.

PCR-based techniques can be used to analyze DNA for translocations, including very small translocations that may not be detected by the use of other techniques. Chromosomal translocations occur when DNA is exchanged between chromosomes. Most commonly, these translocations are balanced (ie, a near equivalent amount of DNA material is transferred between two chromosomes). Because a given translocation may be associated with a specific neoplasm, identification of this genetic change may help in the diagnosis of such tumors. For example, translocations are routinely used in classifying lymphoid neoplasms and are increasingly being identified in other tumor types. In some cases, several translocations are found to be associated with a specific tumor phenotype. One such example, pertinent to the head and neck, is rhabdomyosarcoma (RMS). RMS is the most common pediatric sarcoma,[2] for which cytogenetic studies have become the standard of care. Approximately 35–40% of all RMSs involve the head and neck.[3,4]

A translocation commonly associated with the alveolar subtype of RMS (A-RMS) is t(2;13)(q35;q14), present in 70% of cases. The resulting gene fusion protein, *PAX3-FOX01*, acts as a transcription activator.[5,6] A-RMSs with the *PAX3-FOX01* gene fusion are associated with a worse prognosis.[7] It is important to analyze such tumors for specific translocations in determining the prognosis and in guiding treatment.

In addition, the chimeric proteins associated with specific translocations may also be used to develop targeted therapies in the future. RMS is an excellent example of a tumor type in which advanced molecular techniques have become the standard of care, aid in the diagnosis of the pathology, have the ability to anticipate the probable behavior of the tumor, and guide therapeutic decisions. In all likelihood, these technologies stratify which tumors might be amenable to more aggressive or conservative resection, and which might be best treated with adjuvant chemotherapy or radiation.

PCR-based techniques can be used to detect mutations in oncogenes and tumor suppressor genes.[8] The tumor suppressor gene p53 is commonly mutated in cancers of the oral cavity.[9–12] Such mutations result in loss of function of p53, a protein important in regulating the cell cycle and preventing cellular division. Another major function of p53 is to induce apoptosis (cell death) in damaged cells. Because of its ability to detect such mutations PCR can be used to detect minimal residual disease. Researchers have demonstrated that head and neck squamous cell carcinomas (HNSCCs) with histopathologically negative resection margins that show p53 mutations on molecular assay, or stain positively for p53 by immunohistochemistry (IHC), were found to have an increased risk of recurrence.[13,14] Detection of p53 mutations at surgical margins may help predict treatment failure and could potentially guide therapy. Research into interesting therapeutic approaches includes the possible use of adenovirus-assisted transfer of a functional p53 gene into the DNA of cancer cells.[15–18]

PCR-based techniques can also be used to look for hypermethylation of promoter regions. Hypermethylation of the promoter region of tumor suppressor genes is an early change in the pathogenesis of HNSCC, which can lead to inactivation of tumor suppressor gene function.[19,20] For example, loss of p16 is frequently seen in human cancers, including HNSCC, and may be the result of gene deletion or promoter hypermethylation.[21] These techniques may be helpful in the early detection of cancer or perhaps in monitoring a patient's response to treatment.

In Situ Hybridization and Fluorescent In Situ Hybridization

Detection of specific chromosomal changes, such as translocations, can be accomplished by in situ hybridization (ISH) or fluorescent in situ hybridization (FISH). These are similar techniques wherein a DNA or RNA probe that is complementary to a given sequence is hybridized to the target DNA or RNA. Unlike ISH, FISH uses a fluorescently labeled probe that can be used to determine gene amplification or loss (**Fig. 1**). Some of ISHs common applications in oral pathology are in virology, such as in detection of cytomegalovirus, Epstein-Barr virus (EBV), and human herpes virus 8 within cells.[22–24] Human papilloma virus (HPV) has been implicated in the development of HNSCC, particularly oropharyngeal cancer. In one study, over 70% of oropharyngeal squamous cell carcinomas exhibited positivity for the

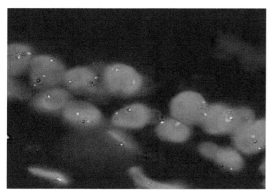

Fig. 1. Dual-color FISH illustrating the MAML2 rearrangement. The association between the translocation at t(11;19)(q21;p13) and mucoepidermoid carcinomas has been documented.[119] (*From* Kathleen Cieply, University of Pittsburgh Medical Center; with permission.)

high-risk subtype, HPV-16, by ISH.[25] The presence of HPV-16 in HNSCC is associated with a more positive outcome.[26,27] Analyzing for the presence of HPV-16 in certain tumors of the head and neck could be important in determining the prognosis and in deciding on the best treatment approach. Some have observed a strong correlation between HPV-16 positivity and deregulation of the p16 tumor suppressor gene, with resultant increased expression of p16. IHC for p16 could potentially be used as a surrogate marker for HPV positivity in HNSCC and high-grade dysplasia.[28,29] Other studies, however, have not shown HPV expression reliably correlating with p16 expression.[30]

Oral hairy leukoplakia is a benign hair-like leukoplakia that develops on the lateral aspect of the tongue of patients infected with HIV or who are otherwise immunocompromised (eg, transplant recipients), although rare cases have been reported in immunocompetent individuals.[31-34] The condition is associated with EBV, a virus known to infect oropharyngeal epithelial cells and B-lymphocytes. Given the serious implications of a diagnosis of oral hairy leukoplakia in a patient thought to be immunocompetent, EBV should be demonstrated for diagnosis in such a patient.[35] There are many ways to detect the presence of EBV in a sample, including IHC, PCR, or ISH. ISH is the preferred method for detecting EBV because it is relatively low cost, fast, simple, and sensitive (**Fig. 2**).[36]

ISH and FISH offer the advantage of examining DNA or RNA within an intact specimen, without requiring fresh tissue, and without the cost associated with karyotyping. However, these techniques are limited to the detection of specific chromosomal changes. The specific gene defects must

be anticipated before testing. Other disadvantages of FISH include instability of the fluorescent signal, the need for a fluorescent microscope, familiarity with fluorescent microscopy, and the lack of a standardized interpretation system.[37]

Microsatellite Instability

Microsatellites are segments of DNA consisting of a repeated sequence of one to six nucleotides. For example, a common repeated unit in humans is cytosine and adenine.[38] Microsatellites can be analyzed by using PCR primers unique to a specific genetic locus. By measuring the size of the PCR product, the number of nucleotide repeats can be calculated.[39] Multiple alleles for a specific microsatellite may exist, in which the different alleles contain a different number of nucleotide repeats. When this occurs, the microsatellite is said to be polymorphic. Because microsatellites occur at thousands of locations within the genome and, because of polymorphism, vary between individuals, PCR-based microsatellite analysis has been popular in forensics (victim identification) and for paternity testing. In addition, microsatellite analysis has also been used as a means of identifying loss of heterozygosity (LOH) in tumors. LOH is described more fully later in this article.

Microsatellite instability (MSI) occurs when one allele gains (insertion) or loses (deletion) repeat units, altering the length of that microsatellite allele. This change can be used to identify a clonal proliferation of tumor cells. Remarkably, in some cancers, multiple microsatellite loci within tumor cells showed similar alterations, hence the name microsatellite "instability." This phenomenon was found to be related to mutations in DNA-mismatch repair genes. These defective genes contribute to carcinogenesis by failing to repair mutations in other genes. Such changes have been associated with hereditary nonpolyposis colorectal cancer syndrome.[40]

Although MSI has been reported in 5% to 55% of HNSCC, its significance in HNSCC tumorigenesis is still not fully understood.[41-44] In one study, low-level MSI was detected in 7.7% of HNSCC, but mismatch repair gene mutations were not present.[45] When present, however, an increase in the frequency of MSI seems to correlate with progression from early dysplasia to HNSCC.[46] In addition, presence of MSI in HNSCC may be associated with more aggressive lesions.[44]

Loss of Heterozygosity

LOH at microsatellite loci is an event found early in the process of carcinogenesis. As such, LOH within these regions could be used as a marker

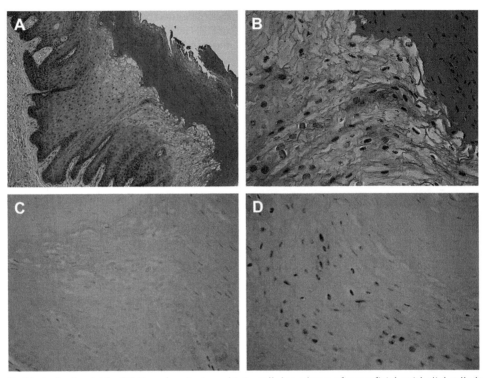

Fig. 2. Oral hairy leukoplakia. (*A*) Hyperkeratosis and intracellular edema of superficial epithelial cells (referred to as "balloon cells") are seen here (hematoxylin-eosin, original magnification ×10). (*B*) At a higher power, chromatin beading within nuclei of epithelial cells is seen (hematoxylin-eosin, original magnification ×40). (*C*) This image demonstrates a negative control for EBER (EBV) by ISH (in situ hybridization, original magnification ×40). (*D*) This image demonstrates positive cells staining EBER (EBV) by ISH (in situ hybridization, original magnification ×40).

to detect tumor cells.[47] LOH seems to be more common than MSI in HNSCC.[41–48] LOH is detected by comparing the ratio of DNA lengths between normal and tumor cells. LOH may impact a tumor suppressor gene, such as p53.[49] Certain regions on chromosomes 3p, 9p, 17p, and 18p commonly show alterations in patients with HNSCC.[48,50–52] Although LOH has been identified in early premalignant lesions, it becomes more prevalent with increased severity of the dysplastic changes and progression to malignancy.[53–56] LOH of microsatellites in key chromosomal regions, such as 3p and 9p21, could be used as a predictor of progression of premalignant lesions to HNSCC.[55–57] An association with LOH at certain loci corresponds with a higher incidence of lymph node metastasis and higher-grade disease.[58,59]

Comparative Genomic Hybridization

Although techniques used to detect LOH are limited to evaluating specific chromosomal areas, comparative genomic hybridization (CGH) allows for evaluation of the entire tumor genome at one time.[60] Tumor DNA is fluorescently labeled with one color, whereas normal DNA is labeled with a different color.[61] The ratio of fluorescence between the two colors is examined and quantified to detect any chromosomal imbalances. CGH allows for identification of both gains and losses in the DNA. It is a powerful tool that can locate the positions of oncogenes or tumor suppressor genes that may be involved in tumorigenesis.

As far as HNSCC is concerned, gains and losses in DNA have been detected on multiple chromosomes, including 3, 5p, and 8q.[52,62–64] The average number of genetic alterations detected in HNSCC, using CGH, is 16.[65] It also seems that the number of alterations correlates with disease progression, with a lower number of genetic changes noted in mildly dysplastic premalignant lesions when compared with severely dysplastic lesions and malignant tumors.[66,67] In addition, it seems that metastasizing HNSCCs harbor more chromosomal imbalances than nonmetastasizing tumors, although further investigation is necessary to confirm this finding.[63,66–69] In one study, fewer chromosomal aberrations were found in young, nonsmoking patients with HNSCC, when compared with more typical HNSCC patients, suggesting that different mechanisms of carcinogenesis may be at play.[70] One drawback of CGH is low resolution, which may prevent detection of balanced chromosomal changes and alterations in small DNA regions.

RNA-BASED TECHNOLOGIES
Reverse Transcriptase PCR

To study RNA using PCR, reverse transcription to complementary DNA (cDNA) must first be performed in a process called reverse transcriptase PCR (RT-PCR). Although RNA is less stable than DNA, it can be used to look for translocations using this method. Another technique known as "real-time RT-PCR" can also be used in analyzing such tumors. It allows for the detection of fusions and can quantitatively assess disease burden over time.[71] Although standard PCR can allow detection of one neoplastic cell per several hundred thousand cells, RT-PCR can permit detection of one neoplastic cell in 1 million.[61,72] This is far more sensitive than FISH or conventional histologic analysis.

DNA Microarrays

Microarrays measure the mRNA levels in tumors rather than detecting mutations in the DNA itself. The microarrays consist of gene-specific probes that can be used to identify activated or repressed genes in various cell populations. The technology behind DNA microarrays involves an arrangement of fluorescently labeled DNA fragments or cDNA, produced by RT-PCR, that can be detected by a laser fluorescent scanner.[73] The use of cDNA provides higher resolution of the genetic changes than other methods.[74] Several commercially available DNA microarrays are currently used in breast pathology.[75] They provide a panel of information about a tumor (eg, estrogen receptor positivity) and consequently may help guide treatment strategies.

Research involving HNSCC has implemented the usage of DNA microarrays, because they provide an automated way to analyze a large amount of data.[76,77] Patterns of gene expression (gene expression signatures) are being studied in various tumors using DNA microarrays (**Fig. 3**). Ziober and colleagues[78] discovered a 25-gene signature for oral squamous cell carcinoma. Such a gene signature could assist in the diagnosis of HNSCC, could be used for saliva-based

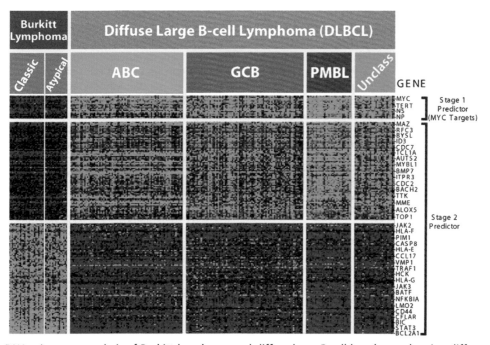

Fig. 3. DNA-microarray analysis of Burkitt lymphoma and diffuse large B-cell lymphoma showing differences in gene expression patterns. Colors indicate levels of expression: green indicates genes that are overexpressed in normal cells compared with lymphoma cells; and red indicates genes that are overexpressed in lymphoma cells compared with normal cells. (*From* Dave SS, Fu K, Wright GW, et al. Molecular diagnosis of Burkitt's lymphoma. N Engl J Med 2006;354:2431–42; with permission. Copyright © 2006 Massachusetts Medical Society.)

rapid screening of patients for oral squamous cell carcinoma, and could lead to the development of new treatment approaches and prevention strategies.[78,77] Studying the patterns of gene expression in HNSCC also helps to gain a better understanding of the interactions between tumor cells and surrounding tissues, and the events leading to metastatic progression of HNSCC. DNA microarray technology may also prove to be an invaluable tool in the research and development of targeted drug therapies and prevention strategies.

MicroRNA Microarrays

MicroRNAs (mirs) are small RNA molecules that regulate the posttranscription expression of several genes that control cellular differentiation, proliferation, and apoptosis.[80–82] It has been shown that increased or decreased mir expression is linked to carcinogenesis, and each cancer exhibits a unique mir profile, or mir signature.[83–85] Mir expression can be evaluated using microarray technology. This technology has been used to evaluate the mir expression signature of HNSCC.[80] Mirs are retrievable from formalin-fixed, paraffin-embedded tissue, with good correlation to fresh frozen tissue samples.[86]

One microRNA, *mir-21*, is significantly upregulated in a variety of human tumors, such as pancreatic and breast cancer.[87–89] *Mir-21* was also found to be overexpressed in HNSCC.[80] It is thought that overexpression of *mir-21* promotes cellular proliferation by impaired regulation of *bcl-2* (an antiapoptotic protein) and tropomyosin-1 (a tumor suppressor gene).[89,90] In addition to their use in characterizing tumors, mirs could also prove useful in determining prognosis or in providing potential targets for drug therapies.

PROTEIN-BASED TECHNOLOGIES
Immunohistochemistry

IHC is a standard technique used in pathology to aid in the diagnosis of poorly differentiated neoplasms. IHC uses antibodies against proteins, or antigens, which can help in identifying the predominant cell type within a tumor (eg, epithelial cells, fibroblasts, B-lymphocytes).[91] Typically, neoplasms demonstrate a specific pattern of reactivity to various antigens, and a panel of immunohistochemical stains is frequently ordered. Epithelial tumors, for example, stain with cytokeratins, but are negative for vimentin. Advantages of IHC include (1) widespread availability of commercial stains, (2) relatively low cost, and (3) the ability to perform the stain on formalin-fixed tissue. The usefulness of the stain is dependent on successful techniques and procedures,

however, and stains can be misinterpreted by the pathologist, leading to a wrong diagnosis. Furthermore, IHC is of limited use in hard tissues decalcified in nitric acid.

In addition to its diagnostic value, IHC may also prove useful in assessing risk and guiding treatment. For example, histopathologically negative margins of resection that stain positive for *p53* mutations are associated with an increased risk of tumor recurrence in HNSCC.[13,14] Another possible use of IHC involves tissue microarrays. Cores of tissue ranging from 0.6 to 3 mm are obtained from several areas within the specimen (or from several specimens) and can be analyzed simultaneously on a single slide for immunohistochemical properties. Automated analysis of tissue microarrays is now available from several companies.[92]

Proteomics

Proteomics is the identification and characterization of proteins by mass spectrometry. There are two principle ways in which this can be carried out: bottom-up and top-down. The bottom-up approach relies on a cleaved protein mixture, resulting in protein fragments that can be analyzed and identified using mass spectrometry.[92–95] This approach often yields incomplete protein sequences, making interpretation of the results difficult. Top-down proteomics is a relatively new approach in which intact proteins are directly fragmented and then analyzed, decreasing the potential for interpretation errors.[93,96] Proteomic analysis can be carried out using blood or saliva samples, or paraffin-embedded tissue.[97]

One of the values of proteomics is that it can identify the various proteins that could be expressed by altered or mutated genes (proteomic signature). A variety of proteins are found to be overexpressed in HNSCC, such as enolase-α, annexin-1, and annexin-2.[97,98] Proteomics could be used to (1) identify specific protein markers found in HNSCC to be used in establishing a diagnosis and determining prognosis, (2) predict the function of certain proteins, (3) elucidate mechanisms of carcinogenesis or pathogenesis, (4) identify novel therapeutic targets, (5) determine drug efficacy and monitor response to treatment, and (6) monitor patients for relapse.

MICROFLUIDIC ANALYSIS

Saliva is an easily obtained bodily fluid containing exfoliated normal and potentially abnormal cells, making it ideal for head and neck cancer screening. Saliva could also be used to evaluate patients' response to treatment and to monitor for relapse, particularly because it allows for repeated, noninvasive, procurement of samples.[93] The p16 and p53 tumor suppressor genes are mutated in approximately 70% and 40% of all HNSCC, respectively.[99] Those mutations can act as markers for the presence of cancerous cells. In one study, Boyle and colleagues[100] used saliva specimens of seven patients with HNSCC to screen for p53 mutations. Tumor cells harboring such mutations were demonstrated in five (71%) of the patients. Using gene mutations as markers for HNSCC, microfluidic analysis could be used to screen patients for oral cancer.

Saliva could also be used to detect promoter region hypermethylation of cancer-related genes, a process that occurs early in carcinogenesis. In one study, methylation-specific PCR was used to detect promoter hypermethylation in both tissue and saliva samples of patients with HNSCC.[101] In the study, p16 (a tumor suppressor gene), MGMT (a DNA repair gene), and DAP-K (a metastasis suppressor gene) were found to be hypermethylated in over half of the tumor specimens. Of the methylated tumors, 65% also showed hypermethylation in the matched saliva DNA. The p16 showed the highest frequency of hypermethylation. Matched saliva samples were more frequently positive in tumors located within the oral cavity, compared with tumors located elsewhere in the head and neck. It was suggested that detection of promoter hypermethylation of cancer-related genes in the saliva of HNSCC patients may potentially be useful in early detection of cancer and in monitoring for disease recurrence.

Nunes and colleagues[102] compared detection of LOH at microsatellite loci in cytologic brushings of tumors with detection of LOH in mouth washes of patients with oral and oropharyngeal cancer. They found that 84% of salivary samples contained microsatellite allele losses, when LOH was also demonstrated in tumor brushings. None of the normal controls showed such genetic alterations. In a different study, 25 microsatellite markers were evaluated for LOH. Forty-nine percent of patients with oral squamous cell carcinoma showed LOH in salivary samples compared with 86% of the tumors when directly analyzed.[50]

In one recent study, the presence of HPV DNA in saliva samples of convalescent HNSCC patients was a negative prognostic indicator.[103] Surveillance of HPV-16 in saliva has been suggested as a possible, readily available, and noninvasive method to determine the prognosis and risk of recurrence of HPV-related HNSCC.

Finally, saliva microfluidic analysis could be used to identify gene or protein signatures.[78] Microfluidic diagnostic ("lab-on-a-chip") systems are currently being developed for various uses, including disease diagnostics.[79] Such devices are already used for rapid HIV screening[104–106] and may potentially provide a rapid screening tool to detect oral cancer at an earlier stage or to assess for recurrent disease. Analysis of salivary samples could offer a convenient, easily obtainable, and noninvasive way to diagnose and screen for HNSCC or other tumors.

TARGETED DRUG THERAPIES AND EPIDERMAL GROWTH FACTOR RECEPTOR

New molecular technologies will most likely prove to be invaluable in the research and development of targeted drug therapies aimed at treating HNSCC. In other disciplines, such as breast oncology, molecular technology has become integral to the diagnosis and chemotherapeutic regimen. Currently used technologies include IHC, FISH, and DNA microarrays. Estrogen receptor, progesterone receptor, and human epidermal growth factor receptor 2 (HER2) status is routinely assessed for breast tumors and serve as prognostic factors in predicting outcome. Drugs aimed at molecular targets are also being developed and used in the treatment of breast cancer. HER2, which is overexpressed in 20% of breast cancers, is the target of trastuzumab (Herceptin). Treatment with trastuzumab, a recombinant monoclonal antibody against HER2, significantly improved disease-free survival in patients with HER2-positive tumors.[107] Molecular diagnostics may lead to this type of targeted therapy for HNSCC.

In HNSCC one potential target is epidermal growth factor receptor (EGFR), which is commonly overexpressed in HNSCC; high levels are associated with a poor prognosis.[79,108–110] Therapies targeting EGFR include monoclonal antibodies against the receptor (eg, cetuximab) and tyrosine kinase inhibitors (eg, erlotinib, gefitinib). Although the standard of care still remains platinum-based (cisplastin) chemoradiotherapy, cetuximab may be beneficial in HNSCC patients with recurrent or metastatic disease no longer responsive to platinum agents, or in conjunction with radiotherapy in patients with advanced disease.[111–113] Tyrosine kinase inhibitors may also prove to be beneficial in treating patients with advanced, recurrent, or metastatic disease.[114–116] Another approach to treatment could involve EGFR gene therapy. In one recent study, a phase I clinical trial was conducted evaluating the use of intratumoral EGFR antisense injections in patients with advanced HNSCC unresponsive to standard therapy.[117] The authors concluded that this therapeutic approach was safe and may be beneficial in some patients with refractory disease.

SUMMARY

At present, the use of molecular techniques in head and neck pathology is still primarily research-based, helping to gain much valuable insight into the pathogenesis of various diseases, including oral squamous cell carcinoma. Such techniques are becoming increasingly important, however, in the clinical practice of pathology, oncology, and surgery. Identification of certain gene mutations or translocations may provide information essential in establishing a definitive diagnosis, predicting the behavior of a tumor, or in determining long-term prognosis. The mortality rates for HNSCC are still poor despite advances in surgery, chemotherapy, and radiotherapy.[118] One role of molecular techniques is to aid in refining treatment approaches and prevention strategies. In addition, these techniques will become increasingly important in the research and development of targeted drug therapy. Finally, specific mutations and other genetic changes, and the resultant protein signatures, can act as markers of carcinogenesis, enabling the development of screening tools for the early detection and treatment of oral cancer.

REFERENCES

1. Saiki RK, Scharf S, Faloona F, et al. Enzymatic amplification of beta-globin genomic sequences and restriction site analysis for diagnosis of sickle cell anemia. Science 1985;230(4732):1350.
2. Herzog CE, Herzog CE. Overview of sarcomas in the adolescent and young adult population. J Pediatr Hematol Oncol 2005;27(4):215.
3. Barnes L, Eveson JW, Reichart P, et al, editors. Pathology and genetics of head and neck tumours. Lyon (France): IARC Press; 2005. p. 38–40.
4. Gillespie MB, Marshall DT, Day TA, et al. Pediatric rhabdomyosarcoma of the head and neck. Curr Treat Options Oncol 2006;7(1):13.
5. Kushner BH, LaQuaglia MP, Cheung NK, et al. Clinically critical impact of molecular genetic studies in pediatric solid tumors. Med Pediatr Oncol 1999; 33(6):530.
6. Gallego Melcon S, Sanchez de Toledo Codina J. Molecular biology of rhabdomyosarcoma. Clin Transl Oncol 2007;9(7):415.
7. Sorensen PH, Lynch JC, Qualman SJ, et al. PAX3-FKHR and PAX7-FKHR gene fusions are prognostic indicators in alveolar rhabdomyosarcoma: a report from the children's oncology group. J Clin Oncol 2002;20(11):2672.
8. Sidransky D, Boyle J, Koch W. Molecular screening: prospects for a new approach. Arch Otolaryngol Head Neck Surg 1993;119(11):1187.
9. Sauter ER, Cleveland D, Trock B, et al. p53 is over-expressed in fifty percent of pre-invasive lesions of head and neck epithelium. Carcinogenesis 1994; 15(10):2269.
10. Kropveld A, Rozemuller E, Leppers F, et al. Sequencing analysis of RNA and DNA of exons 1 through 11 shows p53 gene alterations to be present in almost 100% of head and neck squamous cell cancers. Lab Invest 1999;79:347.
11. Gasco M, Crook T, Gasco M, et al. The p53 network in head and neck cancer. Oral Oncol 2003;39(3): 222.
12. Somers KD, Merrick MA, Lopez ME, et al. Frequent p53 mutations in head and neck cancer. Cancer Res 1992;52(21):5997.
13. Brennan JA, Mao L, Hruban RH, et al. Molecular assessment of histopathological staging in squamous-cell carcinoma of the head and neck. N Engl J Med 1995;332(7):429.
14. Ball VA, Righi PD, Tejada E, et al. p53 immunostaining of surgical margins as a predictor of local recurrence in squamous cell carcinoma of the oral cavity and oropharynx. Ear Nose Throat J 1997;76(11):818.
15. Liu TJ, el-Naggar AK, McDonnell TJ, et al. Apoptosis induction mediated by wild-type p53 adenoviral gene transfer in squamous cell carcinoma of the head and neck. Cancer Res 1995; 55(14):3117.
16. Clayman GL, el-Naggar AK, Lippman SM, et al. Adenovirus-mediated p53 gene transfer in patients with advanced recurrent head and neck squamous cell carcinoma. J Clin Oncol 1998;16(6):2221.
17. Bischoff JR, Kirn DH, Williams A, et al. An adenovirus mutant that replicates selectively in p53-deficient human tumor cells. Science 1996;274(5286): 373.
18. Ganly I, Kirn D, Eckhardt G, et al. A phase I study of Onyx-015, an E1B attenuated adenovirus, administered intratumorally to patients with recurrent head and neck cancer. Clin Cancer Res 2000;6(3):798.
19. Baylin SB, Herman JG, Graff JR, et al. Alterations in DNA methylation: a fundamental aspect of neoplasia. Adv Cancer Res 1998;72:141.
20. Sanchez-Cespedes M, Esteller M, Wu L, et al. Gene promoter hypermethylation in tumors and serum of head and neck cancer patients. Cancer Res 2000;60(4):892.
21. Herman JG, Merlo A, Mao L, et al. Inactivation of the CDKN2/p16/MTS1 gene is frequently

associated with aberrant DNA methylation in all common human cancers. Cancer Res 1995; 55(20):4525.

22. Jones AC, Freedman PD, Phelan JA, et al. Cytomegalovirus infections of the oral cavity: a report of six cases and review of the literature. Oral Surg Oral Med Oral Pathol 1993;75(1):76.

23. Cathomas G. Human herpes virus 8: a new virus discloses its face. Virchows Arch 2000;436(3):195.

24. Shimakage M, Horii K, Tempaku A, et al. Association of Epstein-Barr virus with oral cancers. Hum Pathol 2002;33(6):608.

25. D'Souza G, Kreimer AR, Viscidi R, et al. Case-control study of human papillomavirus and oropharyngeal cancer. N Engl J Med 2007; 356(19):1944.

26. Westra WH, Taube JM, Poeta ML, et al. Inverse relationship between human papillomavirus-16 infection and disruptive p53 gene mutations in squamous cell carcinoma of the head and neck. Clin Cancer Res 2008;14(2):366.

27. Charfi L, Jouffroy T, de Cremoux P, et al. Two types of squamous cell carcinoma of the palatine tonsil characterized by distinct etiology, molecular features and outcome. Cancer Lett 2008; 260(1–2):72.

28. Cunningham LL Jr, Pagano GM, Li M, et al. Overexpression of p16INK4 is a reliable marker of human papillomavirus-induced oral high-grade squamous dysplasia. Oral Surg Oral Med Oral Pathol Oral Radiol Endod 2006;102(1):77.

29. Ansari-Lari MA, Staebler A, Zaino RJ, et al. Distinction of endocervical and endometrial adenocarcinomas: immunohistochemical p16 expression correlated with human papillomavirus (HPV) DNA detection. Am J Surg Pathol 2004;28(2):160.

30. Greer RO, Meyers A, Said SM, et al. Is p16(INK4a) protein expression in oral ST lesions a reliable precancerous marker? Int J Oral Maxillofac Surg 2008;37(9):840.

31. Greenspan D, Greenspan JS, Conant M, et al. Oral "hairy" leucoplakia in male homosexuals: evidence of an association with both papillomavirus and herpes-group virus. Lancet 1984;2(8407):831–4.

32. Greenspan JS, Greenspan D, Lennette ET, et al. Replication of Epstein-Barr virus within the epithelial cells of oral "hairy" leukoplakia, an AIDS-associated lesion. N Engl J Med 1985;313(25):1564–71.

33. Seymour RA, Thomason JM, Nolan A. Oral lesions in organ transplant patients. J Oral Pathol Med 1997;26(7):297.

34. Eisenberg E, Krutchkoff D, Yamase H. Incidental oral hairy leukoplakia in immunocompetent persons. A report of two cases. Oral Surg Oral Med Oral Pathol 1992;74(3):332–3.

35. Braz-Silva PH, Rezende NP, Ortega KL, et al. Detection of the Epstein–Barr Virus (EBV) by in situ hybridization as definitive diagnosis of hairy leukoplakia. Head and Neck Pathol 2008;2:19.

36. Mabruk MJ, Antonio M, Flint SR, et al. A simple and rapid technique for the detection of Epstein-Barr virus DNA in HIV-associated oral hairy leukoplakia biopsies. J Oral Pathol Med 2000; 29(3):118.

37. Gallegos Ruiz MI, Floor K, Vos W, et al. Epidermal growth factor receptor (EGFR) gene copy number detection in non-small-cell lung cancer; a comparison of fluorescence in situ hybridization and chromogenic in situ hybridization. Histopathology 2007; 51(5):631.

38. de la Chapelle A. Microsatellite instability. N Engl J Med 2003;349(3):209.

39. Schlotterer C. Evolutionary dynamics of microsatellite DNA. Chromosoma 2000;109(6):365.

40. de la Chapelle A. Genetic predisposition to colorectal cancer. Nat Rev Cancer 2004;4(10):769.

41. El-Naggar AK, Hurr K, Huff V, et al. Microsatellite instability in preinvasive and invasive head and neck squamous carcinoma. Am J Pathol 1996; 148(6):2067.

42. Field JK, Kiaris H, Howard P, et al. Microsatellite instability in squamous cell carcinoma of the head and neck. Br J Cancer 1995;71(5):1065.

43. Ishwad CS, Ferrell RE, Rossie KM, et al. Microsatellite instability in oral cancer. Int J Cancer 1995; 64(5):332.

44. Partridge M, Emilion G, Pateromichelakis S, et al. Allelic imbalance at chromosomal loci implicated in the pathogenesis of oral precancer, cumulative loss and its relationship with progression to cancer. Oral Oncol 1998;34(2):77.

45. Koy S, Plaschke J, Luksch H, et al. Microsatellite instability and loss of heterozygosity in squamous cell carcinoma of the head and neck. Head Neck 2008;30(8):1105.

46. Ha PK, Pilkington TA, Westra WH, et al. Progression of microsatellite instability from premalignant lesions to tumors of the head and neck. Int J Cancer 2002;102(6):615.

47. Nawroz H, van der Riet P, Hruban RH, et al. Allelotype of head and neck squamous cell carcinoma. Cancer Res 1994;54(5):1152.

48. El-Naggar AK, Hurr K, Batsakis JG, et al. Sequential loss of heterozygosity at microsatellite motifs in preinvasive and invasive head and neck squamous carcinoma. Cancer Res 1995;55(12):2656.

49. Nogueira CP, Dolan RW, Gooey J, et al. Inactivation of p53 and amplification of cyclin D1 correlate with clinical outcome in head and neck cancer. Laryngoscope 1998;108(3):345.

50. El-Naggar AK, Mao L, Staerkel G, et al. Genetic heterogeneity in saliva from patients with oral squamous carcinomas: implications in molecular diagnosis and screening. J Mol Diagn 2001;3(4):164.

51. Beder LB, Gunduz M, Ouchida M, et al. Genome-wide analyses on loss of heterozygosity in head and neck squamous cell carcinomas. Lab Invest 2003;83(1):99.

52. Squire JA, Bayani J, Luk C, et al. Molecular cytogenetic analysis of head and neck squamous cell carcinoma: by comparative genomic hybridization, spectral karyotyping, and expression array analysis. Head Neck 2002;24(9):874.

53. Califano J, van der Riet P, Westra W, et al. Genetic progression model for head and neck cancer: implications for field cancerization. Cancer Res 1996;56(11):2488.

54. Jiang WW, Fujii H, Shirai T, et al. Accumulative increase of loss of heterozygosity from leukoplakia to foci of early cancerization in leukoplakia of the oral cavity. Cancer 2001;92(9):2349.

55. Mao L, Lee JS, Fan YH, et al. Frequent microsatellite alterations at chromosomes 9p21 and 3p14 in oral premalignant lesions and their value in cancer risk assessment. Nat Med 1996;2(6):682.

56. Roz L, Wu CL, Porter S, et al. Allelic imbalance on chromosome 3p in oral dysplastic lesions: an early event in oral carcinogenesis. Cancer Res 1996;56(6):1228.

57. Rosin MP, Cheng X, Poh C, et al. Use of allelic loss to predict malignant risk for low-grade oral epithelial dysplasia. Clin Cancer Res 2000;6(2):357.

58. Ogawara K, Miyakawa A, Shiba M, et al. Allelic loss of chromosome 13q14.3 in human oral cancer: correlation with lymph node metastasis. Int J Cancer 1998;79(4):312.

59. Bockmuhl U, Schwendel A, Dietel M, et al. Distinct patterns of chromosomal alterations in high- and low-grade head and neck squamous cell carcinomas. Cancer Res 1996;56(23):5325.

60. Patmore HS, Cawkwell L, Stafford ND, et al. Unraveling the chromosomal aberrations of head and neck squamous cell carcinoma: a review. Ann Surg Oncol 2005;12(10):831.

61. Tubbs RR, Stoler MH, editors. Cell and tissue based molecular pathology. Philadelphia: Churchill Livingstone/Elsevier; 2009. Foundations in diagnostic pathology.

62. Baldwin C, Garnis C, Zhang L, et al. Multiple micro-alterations detected at high frequency in oral cancer. Cancer Res 2005;65(17):7561.

63. Bockmuhl U, Petersen S, Schmidt S, et al. Patterns of chromosomal alterations in metastasizing and nonmetastasizing primary head and neck carcinomas. Cancer Res 1997;57(23):5213.

64. Bockmuhl U, Wolf G, Schmidt S, et al. Genomic alterations associated with malignancy in head and neck cancer. Head Neck 1998;20(2):145.

65. Gebhart E, Liehr T. Patterns of genomic imbalances in human solid tumors [review]. Int J Oncol 2000;16(2):383.

66. Tsui IF, Rosin MP, Zhang L, et al. Multiple aberrations of chromosome 3p detected in oral premalignant lesions. Cancer Prev Res (Phila Pa) 2008;1(6):424.

67. Weber RG, Scheer M, Born IA, et al. Recurrent chromosomal imbalances detected in biopsy material from oral premalignant and malignant lesions by combined tissue microdissection, universal DNA amplification, and comparative genomic hybridization. Am J Pathol 1998;153(1):295.

68. Kujawski M, Aalto Y, Jaskula-Sztul R, et al. DNA copy number losses are more frequent in primary larynx tumors with lymph node metastases than in tumors without metastases. Cancer Genet Cytogenet 1999;114(1):31.

69. Kujawski M, Sarlomo-Rikala M, Gabriel A, et al. Recurrent DNA copy number losses associated with metastasis of larynx carcinoma. Genes Chromosomes Cancer 1999;26(3):253.

70. O'Regan EM, Toner ME, Smyth PC, et al. Distinct array comparative genomic hybridization profiles in oral squamous cell carcinoma occurring in young patients. Head Neck 2006;28(4):330.

71. Mercado GE, Barr FG, Mercado GE, et al. Fusions involving PAX and FOX genes in the molecular pathogenesis of alveolar rhabdomyosarcoma: recent advances. Curr Mol Med 2007;7(1):47.

72. Fletcher CD, editor, Diagnostic histopathology of tumors, vol. II. Philadelphia: Churchill Livingstone Elsevier; 2007. p. 1861–83.

73. Shalon D, Smith SJ, Brown PO. A DNA microarray system for analyzing complex DNA samples using two-color fluorescent probe hybridization. Genome Res 1996;6(7):639.

74. Wang N, Wang N. Methodologies in cancer cytogenetics and molecular cytogenetics. Am J Med Genet 2002;115(3):118.

75. Quackenbush J. Microarray analysis and tumor classification. N Engl J Med 2006;354(23):2463.

76. Villaret DB, Wang T, Dillon D, et al. Identification of genes overexpressed in head and neck squamous cell carcinoma using a combination of complementary DNA subtraction and microarray analysis. Laryngoscope 2000;110(3 Pt 1):374.

77. Belbin T. Site-specific molecular signatures predict aggressive disease in HNSCC. Head and Neck Pathol 2008;2:243.

78. Ziober AF, Patel KR, Alawi F, et al. Identification of a gene signature for rapid screening of oral squamous cell carcinoma. Clin Cancer Res 2006;12(20 Pt 1):5960.

79. Ziober BL, Mauk MG, Falls EM, et al. Lab-on-a-chip for oral cancer screening and diagnosis. Head Neck 2008;30(1):111.

80. Chang SS, Jiang WW, Smith I, et al. MicroRNA alterations in head and neck squamous cell carcinoma. Int J Cancer 2008;123(12):2791.

81. Lewis BP, Burge CB, Bartel DP. Conserved seed pairing, often flanked by adenosines, indicates that thousands of human genes are microRNA targets. Cell 2005;120(1):15.

82. Scaria V, Hariharan M, Pillai B, et al. Host-virus genome interactions: macro roles for microRNAs. Cell Microbiol 2007;9(12):2784.

83. Calin GA, Croce CM. MicroRNA signatures in human cancers. Nat Rev Cancer 2006;6(11):857.

84. Croce CM, Calin GA. miRNAs, cancer, and stem cell division. Cell 2005;122(1):6.

85. Mirnezami AH, Pickard K, Zhang L, et al. Micro-RNAs: key players in carcinogenesis and novel therapeutic targets. Eur J Surg Oncol 2009;35(4):339.

86. Xi Y, Nakajima G, Gavin E, et al. Systematic analysis of microRNA expression of RNA extracted from fresh frozen and formalin-fixed paraffin-embedded samples. RNA 2007;13(10):1668.

87. Iorio MV, Ferracin M, Liu CG, et al. MicroRNA gene expression deregulation in human breast cancer. Cancer Res 2005;65(16):7065.

88. Roldo C, Missiaglia E, Hagan JP, et al. MicroRNA expression abnormalities in pancreatic endocrine and acinar tumors are associated with distinctive pathologic features and clinical behavior. J Clin Oncol 2006;24(29):4677.

89. Si ML, Zhu S, Wu H, et al. miR-21-mediated tumor growth. Oncogene 2007;26(19):2799.

90. Zhu S, Si ML, Wu H, et al. MicroRNA-21 targets the tumor suppressor gene tropomyosin 1 (TPM1). J Biol Chem 2007;282(19):14328.

91. Folpe AL, Gown AM. Immunohistochemistry for analysis of soft tissue tumors. In: Weiss SW, editor, editor. Enzinger and Weiss's soft tissue tumors. 5th edition. St. Louis (MO): Mosby; 2008. p. 129–74.

92. Blow N. Tissue preparation: tissue issues. Nature 2007;448:959.

93. Hu S, Wong DT, Hu S, et al. Oral cancer proteomics. Curr Opin Mol Ther 2007;9(5):467.

94. Hu S, Loo JA, Wong DT. Human saliva proteome analysis. Ann N Y Acad Sci 2007;1098:323.

95. Pandey A, Mann M. Proteomics to study genes and genomes. Nature 2000;405(6788):837.

96. Kelleher NL. Top-down proteomics. Anal Chem 2004;76(11):197A.

97. Patel PS, Telang SD, Rawal RM, et al. A review of proteomics in cancer research. Asian Pac J Cancer Prev 2005;6(2):113.

98. Mlynarek AM, Balys RL, Su J, et al. A cell proteomic approach for the detection of secretable biomarkers of invasiveness in oral squamous cell carcinoma. Arch Otolaryngol Head Neck Surg 2007;133(9):910.

99. Nagpal JK, Das BR. Oral cancer: reviewing the present understanding of its molecular mechanism and exploring the future directions for its effective management. Oral Oncol 2003;39(3):213.

100. Boyle JO, Mao L, Brennan JA, et al. Gene mutations in saliva as molecular markers for head and neck squamous cell carcinomas. Am J Surg 1994;168(5):429.

101. Rosas SL, Koch W, da Costa Carvalho MG, et al. Promoter hypermethylation patterns of p16, O6-methylguanine-DNA-methyltransferase, and death-associated protein kinase in tumors and saliva of head and neck cancer patients. Cancer Res 2001;61(3):939.

102. Nunes DN, Kowalski LP, Simpson AJ. Detection of oral and oropharyngeal cancer by microsatellite analysis in mouth washes and lesion brushings. Oral Oncol 2000;36(6):525.

103. Chuang AY, Chuang TC, Chang S, et al. Presence of HPV DNA in convalescent salivary rinses is an adverse prognostic marker in head and neck squamous cell carcinoma. Oral Oncol 2008;44(10):915.

104. Mylonakis E, Paliou M, Lally M, et al. Laboratory testing for infection with the human immunodeficiency virus: established and novel approaches. Am J Med 2000;109(7):568.

105. Kassler WJ, Dillon BA, Haley C, et al. On-site, rapid HIV testing with same-day results and counseling. AIDS 1997;11(8):1045.

106. Stetler HC, Granade TC, Nunez CA, et al. Field evaluation of rapid HIV serologic tests for screening and confirming HIV-1 infection in Honduras. AIDS 1997;11(3):369.

107. Piccart-Gebhart MJ, Procter M, Leyland-Jones B, et al. Trastuzumab after adjuvant chemotherapy in HER2-positive breast cancer. N Engl J Med 2005;353(16):1659.

108. Chung CH, Ely K, McGavran L, et al. Increased epidermal growth factor receptor gene copy number is associated with poor prognosis in head and neck squamous cell carcinomas. J Clin Oncol 2006;24(25):4170.

109. Hitt R, Ciruelos E, Amador ML, et al. Prognostic value of the epidermal growth factor receptor (EGRF) and p53 in advanced head and neck squamous cell carcinoma patients treated with induction chemotherapy. Eur J Cancer 2005;41(3):453.

110. Zimmermann M, Zouhair A, Azria D, et al. The epidermal growth factor receptor (EGFR) in head and neck cancer: its role and treatment implications. Radiat Oncol 2006;1:11.

111. Bonner JA, Harari PM, Giralt J, et al. Radiotherapy plus cetuximab for squamous-cell carcinoma of the head and neck. N Engl J Med 2006;354(6):567.

112. Posner MR, Wirth LJ. Cetuximab and radiotherapy for head and neck cancer. N Engl J Med 2006; 354(6):634.

113. Blick SK, Scott LJ. Cetuximab: a review of its use in squamous cell carcinoma of the head and neck and metastatic colorectal cancer. Drugs 2007; 67(17):2585.

114. Wakeling AE. Epidermal growth factor receptor tyrosine kinase inhibitors. Curr Opin Pharmacol 2002;2(4):382.

115. Rogers SJ, Box C, Chambers P, et al. Determinants of response to epidermal growth factor receptor tyrosine kinase inhibition in squamous cell carcinoma of the head and neck. J Pathol 2009; 218(1):122–30.

116. Cohen EE, Davis DW, Karrison TG, et al. Erlotinib and bevacizumab in patients with recurrent or metastatic squamous-cell carcinoma of the head and neck: a phase I/II study. Lancet Oncol 2009;10(3):247.

117. Lai SY, Koppikar P, Thomas SM, et al. Intratumoral epidermal growth factor receptor antisense DNA therapy in head and neck cancer: first human application and potential antitumor mechanisms. J Clin Oncol 2009;27(8):1235.

118. Jemal A, Siegel R, Ward E, et al. Cancer statistics, 2008. CA a Cancer J Clin 2008;58(2):71.

119. Tonon G, Modi S, Wu L, et al. t(11;19)(q21;p13) Translocation in mucoepidermoid carcinoma creates a novel fusion product that disrupts a Notch signaling pathway. Nat Genet 2003; 33(2):208.

Adhesive Use in Oral and Maxillofacial Surgery

Michael J. Buckley, DMD, MBA, MS[a,b,*],
Eric J. Beckman, PhD[c,d]

KEYWORDS

- Tissue adhesives • Adhesives for bone fixation
- Cyanoacrylates • Fibrin sealants
- Collagen-based sealants
- Synthetic polymer-based materials
- Protein-based sealants

The tissue adhesive market is a vibrant and dynamic sector with emerging technologies and innovative concepts for cutting-edge applications. Presently in oral and maxillofacial surgery, adhesives have a minimal role, but this is changing rapidly. In oral and maxillofacial surgery, closure of soft tissue wounds is primarily done with mechanical devices, such as sutures and staples. To close larger soft tissue wounds or develop large soft tissue flaps in cosmetic and reconstructive procedures, clinicians use mechanical devices and apply drains that help evacuate dead spaces to prevent hematomas and seromas. Similarly bone fixation in oral and maxillofacial surgery is primarily done with external fixation, such as maxillomandibular fixation, or with internal fixation using small bone plates and screws. The emerging adhesives and sealants are likely to have clinical applicability in oral and maxillofacial surgery soon and accelerate this clinical change.

IDEAL PROPERTIES OF TISSUE ADHESIVES

The ideal tissue adhesive must be biodegradable and biocompatible. To be effective, it must have both significant cohesive (covalent bonding of glue molecules to each other) and adhesive (bonding of glue molecules to adjacent tissue) properties. To be biocompatible, tissue adhesives must pass both acute and subacute toxicity tests and have minimal cytotoxicity. The adhesive must have a suitable setting time and be user friendly, requiring little preparation time. It should also have no special storage or shipping requirements. It must be relatively hydrophilic so it readily spreads on wet surfaces at body temperature, and have adequate working time for the given application. The adhesives must be strong, yet flexible, with an elastic modulus similar to that of the tissue being glued. Lastly, the adhesives must have minimal heat generation (exothermic) characteristics and degrade with minimal inflammatory response. At the moment, no adhesives on the market fulfill all of these requirements.

Surgeons have been using tissue sealants and adhesives since the early nineteenth century.[1] There are presently four types of tissue adhesives: fibrin sealants, collagen-based sealants, synthetic polymer-based materials, and protein-based sealants. In 2000, fibrin sealants accounted for 86% of the total tissue sealant market while protein-based sealants accounted for 12% and synthetic polymer-based materials represented 2%.[2]

FIBRIN ADHESIVES

In the early 1940s, the combination of fibrin and thrombin was first used as an adhesive. These

[a] Private Practice, 31 N Maple Avenue, Greensburg, PA 15601, USA
[b] University of Pittsburgh School of Dental Medicine, 3501 Terrace Street, Pittsburgh, PA 15213, USA
[c] Cohera Medical Inc, Pittsburgh, PA, USA
[d] University of Pittsburgh School of Engineering, 3800 O'Hara Street, Pittsburgh, PA 15213, USA
* Corresponding author. Private Practice, 31 N Maple Avenue, Greensburg, PA 15601.
E-mail address: mbuckley@coheramed.com

Oral Maxillofacial Surg Clin N Am 22 (2010) 195–199
doi:10.1016/j.coms.2009.10.008

fibrin sealants and glues were developed and used extensively in the 1960s with donor-preserved and autologous-donated plasma as the source of the coagulation components. In 1977, however, the US Food and Drug Administration (FDA) revoked the license for the commercial use of fibrin sealants and glues from donor-preserved human plasma because of the possibility of disease transmission.[3–5] The fibrin glues presently on the market are Tisseel (Baxter International Inc, Deerfield, Illinois) and Hemaseel (Haemacure Corp, Montreal, Canada). The fibrin glues in head and neck surgery are primarily used as hemostatic agents over large surface areas and are very effective for that use. Fibrin glues, however, require mixing of several different components on the back table, which takes 20 to 40 minutes, before they can be used. Fibrin glues are good hemostatic agents but are poor adhesives as they exhibit a very weak bond. They are, however, entirely biodegradable and biocompatible.[6]

COLLAGEN- AND PROTEIN-BASED SEALANTS

Collagen- and protein-based adhesives and sealants are made up of connective tissue components used as a two-part adhesive by taking advantage of the ability of the components to cross-link upon mixing. Collagen, when cross-linked with glutaraldehyde, forms a protein-based sealant that can seal against both air and fluid leakage. This two-part sealant also creates a weak adhesive bond to adjacent tissue and is sometimes referred to as an adhesive for that reason. Protein-based adhesives (eg, BioGlue [CryoLife, Kennesaw, Georgia]) have several disadvantages: Because they are made from bovine serum albumin, they pose a small risk for transmission of disease and contain a foreign protein that can cause hypersensitization.[7] More importantly, they use glutaraldehyde as the cross-bonding agent, which is a neurotoxin. Degradation of these sealants is very slow and strong inflammatory responses can result. Because of their weak adhesive strength, their use in craniomaxillofacial surgery is primarily in free flap surgery as a sealant around a vascular anastamosis.[8,9]

Another of the two-part sealants, is DuraSeal (Confluent Surgical, Inc, Waltham, Massachusetts), an FDA-approved product for use in dural sealing. When employed for appropriate dural closure, DuraSeal can be used to complete the watertight closure necessary in this tissue. DuraSeal is a polyethylene glycol–based hydrogel that is synthetic, absorbable, and easily applied. It is designed such that each of its two parts contains polyethylene glycol polymers with complementary functional groups at the polymer chain ends. When mixed, these complementary groups react with each other, leading to a rapid cure. Its use as an adhesive, however, is limited because of its poor adhesive strength. DuraSeal is readily degradable (the linkages formed during curing are hydrolytically cleaved) and biocompatible.[10]

CYANOACRYLATES

Cyanoacrylates (superglues) have been used for years as wound-closure materials. Octyl-cyanocrylates and butyl-cyanocrylates have been recently used as skin-closure adhesives with good success. All of the cyanoacrylates operate as adhesives in similar manners. They are applied as mononers, which then rapidly polymerize to a high molecular-weight material.[11–13] The presence of the cyano group on the acrylate monomer enables initiation of polymerization (curing) simply by water or amine groups present on proteins, a characteristic not present in typical acrylates. Conventional superglue (methyl cyanoacrylate) cures to a hard, brittle material, whereas the octyl and butyl analogs used as tissue adhesives form a more resilient material once cured. While exhibiting a strong adhesive bond once cured, cyanoacrylates do not biodegrade to any real extent and can induce a significant inflammatory response given their hydrophobic nature. Their use has generally been limited to superficial wounds. Cyanoacrylate tissue adhesives form a strong bond across tissue-wound edges, enabling normal healing to occur below the seal. They are marketed to replace small sutures in incision and laceration repairs. These adhesives have been shown to save time and provide a flexible water-resistant protective coating that will seal head and neck wounds from water exposure and contamination. They can be used safely in small wounds, but also in larger wounds where subcutaneous sutures are needed and a watertight sealant is appropriate. There is a small exothermic reaction during curing, but the patient does not usually feel the temperature rise. These cyanoacrylates have been shown to have some antimicrobial properties.[14]

POLYURETHANE ADHESIVES

Polyurethane adhesives exhibit a wide range of physical and mechanical properties that make them attractive candidates for biomedical use. Created by the reaction of polyester- or polyether-polyols with polyfunctional isocyanates, polyurethane polymers are frequently used in

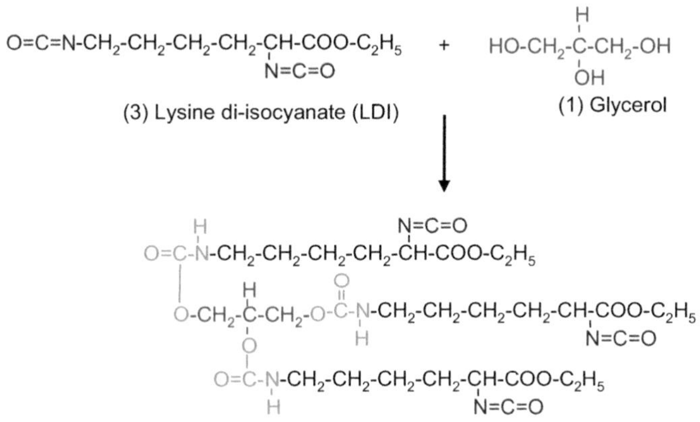

O=C=N-CH$_2$-CH$_2$-CH$_2$-CH$_2$-CH-COO-C$_2$H$_5$ +   HO-CH$_2$-C-CH$_2$-OH
          N=C=O   OH

(3) Lysine di-isocyanate (LDI)   (1) Glycerol

$$O=C-N-CH_2-CH_2-CH_2-CH_2-CH-COO-C_2H_5$$

Fig. 1. Reaction of glycerol and lysine di-isocyanate (LDI). LDI is composed of a lysine core (*black*) with two isocyanate groups (*blue*). One glycerol (*red*) reacts with three LDI molecules to produce an isocyanate-capped glycerol prepolymer. The reaction of the hydroxyl groups on glycerol with the isocyanate groups on LDI produces a urethane linkage (*green*). The resultant prepolymer has three unreacted isocyanate groups remaining.

medical applications, such as heart valves, dialysis membranes, breast implants, and aortic grafts. When employed as an adhesive, a urethane prepolymer generally has an oligomeric (rather than polymeric) structure and contains terminal (ie, at chain ends) isocyanate groups (**Fig. 1**). These groups react readily with hydroxyls and amines found in tissue, forming a strong bond with the surface. In addition, the presence of water leads to rapid curing through the transformation of some of the isocyanate groups to amines, followed by reaction of these amines with nearby isocyanates to create urea crosslinks. Although various adhesive and nonadhesive biodegradable polyurethanes have been synthesized, current available synthetic adhesive components have met with limited commercial success for a number of reasons. For example, a number of such compositions exhibit unacceptable toxicity arising, for example, from the cytotoxicity of the degradation products of the isocyanates used in the synthesis of these adhesives. Isocyanates are generated from the analogous amines, and several of the aromatic amines used to create commercial isocyanates (those used in foam bedding and seating) have been shown to be carcinogenic, rendering such isocyanates entirely unsuitable for use in medical adhesives. In addition, early attempts at using commercial polyisocyanates and polyols in medical adhesives led to cured products that were too hydrophobic to degrade quickly.

Recently in development and beginning initial clinical trials is a lysine-derived urethane tissue adhesive that may prove ideal for fixation of deep wounds. This adhesive is biocompatible, resorbable, and nontoxic and could dramatically improve the field of wound closure and hence significantly advance surgical care. This adhesive is best

used on plainer tissues and will be suitable for reducing or eliminating dead space in large traumatic wounds and for developing soft tissue flaps. Its use in eliminating dead space and preventing seromas and hematomas in cosmetic surgery procedures, such as in face lifts and forehead lifts, will likely be significant. In a recent study using a canine abdominoplasty model (**Fig. 2**), use of the lysine-based urethane adhesive decreased

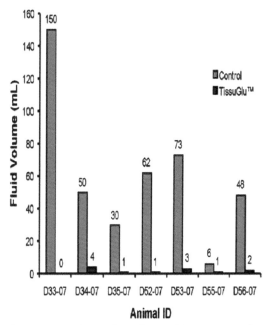

Fig. 2. Comparison of test lysine di-isocyanate adhesive and control in canine abdominoplasty model. (*From* Gilbert TW, Badylak SF, Gusenoff J, et al. Lysine-derived urethane surgical adhesive prevents seroma formation in a canine abdominoplasty model. Plast Reconstr Surg 2008;122:95–102; with permission.)

Time	Control Strain (N/cm^2)	SD	Glue Strain (N/cm^2)	SD
1 hours	0.268	0.213	10.437	5.451
12 hours	0.612	0.185	3.883	0.937
24 hours	0.992	0.13	8.358	6.315
1 week	3.2	1.869	14.472	4.414
2 weeks	19.861	11.553	22.789	14.912
4 weeks	62.866	22	56.571	19.8

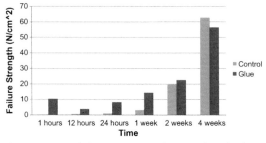

Fig. 3. Strength comparison of TissuGlue (Cohera Medical, Inc, Pittsburgh, Pennsylvania). Tensile strengths were measured for control wounds and wounds with TissuGlue at 1 hour, 12 hours, 24 hours, and 1 week. At all time points, tensile strength of wounds with TissuGlue were stronger than that of a naturally healing wound at 1 week.

wound exudates by 97%, versus the control, with minimal inflammatory response. As shown in **Fig. 3**, tensile strengths were measured for control wounds and wounds with a polyurethane adhesive at 1 hour, 12 hours, 24 hours, and 1 week. At all time points, tensile strengths of the polyurethane-closed wounds were stronger than that of a naturally healing wound at 1 week. Histologic analysis revealed no tissue reaction, minimal inflammation, and no necrosis of muscle-wound tissue. Planar wounds in the head and neck region could greatly benefit from an adhesive with the chemical proprieties and surgical strength to eliminate the dead space.

The various building blocks of the polyurethane adhesives can be blended in different proportions to create adhesives with a useful range of physical properties and cure times. Polyurethane created via moisture curing of the prepolymer simply degrades to an initial hydroxyl-containing compound plus lysine, small amounts of ethanol, and carbon dioxide.

BONE ADHESIVE

A particular problem in oral and maxillofacial surgery is bone fixation of small pieces of bone where use of bone screws and bone plates is impossible or impractical. These applications might include not only small fragments of bone in the craniomaxillofacial region, but also fixation of intracapsular fractures where the use of screws and bone plates is precluded. A bone adhesive strong enough

to hold bony fragments in their original anatomic position and enable osseous union between these fragments would be of great benefit. Presently, a polyurethane adhesive with building blocks has been designed to give significant bony strength, and still allow for osseous union to occur.[15–16]

SUMMARY

Presently, tissue adhesives and sealants have a limited use in oral and maxillofacial surgical procedures.[17] Skin closure occurs regularly with cyanoacrylate adhesives.[18–23] Sealing of dural tears in conjunction with dural closure has been shown to be very successful. With the development of more head and neck reconstructive procedures and cosmetic procedures, demand will increase for better surgical adhesives. Clinical trials are beginning for newly developed adhesives with the chemical characteristics, the safe reabsorptive profile, and the adhesive strength necessary to benefit oral and maxillofacial surgery patients in the near future. Adhesives for bone fixation, while in early development, also show a promising chemical profile and will be of significant benefit to oral and maxillofacial surgical patients.

REFERENCES

1. Currie LJ, Sharpe JR, Martin R. The use of fibrin glue in skin grafts and tissue-engineered skin replacements: a review. Plast Reconstr Surg 2001;108(6): 1713–26.
2. Frost and Sullivan. US market for hemostats-tissue sealants-tissue adhesives and adhesion prevention products. Available at: http://www.frost.com. Accessed May 1, 2009.
3. Carless PA, Anthony DM, Henry DA. Systemic review of the use of fibrin sealant to minimize perioperative allogeneic blood transfusion. Br J Surg 2002;89(6):695–703.
4. Jackson MR, Alving BM. Fibrin sealant in preclinical and clinical studies. Curr Opin Hematol 1999;6(6): 415.
5. Jackson MR. Fibrin sealants in surgical practice: an overview. Am J Surg 2001;182(2 Suppl 1):S1–7.
6. Silver FH, Wang M-C, Pins GD. Review: preparation and use of fibrin glue in surgery. Biomaterials 1995; 16(2):891–903.
7. Streiff MB, Ness PM. Acquired FV inhibitors: a needless iatrogenic complication of bovine thrombine exposure. Transfusion 2002;42(1):18.
8. Passage J, Jalali H, Tam RK, et al. BioGlue surgical adhesive—an appraisal of its indications in cardiac surgery. Ann Thorac Surg 2001;72(2):638–40.

9. Raanani E, Latter DA, Errett LE, et al. Use of BioGlue in aortic surgical repair. Ann Thorac Surg 2001; 72(2):509–14.

10. Dutt SM, Mirza S, Irving RM. Middle cranial fossa approach for repair of spontaneous cerebrospinal fluid otorrhoea using autologous bone pate. Clin Otolaryngol Allied Sci 2001;26(2):117–25.

11. Bruns TB, Simon HK, McLario DJ, et al. Laceration repair using a tissue adhesive in children's emergency department. Pediatrics 1996;98:673–5.

12. Bruns TB, Robinson BS, Smith RJ, et al. A new tissue adhesive for laceration repair in children. J Pediatr 1988;132:1067–70.

13. Brun TB, Worthington JM. Using tissue adhesive for wound repair: a practical guide to Dermabond. Am Fam Physician 2000;61(5):1383–8.

14. Simon HK, McLario DJ, Bruns TB, et al. Long-term appearance of lacerations repaired using a tissue adhesive. Pediatrics 1997;99:193–5.

15. Zhang JY, Doll BA, Beckman EJ, et al. Three-dimensional biocompatible ascorbic acid-containing scaffold for bone tissue engineering. Tissue Eng 2003; 9(6):1143–7.

16. Ganta SR, Piesco NP, Long P, et al. Vascularization and tissue infiltration of a biodegradable polyurethane matrix. J Biomed Mater Res A 2003; 64(2):242–8.

17. Anderson KW, Baker SR. Advances in facial rejuvenation surgery. Curr Opin Otolaryngol Head Neck Surg 2003;11(4):256–60.

18. Charters A. Wound glue: a comparative study of tissue adhesives. Accid Emerg Nurs 2000;8(4):223–7.

19. Doraiswamy NV, Baig H, Hammett S, et al. Which tissue adhesive for wounds? Injury 2004;34(8):564–7.

20. Quinn JV, Drzewiecki A, Li MM, et al. A randomized, controlled trial comparing a tissue adhesive with a suturing in the repair of pediatric facial lacerations. Ann Emerg Med 1993;22:1130–5.

21. Quinn J, Wells G, Sutcliffe T, et al. A randomized trial comparing octylcyanoacrylate tissue adhesive and sutures in the management of lacerations. JAMA 1997;277:1527–30.

22. Singer AJ, Hollander JE, Valentine SM, et al. Prospective randomized, controlled trial of tissue adhesive (2-octylcyanoacrylate) vs. standard wound closure techniques for laceration repair. Acad Emerg Med 1998;5:94–9.

23. Toriumi DM, O'Grady K, Desai D, et al. Use of octyl-2-cyanoacrylate for skin closure in facial plastic surgery. Plast Reconstr Surg 1998;102:2209–19.

Index

Note: Page numbers of article titles are in **boldface** type.

A

Adhesives, use in oral and maxillofacial surgery, **195–199**
    bone adhesives, 199
    collagen and protein-based sealants, 196
    cyanoacrylates, 196
    fibrin adhesives, 195–196
    ideal properties of, 195
    polyurethane adhesives, 196–199
Anastomotic technique, in microvascular surgery, 80–83
    Coupler system, 82–83
Anchorage, skeletal. *See* Skeletal anchorage.
Angiography, for donor site assessment prior to microvascular surgery, computed tomographic (CTA), 79
    magnetic resonance (MRA), 78–79
    for recipient site assessment prior to microvascular surgery, three-dimensional spiral computed tomographic (CTA), 80

B

Bone adhesives, use in oral and maxillofacial surgery, 199
Bone flap shaping, in computer-assisted craniomaxillofacial surgery, 126–129
Bone morphogenetic proteins, in craniomaxillofacial surgery, **17–31**
    biologic activity, 18–19
    carrier materials, 19
    clinical applications, 21–29
    clinical study and safety, 19–21
    history, 17–18

C

Cancer, head and neck, molecular diagnostics for, **183–194**
Cellular approaches, in regenerative medicine, 38–39
Cervical masses, prenatal diagnosis and treatment, 13
Cleft lip and palate, clinical outcomes for primary repair, **43–58**
    cleft lip repair, 44–48
        muscular reconstruction, 46–47
        presurgical orthopedics, 47–48
        primary nasal reconstruction, 44–46
        timing of, 48

    cleft palate repair, 48–54
        double-opposing Z-plasty, 50–52
        growth and, 52–53
        timing of, 53
        two-flap palatoplasty, 50
    prenatal diagnosis and treatment, 11–12
Collagen-based sealants, use in oral and maxillofacial surgery, 196
Color-duplex ultrasonography, for donor site assessment prior to microvascular surgery, 76–77
Comparative genomic hybridization, for head and neck pathology diagnostics, 186–187
Computed tomographic angiography (CTA), for donor site assessment prior to microvascular surgery, 79
    three-dimensional spiral, for recipient site assessment prior to microvascular surgery, 80
Computed tomography (CT), advances in head and neck imaging with, 107–110
Computer-assisted surgery, computer planning and, **135–156**
    intraoperative navigation, 137–153
        cranial reconstruction, 143
        dental/craniofacial implants, 151–153
        maxillo-mandibular reconstruction, 141–143
        orbital reconstruction, 138–141
        orthognathic surgery, 145–148
        temporomandibular joint surgery, 148–151
        tumor resection, 143–145
    craniomaxillofacial, **117–134**
        bone flap shaping, 126–129
        concepts of, 122–124
        distraction osteogenesis, 129
        enhanced three-dimensional diagnostics, 119–121
        imaging, 118–119
        orthognathic surgery, 129–133
        reconstructive surgery, 124–126
        tactile models, 121–122
Congenital anomalies, craniofacial, prenatal diagnosis and treatment, **5–15**
Cook-Swartz Doppler probe system, for postoperative monitoring after microvascular surgery, 85–86
Counseling, prenatal, for parents of a fetus with congenital a anomaly, 9–10
Coupler system, microvascular anastomotic, 82–83
Craniomaxillofacial anomalies, prenatal diagnosis and treatment, **5–15**

Oral Maxillofacial Surg Clin N Am 22 (2010) 201–207
doi:10.1016/S1042-3699(10)00017-8
1042-3699/10/$ – see front matter © 2010 Elsevier Inc. All rights reserved.

Craniomaxillofacial (*continued*)
    cervical masses and oral/pharyngeal masses, 13
    cleft lip and palate, 11–12
    ex utero intrapartum therapy (EXIT), 10–11
    fetal interventions and perinatal therapies, 9–10
        parental support and counseling, 9–10
        procedures and surgery, 10
    interdisciplinary team care, 5–9
        fetal MRI, 8–9
        prenatal care, 6–7
        ultrasonography, 7–8
    micrognathia, 12–13
    other craniofacial anomalies, 13–14
Craniomaxillofacial surgery, advances in head and neck imaging, **107–118**
    bone morphogenetic proteins in, **17–31**
        biologic activity, 18–19
        carrier materials, 19
        clinical applications, 21–29
        clinical study and safety, 19–21
        history, 17–18
    cleft lip and palate surgery, **43–58**
        cleft lip repair, 44–48
            muscular reconstruction, 46–47
            presurgical orthopedics, 47–48
            primary nasal reconstruction, 44–46
            timing of, 48
        cleft palate repair, 48–54
            double-opposing Z-plasty, 50–52
            growth and, 52–53
            timing of, 53
            two-flap palatoplasty, 50
    computer planning and, **135–156**
        intraoperative navigation, 137–153
            cranial reconstruction, 143
            dental/craniofacial implants, 151–153
            maxillo-mandibular reconstruction, 141–143
            orbital reconstruction, 138–141
            orthognathic surgery, 145–148
            temporomandibular joint surgery, 148–151
            tumor resection, 143–145
        stereolithographic models, 138
        surgical simulation, 138–139
    computer-assisted, **117–134**
        bone flap shaping, 126–129
        concepts of, 122–124
        distraction osteogenesis, 129
        enhanced three-dimensional diagnostics, 119–121
        imaging, 118–119
        orthognathic surgery, 129–133
        reconstructive surgery, 124–126
        tactile models, 121–122
    endoscopic techniques, **169–182**

        orthognathic surgery, 172–174
            LeFort I osteotomy, 173–174
            sagittal split osteotomy, 172–173
            vertical ramus osteotomy, 173
        removal of foreign bodies, 179
        sialoendoscopy, 174–176
        temporomandibular joint surgery, 176–178
        trauma, 169–172
            frontal sinus fracture, 172
            mandibular angle fracture, 171–172
            orbital floor fractures, 169–171
            subcondylar fracture, 171–172
    microvascular surgery, technology in, **73–90**
        history of free-tissue transfer and, 73–75
        intraoperative anastomotic technique, 80–83
        postoperative flap monitoring, 83–88
        preoperative imaging assessment, 75–80
            donor site assessment, 76–79
            recipient site assessment, 79–80
    orbital surgery, **59–71**
        endoscopic and advanced imaging techniques for, 68–69
        medial orbital wall fractures, 64–66
        orbital floor fractures, 59–64
        orbital roof fractures, 66–68
    prenatal diagnosis and treatment of craniomaxillofacial anomalies, **5–15**
    regenerative medicine for, **33–42**
        basic principles of, 34–38
            bone regeneration, 34–35
            growth factors, 38
            scaffolds, 35–37
        cellular approaches, 38–39
            differentiated osteoblasts, 40
            mesenchymal stem cell technology, 39–40
        new interdisciplinary field of, 34
        vascular regeneration, 39–40
    temporary skeletal anchorage devices for orthodontics, **91–105**
        basic mechanics of, 92–94
        clinical indications for, 95–100
            closure of anterior open bite, 96–97
            mesial or distal movement of teeth with maximum anchorage, 95–96
            orthopedic growth modification, 97–100
            uprighting or intruding molar teeth, 96
        devices for, 94–95
        history of, 92
        outcomes and complications, 103–104
        postoperative regimen, 101–103
        surgical procedures, 100–101
            placement of miniscrews for skeletal anchorage, 101
            placement of skeletal anchorage plates, 100–101
    transcranial endoscopic, of the ventral skull base, **157–168**

controversies, 167
intraoperative strategies, 160–162
preoperative evaluation, 159–160
principles of, 157–159
reconstruction, 164–167
surgical approaches, 162–164
coronal plane modules, 163–164
sagittal plane modules, 162–163
Craniosynostosis, prenatal diagnosis and treatment,
13–14
Cyanoacrylates, use in oral and maxillofacial
surgery, 196

D

Dental implants, computer planning and
intraoperative navigation, 151–153
Dermoids, central, prenatal diagnosis and
treatment, 14
Diagnostics, molecular. See Molecular diagnostics.
Distraction osteogenesis, computer-assisted, 129
DNA microarrays, for head and neck pathology
diagnostics, 187–188

E

Encephaloceles, prenatal diagnosis and
treatment, 14
Endonasal surgery, techniques in oral and
maxillofacial surgery, 169–182
transcranial, of the ventral skull base, 157–168
controversies, 167
intraoperative strategies, 160–162
preoperative evaluation, 159–160
principles of, 157–159
reconstruction, 164–167
surgical approaches, 162–164
coronal plane modules, 163–164
sagittal plane modules, 162–163
Endoscopic techniques, for orbital fracture
repair, 68–69
in oral and maxillofacial surgery, 169–182
orthognathic surgery, 172–174
LeFort I osteotomy, 173–174
sagittal split osteotomy, 172–173
vertical ramus osteotomy, 173
removal of foreign bodies, 179
sialoendoscopy, 174–176
temporomandibular joint surgery, 176–178
trauma, 169–172
frontal sinus fracture, 172
mandibular angle fracture, 171–172
orbital floor fractures, 169–171
subcondylar fracture, 171–172
transcranial endonasal surgery of ventral skull
base, 157–168

Epidermal growth factor receptor, targeted drug
therapies for head and neck cancers, 189–190
Evidence-based surgery, outcomes research and,
1–4
definition, 1–2
model for, 2–3
use to enhance surgical practice and
healthcare processes, 2
Ex utero intrapartum therapy (EXIT), for newly born
child with congenital anomaly, 10–11

F

Fetal diagnosis. See Prenatal diagnosis.
Fibrin adhesives, use in oral and maxillofacial
surgery, 195–196
Fluorescence in situ hybridization, for head and neck
pathology diagnostics, 184–185
Foreign bodies, endoscopic techniques for removal,
179
Fractures, endoscopic surgery for oral and
maxillofacial, 169–172
frontal sinus, 172
mandibular angle, 171–172
orbital floor, 169–171
subcondylar, 171–172
orbital, surgical repair of, 59–71
medial orbital wall, 64–66
orbital floor, 59–64
orbital roof, 66–68
Free tissue transfer, microvascular surgery,
technology in, 73–90
Frontal sinus fractures, endoscopic surgery for, 172

G

Gliomas, congenital, prenatal diagnosis and
treatment, 14
Grafting, bone morphogenetic proteins in
craniomaxillofacial surgery, 17–31
Growth, outcomes in cleft lip and palate care, 52–53
Growth factors, in regenerative medicine, 38

H

Head, advances in imaging of, 107–118
Heterozygosity, loss of, for head and neck pathology
diagnostics, 185–186

I

Imaging, advanced techniques for orbital fracture
repair, 68–69
head and neck, advances in, 107–118
computed tomography, 107–110
magnetic resonance imaging, 110–114
nuclear medicine, 114

Imaging (*continued*)
    in computer-assisted craniomaxillofacial surgery,
        118–119
    in preoperative assessment for microvascular
        surgery, 75–80
        donor site assessment, 76–79
        recipient site assessment, 79–80
    prenatal, 7–9
        fetal MRI, 8–9
        ultrasonography, 7–8
Immunohistochemistry, for head and neck pathology
    diagnostics, 188
Implants, dental/craniofacial, computer planning and
    intraoperative navigation, 151–153
Implants, orbital, for repair of medial wall orbital
    fractures, 65–66
    for repair of orbital floor fractures, 60–63
In situ hybridization, for head and neck pathology
    diagnostics, 184–185
Intraoperative navigation. *See* Navigation,
    intraoperative.

L

LeFort osteotomy, endoscopic techniques for,
    173–174
Lip, cleft, clinical outcomes for primary repair of,
    44–48
        muscular reconstruction, 46–47
        presurgical orthopedics, 47–48
        primary nasal reconstruction, 44–46
        timing of, 48
    prenatal diagnosis and treatment, 11–12
Loss of heterozygosity, for head and neck pathology
    diagnostics, 185–186

M

Magnetic resonance angiography (MRA), for donor
    site assessment prior to microvascular surgery,
    77–79
Magnetic resonance imaging (MRI), advances in
    head and neck imaging with, 107–110
    fetal, prenatal diagnosis of fetal anomalies with,
        8–9
Mandibular angle fractures, endoscopic surgery for,
    170–171
Masses, cervical and oral/pharyngeal, prenatal
    diagnosis and treatment, 13
Mesenchymal stem cell technology, in regenerative
    medicine, 38–39
Microarrays, for head and neck pathology
    diagnostics, DNA, 187–188
        microRNA, 188
Microfluidic analysis, for head and neck pathology
    diagnostics, 188–189

Micrognathia, prenatal diagnosis and treatment,
    12–13
MicroRNA microarrays, for head and neck pathology
    diagnostics, 188
Microsatellite instability, for head and neck pathology
    diagnostics, 185
Microvascular surgery, technology in, **73–90**
    history of free-tissue transfer and, 73–75
    intraoperative anastomotic technique, 80–83
    postoperative flap monitoring, 83–88
    preoperative imaging assessment, 75–80
        donor site assessment, 76–79
        recipient site assessment, 79–80
Miniscrews, for skeletal anchorage devices,
    placement of, 101
Molecular diagnostics, for head and neck pathology,
    183–194
    DNA-based technologies, 183–187
        comparative genomic hybridization,
            186–187
        in situ hybridization, 184–185
        loss of heterozygosity, 185–186
        microsatellite instability, 185
        polymerase chain technology, 183–184
    microfluidic analysis, 188–189
    protein-based technologies, 188
        immunohistochemistry, 188
        proteomics, 188
    RNA-based technologies, 187–188
        DNA microarrays, 187–188
        microRNA microarrays, 188
        reverse transcriptase PCR, 187
    targeted drug therapies and epidermal growth
        factor receptor, 189–190
Monitoring, postoperative, of flaps in microvascular
    surgery, 82–88
Muscular reconstruction, in cleft lip repair, 46–47

N

Nasal reconstruction, primary, for cleft lip repair,
    44–46
Nasoalveolar molding, presurgical, in cleft lip repair,
    47–48
Navigation, intraoperative, in computer-assisted
    craniomaxillofacial surgery, 137–153
        cranial reconstruction, 143
        dental/craniofacial implants, 151–153
        maxillo-mandibular reconstruction, 141–143
        orbital reconstruction, 138–141
        orthognathic surgery, 145–148
        temporomandibular joint surgery, 148–151
        tumor resection, 143–145
Neck, advances in imaging of, **107–118**
Nuclear medicine, head and neck imaging
    with, 114

O

Oncology, molecular diagnostics for head and neck pathology, **183–194**
 transcranial endoscopic surgery of ventral skull base, **157–168**
Oral cancer, molecular diagnostics for, **183–194**
Oral masses, prenatal diagnosis and treatment, 13
Orbital surgery, **59–71,** 138–141
 computer planning and intraoperative navigation, 138–141
 endoscopic and advanced imaging techniques for, 68–69
 endoscopic surgery for orbital floor fractures, 169–170, 64–66
 medial orbital wall fractures, 64–66
  orbital implants, 65–66
  surgical approaches, 64–65
  surgical incision, 66
 orbital floor fractures, 59–64
  fixation methods and wound closure, 63–64
  indications for repair, 59
  orbital implants, 60–63
  surgical incisions, 60
  timing of repair, 59–60
 orbital roof fractures, 66–68
  surgical incision, 66–68
Orthodontics, temporary skeletal anchorage, **91–105**
 basic mechanics of, 92–94
 clinical indications for, 95–100
  closure of anterior open bite, 96–97
  mesial or distal movement of teeth with maximum anchorage, 95–96
  orthopedic growth modification, 97–100
  uprighting or intruding molar teeth, 96
 devices for, 94–95
 history of, 92
 outcomes and complications, 103–104
 postoperative regimen, 101–103
 surgical procedures, 100–101
  placement of miniscrews for skeletal anchorage, 101
  placement of skeletal anchorage plates, 100–101
Orthognathic surgery, computer planning and intraoperative navigation, 145–148
 computer-assisted, 129–133
 endoscopic techniques for, 172–174
  LeFort I osteotomy, 173–174
  sagittal split osteotomy, 172–173
  vertical ramus osteotomy, 173
Orthopedics, growth modification, skeletal anchorage devices for, 97–100
 presurgical, in cleft lip repair, 47–48
Osteoblasts, differentiated, in regenerative medicine, 39
Osteotomy, endoscopic techniques for, 172–174

 LeFort, 173–174
 sagittal split, 172–173
 vertical ramus, 173
Outcomes research, **1–4**
 definition, 1–2
 model for, 2–3
 use to enhance evidence-based surgical practice and healthcare processes, 2

P

Palate, cleft, clinical outcomes for primary repair of, 48–54
  double-opposing Z-plasty, 50–52
  growth and, 52–53
  timing of, 53
  two-flap palatoplasty, 50
 prenatal diagnosis and treatment, 11–12
Palatoplasty, double-opposing Z-plasty, 50–52
 two-flap, 50
Parents, of a fetus with a congenital anomaly, prenatal support and counseling for, 9–10
Patient-oriented research, enhancing evidence-based surgery with, **1–4**
Perivascular cells, in regenerative medicine, 39
Pharyngeal masses, prenatal diagnosis and treatment, 13
Planning, computer. See Computer-assisted surgery.
Polymerase chain reaction (PCR), for head and neck pathology diagnostics, 183–184
  reverse transcriptase, 187
Polyurethane adhesives, use in oral and maxillofacial surgery, 196–197
Positron emission tomography (PET), advances in head and neck imaging with, 114
Prenatal care, diagnosis of fetal anomalies during, 6–7
Prenatal diagnosis, of craniomaxillofacial anomalies, **5–15**
  interdisciplinary team care, 5–9
   fetal MRI, 8–9
   prenatal care, 6–7
   ultrasonography, 7–8
Preoperative assessment, imaging, for microvascular surgery, 75–80
  donor site assessment, 76–79
  recipient site assessment, 79–80
Protein-based sealants, use in oral and maxillofacial surgery, 196
Protein-based technologies, for head and neck pathology diagnostics, 188
Proteomics, for head and neck pathology diagnostics, 188

Q

Quality assurance, outcomes research and evidence-based surgery, **1–4**

Quality (*continued*)
definition, 1–2
model for, 2–3
use to enhance surgical practice and
healthcare processes, 2

R

Reconstructive surgery, computer planning and
intraoperative navigation in, 138–143
cranial, 143
maxillo-mandibular, 141–143
orbital, 138–141
computer-assisted craniomaxillofacial, 124–126
Regenerative medicine, for craniomaxillofacial
surgery, **33–42**
basic principles of, 34–38
bone regeneration, 34–35
growth factors, 38
scaffolds, 35–37
cellular approaches, 38–39
differentiated osteoblasts, 40
mesenchymal stem cell technology, 39–40
new interdisciplinary field of, 34
vascular regeneration, 39–40
Research, outcomes, **1–4**
definition, 1–2
model for, 2–3
use to enhance evidence-based surgical practice
and healthcare processes, 2

S

Sagittal split osteotomy, endoscopic techniques for,
172–173
Scaffolds, in regenerative medicine, 35–37
Sialoendoscopy, 174–176
Skeletal anchorage, for orthodontics, temporary
devices for, **91–105**
basic mechanics of, 92–94
clinical indications for, 95–100
closure of anterior open bite, 96–97
mesial or distal movement of teeth with
maximum anchorage, 95–96
orthopedic growth modification, 97–100
uprighting or intruding molar teeth, 96
devices for, 94–95
history of, 92
outcomes and complications, 103–104
postoperative regimen, 101–103
surgical procedures, 100–101
placement of miniscrews for skeletal
anchorage, 101

placement of skeletal anchorage plates,
100–101
Skull base, ventral, transcranial endonasal surgery of,
157–168
controversies, 167
intraoperative strategies, 160–162
preoperative evaluation, 159–160
principles of, 157–159
reconstruction, 164–167
surgical approaches, 162–164
coronal plane modules, 163–164
sagittal plane modules, 162–163
Stem cell technology, mesenchymal, in regenerative
medicine, 38–39
Stereolithography, for recipient site assessment prior
to microvascular surgery, 79–80
Subcondylar fractures, endoscopic surgery for,
171–172
Surgery, craniomaxillofacial. *See* Craniomaxillofacial
surgery.
endonasal. *See* Endonasal surgery.
evidence-based surgery, outcomes research and,
1–4
definition, 1–2
model for, 2–3
use to enhance surgical practice and
healthcare processes, 2
prenatal, for fetal congenital anomaly, 10

T

Tactile model technology, in computer-assisted
craniomaxillofacial surgery, 121–122
Targeted drug therapies, for head and neck cancers,
189–190
Temporomandibular joint (TMJ) surgery, computer
planning and intraoperative navigation, 148–151
endoscopic techniques for, 176–179
Tissue adhesives, use in oral and maxillofacial
surgery, **195–199**
bone adhesives, 199
collagen and protein-based sealants, 196
cyanoacrylates, 196
fibrin adhesives, 195–196
ideal properties of, 195
polyurethane adhesives, 196–199
Tissue engineering, cellular approaches in
regenerative medicine, 38–39
Transcranial endoscopic surgery, of ventral skull
base, **157–168**
Trauma, endoscopic surgery for oral and
maxillofacial, 169–172
frontal sinus fracture, 172
mandibular angle fracture, 171–172

orbital floor fractures, 169–171
subcondylar fracture, 171–172
Tumor resection, computer planning and
   intraoperative navigation, 143–145
Two-flap palatoplasty, 50

U

Ultrasonography, color-duplex, for donor site
   assessment prior to microvascular surgery, 76–77
prenatal diagnosis of fetal anomalies with, 7–8

V

Vascular regeneration, in regenerative medicine,
   39–40
Ventral skull base. See Skull base, ventral.
Vertical ramus osteotomy, endoscopic techniques
   for, 173

Z

Z-plasty, double-opposing, 50–52

Moving?

Make sure your subscription moves with you!

To notify us of your new address, find your **Clinics Account Number** (located on your mailing label above your name), and contact customer service at:

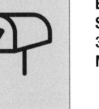

Email: journalscustomerservice-usa@elsevier.com

800-654-2452 (subscribers in the U.S. & Canada)
314-447-8871 (subscribers outside of the U.S. & Canada)

Fax number: 314-447-8029

Elsevier Health Sciences Division
Subscription Customer Service
3251 Riverport Lane
Maryland Heights, MO 63043

*To ensure uninterrupted delivery of your subscription, please notify us at least 4 weeks in advance of move.

Printed and bound by CPI Group (UK) Ltd, Croydon, CR0 4YY

03/10/2024

01040353-0008